# SELF IN RELATIONSHIPS

# SELF IN RELATIONSHIPS

## Perspectives on Family Therapy from Developmental Psychology

*Astri Johnsen, Rolf Sundet, Vigdis Wie Torsteinsson*

Foreword by
*Daniel Stern*

Systemic Thinking and Practice Series

Series Editors
*David Campbell & Ros Draper*

Routledge
Taylor & Francis Group
LONDON AND NEW YORK

First published 2004 by Karnac Books Ltd.

Published 2024 by Routledge
4 Park Square, Milton Park, Abingdon, Oxon OX14 4RN

and by Routledge
605 Third Avenue, New York, NY 10158

*Routledge is an imprint of the Taylor & Francis Group, an informa business*

First issued in paperback 2019



Translated by Susi Enderud.

Norwegian edition: *Samspill og selvopplevelse,* published by Universitetsforlaget AS, Oslo, 2000.

Translation subsidy from NORLA—Non-fiction.

**British Library Cataloguing in Publication Data**

A C.I.P. for this book is available from the British Library

ISBN: 978-1-85575-951-0 (pbk)
ISBN: 978-0-367-32678-4 (hbk)

Edited, designed, and produced by Communication Crafts

# CONTENTS

SERIES EDITORS' FOREWORD ix
ABOUT THE AUTHORS xi
FOREWORD *by Daniel N. Stern* xiii
PREFACE TO THE ENGLISH EDITION xix
PREFACE xxiii

**Introduction**
*Astri Johnsen, Rolf Sundet, Vigdis Wie Torsteinsson* 1

PART I
**A theoretical survey**

1 Daniel Stern's model of self-development
*Astri Johnsen, Rolf Sundet, Vigdis Wie Torsteinsson* 11

2 Perspectives on the concept of self
*Vigdis Wie Torsteinsson* 35

3 Intersubjectivity as a philosophical and psychological concept
*Vigdis Wie Torsteinsson* 61

PART II
**Relation-oriented therapy and modern developmental psychology: clinical implications**

4 Understanding each other—what does that mean? On emotional exchange, self-experience, and interplay
*Astri Johnsen, Vigdis Wie Torsteinsson* 89

5 The traces of experiences and the significance of time in narrative therapy
*Astri Johnsen* 114

6 Self-experience, key metaphors, and family premises: the relation between common and individual stories
*Astri Johnsen* 136

7 Senses of self and interplay as a metaphor for therapy with adolescents
*Rolf Sundet* 155

8 Differences and similarities: the relationship between siblings
*Astri Johnsen* 180

9 Together or alone: a both/and approach in work with eating disorders
*Astri Johnsen* 197

PART III
**What now? Theoretical perspectives and reflections**

10 Involved thinking and concept formation as an aid in therapy
*Rolf Sundet* 215

**11** Opposite and dilemma: reflection on therapy as a meeting place between psychoanalysis and family therapy
*Rolf Sundet* 235

**12** To know or not to know—or how do we know that we know?
*Vigdis Wie Torsteinsson* 256

**13** On understanding relation and ethics: an ethical perspective on the narrative self
*Vigdis Wie Torsteinsson* 278

*REFERENCES* 299

*INDEX* 313

# SERIES EDITORS' FOREWORD

For some years, a small group of family therapists in Norway have been concerned that the primary model of human development that informed family therapy was a non-systemic, non-relational model based on the child's progression through stages of internal cognitive, perceptual, and emotional development. Although relationships were central to these models, these were not relational theories. They did not theorize about the developing capacity to create and maintain relationships. But then Daniel Stern arrived with his major contribution, *The Interpersonal World of the Infant* (1985), which places the development of the self firmly in the context of relationship. Therefore, armed with Stern's research-based theories, the Norwegians were able to re-visit their own family therapy practice in order to apply this relational theory of development to their work.

It is unusual to find a group such as these three authors who are both gifted clinicians and clear theorizers, and they are taking the family therapy field into new territory with this book. Stern's work is clearly elucidated in the early chapters, and then the authors launch into their own clinical applications of his ideas, some of which are direct transpositions, but some use Stern as more of an inspiration to go further afield and explore new models of therapeutic work. The chapters offer a very wide variety of new ideas in the field, including discussions based on the work of Ricoeur, Husserl, and Stierlin, but the abiding strength of the book remains the ability of these authors to try new approaches to clinical problems—such as eating disorders—based on fresh theoretical perspectives. In fact, Daniel Stern, who has written the Foreword to the book, says his great wish in producing his highly acclaimed model was that someone would be able to take his ideas and translate them into practice—and that is exactly what we have here.

It has been a privilege to be part of the conception of this book and to steer it from its original publication in Norwegian to this English edition. Our Series has always tried to present new and exciting ideas in the field, and it is a particular pleasure to bring this creative effort to English readers.

*David Campbell*
*Ros Draper*
London, November 2003

# *ABOUT THE AUTHORS*

All three authors lead training programmes in family therapy and are both experienced teachers and therapists.

**Astri Johnsen** (born 1944) is a specialist in clinical psychology at the Nic Waal Institute for Child, Adolescent, and Family Therapy in Oslo. She is the director of the Institute for Family Therapy, Oslo. Astri Johnsen has written books about women and illness, short-term family therapy, and eating disorders and has also published several articles on related issues.

**Rolf Sundet** (born 1954) is a specialist in clinical psychology at the Centre for Child and Adolescent Psychiatry in Oslo. He has published several articles within the field of family therapy, focusing on clinical and theoretical issues. Rolf Sundet also works with organizational development.

**Vigdis Wie Torsteinsson** (born 1953) is a specialist in clinical psychology at the Nic Waal Institute in Oslo. She has made contributions to several anthologies on therapy and has written articles about both family therapy and the philosophy of science, and she is also an editor of the journal *Focus on the Family*.

# FOREWORD

*Daniel N. Stern*

First, a note of warning to the reader. The authors have relied heavily on many of the ideas in my book *The Interpersonal World of the Infant* (Stern, 1985, 2000). It has been a source of deep gratification for me to find these ideas useful to others who then carry them further. This is particularly so because when I finished that book I could only hope that the notions put forward would prove helpful in clinical situations beyond the ones I knew. I imagined it would take some time of trying and adjusting for this to show. Now, eighteen years later, I find that Astri Johnsen, Rolf Sundet, and Vigdis Wie Torsteinsson have done what I dreamt might happen. They have used the ideas, as well as many ideas from others, to inform a relation-oriented form of therapy. They have done it with a deep understanding of the notions involved, with great imagination, and with exquisite clinical sensibility.

You see now why a warning was necessary.

But why were the ideas in the *Interpersonal World,* which were developmental and largely about the development of the sense of self in infancy and young childhood, taken up and used for a relation-oriented therapy with adolescents and adults that identifies itself with the family therapy tradition? I had not imagined that. However, it makes perfect sense, because both developmental studies and relation-oriented therapies must deal with several similar issues and questions that occupy the centre ground.

The first consideration is how to integrate, or describe the dialogue between, on the one hand, the intrapsychic–the self–the private–the individually unique, with, on the other hand, the interpsychic–interpersonal–social–cultural–relational–linguistic. For both developmentalists and relation-oriented therapists, this is a key issue. The dilemma is that one cannot, a priori, give one side or the other greater weight—anyway, not when one looks closely at the phenomena. The therapeutic approach that evolves will take its form, in great part, on how the problem is posed and how the integration is attempted, not on how it is resolved. The authors of this book are very careful never to attempt closure of this problem. And part of the richness of the book results exactly from its pursuit of the problem rather than from deciding on an answer. In fact, they demonstrate how the multiple posings of the problem can be the essence of the therapeutic process.

One consequence of this approach is not a *how to* book, nor the delineation of a new encompassing, systematic technique. Rather, what emerges is a vision and possibilities for conducting the therapeutic process. Our vision gets altered.

This central question naturally leads the authors to an exploration of self and intersubjectivity as central aspects of their theoretical reflections and clinical observations.

A second similar question faced by developmentalists and relation-oriented therapists and theoreticians alike concerns bringing together the implicit nonverbal with the explicit verbal. This dialogue strikes one immediately in developmental considerations. However, it is just as pervasive in relational therapies, where the implicit nonverbal agendas are at every moment intertwined with the explicit, verbal, narrative agendas. At times, these two agendas are at odds; more often they are confluent, or complementary, or orthogonal, or simply parallel. In any event, they both must be taken into account. And again, which has more weight is undecidable a priori. The clinical task is to follow their dialogue.

It is no wonder, then, that a relation-oriented therapy found a parallel and a help in a developmental view that focused on the different domains of the sense of self, some of which were inevitably nonverbal and implicit.

In part I, which is the theoretical survey, the authors have the problem of how to explain needed but difficult and nuanced concepts to the reader. They come up with a remarkably simple and effective technique. In chapter 2, devoted to the self, we quickly meet Signe, an adolescent girl, who formulates, in the clinical situation, the central questions but in her own words—how to be herself? what/who is herself? which is her authentic self? would she lose herself in conforming? and so on. Each of her questions picks up major points in the theories and arguments of the most influential philosophers and psychologists of these issues. The effect is one of Signe entering into a real dialogue with these minds from the past and present. The issues come alive and become readily comprehensible.

In chapter 3 we see this plan again, but now about intersubjectivity. The author mixes an excellent discussion of the major philosophical and psychological issues without simplifying them. Then we are introduced to Yngvild, a 13-year-old girl with compulsive and eating problems. Yngvild instantiates the major questions raised, with statements like (to her mother) "You can't know how I feel! No one can know it. You say that you understand, but I know that you don't!" At times it feels like Yngvild and the great philosopher, Husserl, are having a real discussion. The clinical world becomes richer. And the theoretical world becomes more accessible.

In Part II, the authors bring together the main strands to weave a coherent picture of relation-oriented therapy: self-experience; experience of the other; the process of relating, including intersubjectivity; the nature and importance of narrativization and metaphors; and the family, systemic context. The clinical case material is well chosen.

What emerges is a vision of what therapy can be like.

In chapter 7, devoted to the difficult task of treating adolescents, Rolf Sundet does a remarkable job in using the model of the *emergent self* as a guideline for this clinical challenge. Instead of seeing adolescents as disorganized, defensive, uncooperative, hardly verbal, and so on (our usual emotional view, if not the cognitive one we try to work with), he pictures them as in a phase of putting together an emergent self. It is not simply a reorganization but a creation. This shift in focus opens up new clinical paths (including different countertransferential stances) to follow and has technical implications including, importantly, greater tolerance and appreciation of the adolescent.

Astri Johnsen accomplishes similar rotations of our clinical vision in her chapters in Part II.

In Parts II and III there are two themes that emerge with increasing strength. The first is the insistence on a phenomenological approach. The second is the importance of the micro-processes that make up therapy (and living). These themes are highly related. Let us take up the first.

The authors try to maintain a constant phenomenological perspective on clinical material. This is evident in Johnsen's chapters on eating disorders and on siblings. It is always how the relational is construed to create the inner landscape that is in clinical focus. It is equally evident in Sundet's chapter on thinking and concept formation, and in Torsteinsson's chapter on problems of knowing. The tension between the phenomenological and the objective and the abstract is maintained. The authors speak of dilemmas and fields of existential tension created by their largely phenomenological approach. This comes as a great relief because the reader is not forced or led to make impossible choices. The complexity of our therapeutic work is not compromised. In fact, much of the therapeutic endeavour is seen as occurring within these fields of tensions.

An inevitable consequence of the authors' appreciation of the phenomenological is their attention to the micro-processes of therapy or of any intimate interaction. This marriage of the phenomenological view with the micro-descriptive or micro-process view fascinates me. Clinically meaningful events happen in the present moment, the here-and-now. The nodal events are of short duration. There is no way to avoid the micro-scale of relating. That is where life is directly lived. That is where *it* happens. Everything else is explanation, abstraction, narrative. (Granted, this everything else is very useful, even indispensable, but it is once-removed from phenomenology.)

These realities have been occupying me, too, these past years and have resulted in a new book, *The Present Moment in Psycho-*

*therapy and Everyday Life* (Stern, in press). I find it encouraging that the authors of this book and I, starting from different points, are converging on what constitute interesting issues at this point in time.

An interesting consequence of taking a phenomenological and micro-descriptive view of the therapeutic process is that when one is acting within the process—that is, while the session is still unfolding in the present—one is struck by how unpredictable, sloppy, improvised, and meandering is the process. What happens did not have to happen that way, or even at all. Sundet's chapter on "opposite and dilemma" and Torsteinsson's on knowing exemplify this very well. The dialogue between clinical theory and practice at the local level of micro-processes is perhaps the most tricky field of tension we have to deal with. This dilemma transcends the dialogues between psychoanalysis and family therapy, for example, and should not be confused with it. It is everywhere.

Here, too, there is a remarkable confluence between the authors of this book and a group of us working on the process of change in psychotherapy, under the name of the Boston Change Process Study Group (2002, 2003; see also Stern, 2003; Stern et al., 1998; Tronick et al., 1998). We have been struck by the sloppiness of the therapeutic process at the local micro-level, yet we see this sloppiness as a source of great potential creativity in the co-creative, intersubjective process of therapy, and not as noise or errors in the system, nor as the irruption of unconscious material requiring explanation.

These various fields of tension—verbal/nonverbal; intrapsychic/interpsychic; individual self/social self; theory/practice—can all be subsumed under another broad and deep field of tension: the grand dilemma between meaning and experience. Or, perhaps more accurately, between "understanding" experience and "more deeply appreciating" experience. Experiences (like music) can become more deeply appreciated without "understanding" them any better. So can some interactive patterns. At times this strikes me as being at the heart of so many of these other unfinishable dialogues.

In summary, this book brings together philosophy, psychology, and clinical practice and lets them interact with clarity and a growing sense of integration. This is done in such a manner that the book should have almost equal value for family therapy (where it started), psychoanalysis (where it also found inspiration), and, in fact, for any form of psychotherapy that deals with subjective experience, relatedness, and narrativity. It is a book that alters the vision and reorients the position with regard to the main issues we encounter in both theory and practice.

# PREFACE TO THE ENGLISH EDITION

To read this book in a different language gives us the opportunity to reflect upon it and to offer some of these reflections to our English-speaking readers. Reading this book in its translation, we are reminded that for us, in our context, it was actually quite a daring move to turn our attention to developmental psychology. Today we are proud of that move. We now experience family therapy and our context differently. The field looks different, and we realize that we have more friends and distant relatives than we thought we had when we started this work. We see an increased interest in relations and relationships within the general field of psychotherapy, as well as an interest in pursuing different ways of thinking about relations in the domain of family therapy, to which we ourselves still primarily relate. Many of the critical comments—especially from family therapists—of Daniel Stern's work which we refer to have been met by his later work. It is also important to acknowledge that these critical comments have been important challenges that have expanded our thinking. They have increased our interest in pursuing the consequences and possibilities connected to the ideas put forth in this book. We have had to rethink our relationship to developmental psychology and have ended up with a strong conviction that it is of central importance to have this knowledge as part of our luggage as therapists.

At the same time, we see that the ideas in this book have helped us to establish and maintain a critical gaze upon ideas that have been important for us for years. The ideas connected with the concepts of constructivism and constructionism—specifically the ideas of social constructionism—were increasingly felt as constraints on our investigations of practice and theory. We have been and still are concerned with the central position of language in our field and the possibility that this "centre" may turn into a new kind of reductionism that reduces everything to language. At the same time, we are still fascinated with constructionist ideas in a broad sense, and how language can be kept as a tool for therapists, without being elevated to a centre providing answers to every possible philosophical and ethical question. Reducing language to a phenomenon among other phenomena leaves space for these other phenomena. A main interest for us has been the topic of affects, emotions, and feelings. These are phenomena that exemplify for us what non-language can be. Having an eye for coordinations between family members that cannot be seen as language has opened up new avenues in therapy for us. In addition, it has opened up a new interest in and a respect for language. We see and acknowledge that eventually we have to put these phenomena into words and, as such, necessarily transform them. This is one of the most challenging and exiting paradoxes of therapy for us: to meet and know non-language through language.

The ideas from postmodern thinking that transcend oppositional thinking and allow for a diversity through supplementary forms of thinking have, in this connection, been of valuable help to us. This has inspired us to go in for widening the scope of this book. We have been fascinated by the thought of bringing into contact different ideas from philosophy, behavioural genetics, developmental psychology, systemic family therapy, psychoanalysis, research on psychotherapy, and postmodern, post-structuralist, constructionist, and narrative ideas. This opens up vast areas of knowledge, while at the same time raising questions about in what way and to what use such knowledge might be put for therapists. We need to keep reminding ourselves of a growing concern that these vast fields of knowledge might actually be a hindrance to therapeutic work, because they might distance us from our clients and their perspectives and ideas.

Like many other therapists in our field, we are interested in the possibilities of the narrative metaphor. The developmental psychology of Daniel Stern has given us opportunities to remain in connection with non-language. His focus on the sense of the narrative self opens up further opportunities to stay in contact with and work within the field of modern family therapy. For us this is a comforting thought, because in addition to the work of Daniel Stern, the field of family therapy, with all its critical creativity and keen development of important theoretical and practical ideas, has been the scaffolding that has helped us survive as therapists.

Since the original publication of this book, we have been strengthened in our view that relationships are of central importance. The therapeutic relationship is, for us, just a special case of ordinary human relationships. This has implied a shift in perspective. From being trained in a tradition that saw the therapeutic relationship as a metaphor for "the good and nurturing relationship in general" and, as such, as a measuring-rod for what a good parent–child relationship was supposed to look like, we have now turned this upside down. Today we see the ordinary parent–child relationship as a leading metaphor for therapists. This brings the work of parents to the foreground and gives us the opportunity to honour the thousands of generations of parents who have made it possible for us all to be here. But, most importantly, it serves as a reminder to honour the parents we meet in therapy. Clinical research on therapy seems to us to parallel this through the increased importance of clients in generating results in therapy. It is good to meet families, to get to know their ways of relating to each other and to us, and to think about how this can be a metaphor and help for how we should conduct ourselves in relation to them. We believe that participating in relationships both as persons and as therapists, as well as reflecting upon these relationships, is of central importance in bringing about the change processes that therapy sometimes inspires. Therefore the dual concepts of reflection and participation, detachment and involvement, point to central concerns of this book.

Lastly, we would again like to acknowledge Daniel Stern and his work. It has opened up avenues for us that have led us to all the areas of knowledge we are concerned with in this book. Maybe—and most importantly—by embracing postmodern ideas in connection with the work of Daniel Stern, we have paradoxically been led back to science in general, and to psychology specifically, as a source of inspiration. The gap between academic and clinical psychology that once seemed impossible to cross is today a source of creativity in our therapeutic endeavours. For this we will forever be grateful to Daniel Stern.

*Astri Johnsen, Rolf Sundet, Vigdis Wie Torsteinsson*
Oslo, November 2003

# PREFACE

The idea of initiating a dialogue between modern developmental psychology and systems family therapy was conceived in the bunker-like building of the Nic Waal Institute around 1990. Somewhat exhausted after the epistemology debate in the 1980's and satiated with the systems conceptual apparatus, we looked around for a psychological theory that might be relevant to family therapy. Daniel Stern's self-developmental model, conveyed enthusiastically to us by the Norwegian psychologist Bjørg Røed Hansen, became the point of departure for a collaborative project exploring modern developmental theory and its implications for the work with children, adolescents, and families. The collaboration between the book's three authors has made it possible for us to combine theoretical diversity and philosophical knowledge with clinical experience. After having presented our ideas at congresses (Fyn in 1993; Oslo in 1994; Vesterås in 1996; Oslo in 1996; Petenasco, Italy, in 1997), at seminars, and in other teaching contexts in Norway, Sweden, and Denmark, we were encouraged to write on the subject. Bjørg Roed Hansen has been an important source of inspiration, and for this we would like to extend our thanks to her. Of great importance to us has also been the feedback we received for our project from Daniel Stern, David Campbell, and Luigi Boscolo.

All three authors are working within the field of child and adolescent psychiatry. We would like to thank the Nic Waal Institute, the Buskerud Central Hospital, the Centre for Child and Adolescent Psychiatry, and the new Regional Centre, the R-BUP, for providing a stimulating professional milieu and for giving us opportunities at times to re-allocate our working hours for writing. This help has been most necessary.

We would also like to thank the clients and their families who have shared their experiences with us, and thus also with the readers. Needless to say, their anonymity has been preserved according to prevailing rules.

We were full of enthusiasm about this dialogue, our associations proliferated, and there was a stream of ideas, but reality caught up with us in terms of what was realistic in this project.

This book was written thanks to the notion of the authors that work and leisure time are one and the same.

*Astri Johnsen, Rolf Sundet, Vigdis Wie Torsteinsson*
Oslo, August 1999

# SELF IN RELATIONSHIPS

"It is a pity that nowadays we cannot learn anything to last a lifetime," Eduard exclaimed. "Our forefathers relied on what they were taught in their youth; *we* have to learn something different every five years or so in order not to fall completely behind the times."

Johan Wolfgang von Goethe, *Elective Affinities*

# Introduction

## Important phenomena in relation-oriented therapies

*Astri Johnsen, Rolf Sundet, Vigdis Wie Torsteinsson*

Within the field of family therapy, there is currently a discussion about the type of knowledge that can be considered as relevant. The field has been mostly dominated by systemic theory and social constructionism, with a critical attitude towards psychological theory. At the same time, there has been a higher demand for psychological theory and phenomena-related concepts. The issues appearing increasingly on the agenda have been the individual's place in the system, the significance of the concept of the self, and the connection between the self and the relation, as well as questions about the significance of feelings, the role of ethics, and so forth. When teaching, we are continually confronted with these issues and with a demand for a theory for them. In clinical practice, too, we are faced with these approaches to problems that pose a challenge to our understanding and our methods. One may mention the following examples: How have we confronted the issue of what it means to understand each other, or that of the difference between regulating, sharing, and conveying feelings? How are preverbal experiences conveyed and understood? How are we to understand that siblings growing up in the same family turn out so differently? How are we, while keeping the totality in mind, to take care of the individual's experience of himself/herself and others? The knowledge acquired from modern developmental theory and the research on children and families can be useful in regard to these questions, and we have observed an increasing need for knowledge in this field. The aim of this book is therefore to meet this need.

## *Phenomena and concepts*

Daniel Stern's main focus in his research has been on what may be called phenomena-related descriptions. He wished to explore the topics that in some way are always part of our relational lives.

First of all, this means that micro-interactions are brought into focus—not the significant events. In this way, these phenomena can be approached using many different theoretical concepts.

Concepts are meant to contribute to a better understanding. However, therapy concerns something more than understanding. It is about being together in ways that enable our clients to choose new alternatives for their actions and new ways of experiencing. In this book we invite our readers to explore different ways of understanding therapy, metaphors, and images regarding this type of work. A recurring topic is the relationship, especially that between child and caregiver. In this perspective, the conceptual development deals with the ability to create new forms of companionship or relationships that are of importance to clients. This is our understanding of the term "relation-oriented therapy". The book is about understanding and reflection, but also about spontaneous companionship—the experience of the here-and-now—and about touching and letting oneself be touched by the individual or the individuals one is with in the therapy-room, as an example in chapter 10 shows.

## *Theoretical meeting places*

This book presents many meeting places—between systemic theory, developmental theory, psychoanalysis, and philosophy.

Many of the key figures in family theory had their roots in psychoanalysis (Jackson, Watzlawick, Minuchin, the Milan group, Stierlin, and others). Modern psychoanalytic theory, represented by Heinz Kohut and his successors, has provided interesting contributions to an understanding of the self (Karterud & Monsen, 1997) and affects, and an interest in narrative understanding. It suffices to mention Donald Spence's book *Narrative Truth and Historical Truth* (1982) as a relevant source for all who are interested in narrative thinking and method.

The discussion about the relation between psychoanalysis and systemic family therapy has flared up again. A 1997 issue of the British *Journal of Family Therapy* includes a discussion about the relation between psychoanalysis and systemic family therapy, and one of the articles addresses the issue of whether "psychoanalysis can be of use to systemic therapists" (Speed, 1997, p. 233). Several of the articles discuss the significance of the therapeutic relationship (Flaskas, 1997), the importance of being understood (Pocock, 1997), and—in this context—the concept of empathy.

The question is whether this is merely a repetition of earlier discussions, or whether there actually exists a new basis for this type of discussion. Our book argues in favour of the usefulness for family therapists of modern developmental psychology as represented by Daniel Stern, and we believe that, considering the interest shown by psychoanalysis for the narrative perspective, this may promote a mutual enrichment of these two traditions.

One of our concerns is to discover if we can get new ideas by turning our attention to developments in the fields of psychoanalysis and family therapy. Our main interest has been directed towards family therapy. We have discovered, while working with the material we are presenting here, that there have been changes within both psychoanalysis and family therapy that we believe can enrich both these theoretical fields. The idea is not to integrate but, rather, to bring about a mutual curiosity in these two areas, which may result in dialogues with each other and create reservoirs for ideas and practices that have been found to be useful. Chapter 11 discusses some of the dilemmas and contradictions that may arise between psychoanalysis and family therapy.

One of the main messages of the book is that family therapists can benefit from knowledge about children's development and the development of their social understanding. The developmental theories usually adopted by clinicians, such as those of Freud, Erikson, Bowlby, and Piaget, have been met with scepticism by many family therapists—for example, Lynn Hoffman (1993). There are some good and some poor reasons for this. Several theories are pathology-oriented, with little emphasis on the resources with which family therapists are concerned. The past is considered as a dark shadow to be explored and worked through. In short, the views on the development of small children, as advocated by several of these theories, have not been of current interest and therefore have been irrelevant for many family therapists. As an exception, one may mention John Byng-Hall's interest in Bowlby's attachment theory (Byng-Hall, 1991, 1995a). Luigi Boscolo has also stated that "we all carry a Bowlby inside us" (Boscolo, personal communication 1996) and that we are influenced by the luggage of earlier knowledge (Boscolo & Bertrando, 1996).

Daniel Stern holds a distinctive position both as an infant researcher and as a psychoanalyst. The point of departure in his study is the clinical infant as constructed by psychoanalysts and the observed infant founded on direct observation (Stern, 1985). Based on these two positions, he creates a working hypothesis about the subjectively experiencing infant. In modern self-psychology, which is based on Heinz Kohut, it is first and foremost Joseph Lichtenberg who has integrated modern infant research (Hartmann, 1997). We claim that Stern's theory of the self and relations is two sides of the same coin and is more relevant to systemic family therapists than is modern self-psychology. Chapter 1 presents Stern's model of self-development, discussing its relevance to family therapy and the criticism levelled against it from social-constructionist quarters.

Daniel Stern's theory on the development of the senses of self is the scarlet thread running through this book. The implications of his theory for work with individuals, couples, and families are described and discussed in separate chapters (chapters 5, 6, and 7). We consider his understanding of the significance of relations for regulating, mediating, and sharing feelings to be of great clinical importance. This is especially discussed in chapter 4, but further chapters also demonstrate the relevance to therapeutic work of his understanding of affect regulation and affect attunement (chapters 5, 7, and 9), as well as his emphasis on both preverbal and verbal experiences. In conformity with Jerome Bruner (1990a), he maintains that the tendency to organize experiences in narratives arises very early in development, and before the development of verbal language. In the discussion about narratives and self-experience, we will, in addition to Stern and Bruner, also use theoretical concepts from psychoanalysis (Donald Spence), from social constructionism (Kenneth Gergen), and from philosophy (Paul Ricoeur) (see chapters 2, 3, 5, and 13).

Judy Dunn's study of children's social understanding and of close relationships (among them, sibling relationships) has been another important source of inspiration for our exploration of the relation between developmental psychology and family therapy. Her studies of small children in their natural environment challenge our traditional conception of children. Among other things, she challenges the theory about the unique position in development held by attachment (Dunn, 1993). In Dunn's opinion, attachment research has been important for elucidating aspects in the parent–child relationship and for forming hypotheses about the processes that are crucial for subsequent attachment. This research has, however, set a narrow frame around the insight into children's social understanding and close relationships. Already from the age of 2 to 3 years, children's relationships are multidimensional and complex. They contain a number of different dimensions, such as sharing feelings, sharing humour, harmony in communication, and balancing control and power.

The idea of the egocentric child should also be revised. Modern infant research presents us with a competent and social small being who tries very early to understand the feelings and intentions of others. Infants' understanding of others evolves parallel with their experience of themselves. This view on children stands in sharp contrast to other developmental theories that maintain that children are late in developing an ability to understand the perspectives of others. Judy Dunn's studies are in line with the modern perspective on children. She supplements these studies with a study of close relationships, not only with friends but also with siblings. Together with the behavioural geneticist Robert Plomin, Dunn has done research on the influence of the environment on the individual, as well as on the conditions within the family that cause siblings to turn out differently—an interesting contribution to the understanding of the individual within the system (Dunn & Plomin, 1991). Their findings are presented in chapter 8, which deals especially with sibling relations and sibling differences and with the importance of sibling relations for children's development and for therapeutic practice. Chapter 9 demonstrates how the theories of both Dunn and Stern have been crucial for the evolution of a model for working with eating disorders.

In the field of family therapy, there has always been a lively debate on how to make use of knowledge. The great turning point as regards viewing knowledge as an effective agent in therapeutic relationships came simultaneously with the transition to second-order cybernetics.

After this, family therapeutic methods were primarily based on a recognition of the client's own understanding of his/her situation. The expression "not-knowing position" stood for a wish not to assume the role of an expert on the lives of others. The therapeutic process was defined as a co-construction of new meaning, made possible through the therapeutic dialogue.

This has also generated scepticism towards traditional forms of knowledge, because *knowledge* has been synonymous with *answer*, thus assigning the role of an expert to the therapist. The reasons for these viewpoints are the postmodernistic basic assumptions about an infinite number of possible descriptions of reality and the problems of giving precedence to one of the descriptions.

One key focus in this book is to question this link between being inspired and using knowledge, and being the expert in the sense of a know-all person. We would also maintain that knowledge is necessary for posing good questions. Issues concerning the relation between knowledge and truth, between empiricism and the concept of objectivity, are discussed in chapter 12.

### *The community of diversity*

The concept of intersubjectivity has in recent years become increasingly included in the theory of therapy. From the perspective of individual psychology, this concept suggests a possible meeting of two delimited individuals—what they contain and what place they hold in the therapeutic understanding.

From a family-therapeutic viewpoint, the concept of intersubjectivity comes in addition to the joint concepts on which understanding is based. We propose that this concept is an important extension, making it possible to focus on the individual's role in the relational context (see chapter 3). Moreover, this is the point of departure for an understanding of the ethical perspectives presented in chapter 13.

Stern speaks of the limitations of language. This may be exemplified by the possibly banal fact that we are forced to discuss the nonverbal aspect of language in this type of text. The universe of the infant is a nonverbal universe. Stern points out that it is a universe of spontaneous experience. We seek to grasp this universe through language, but we are fated to fail because language removes us from the experience: we are no longer within the experience—we are pointing at it. At the same time, however, the above text is actually a type of verbalization of the relation between the verbal and the nonverbal. Perhaps other texts are possible, and there may be a different approach to the problem. It is our intent not to solve this issue or to supply an answer, but to point at the dilemmas facing therapists with regard to verbalization and nonverbalization.

Dialogue, communication, conversation, and talk are concepts that are often used in today's therapy language. With this book we seek to encourage a dialogue about the theories that happened to be standing on each side of a front line during a few turbulent decades. We also hope to encourage communication between theory and practice and to share with our readers our experience of letting ourselves be inspired by modern developmental theory. Curiosity and self-reflection emerge already early in life, according to modern developmental theory. Working with this material has intensified and stimulated our curiosity, elucidated a number of problems, but also raised new issues. We also wish through this book to stimulate the appetite of the reader—and her/his curiosity.

A book of this type necessarily reflects the preferences of its authors with regard to problems, topics, and theories. We have also had to select from among the diversity of our ideas to concentrate on the totality. Several of Stern's concepts are repeated and explained anew in different chapters in connection with their uses in particular therapeutic contexts (see especially chapters 4, 6, 7, and 9).

The field of family therapy is concerned with narratives. Stern is also interested in the way the stories come into being. The point of creating a story is to create a chance to act. This book contains many stories about a number of similar topics. We hope this will give our readers diverse and new chances to act in clinical practice. We also hope that it will increase the understanding of clinical phenomena, as well as give us a new understanding of ourselves and others.

The groups at which this book is targeted are postgraduate students at universities and in colleges and health workers in advanced training. The book is also suitable as a textbook for different specialist and family therapy courses. We believe that many clinicians will recognize themselves in the issues that have been raised. It is our hope that the book will make readers reflect on their own work and that it will be a source of pleasure to all those who in different ways are involved with human relationships.

*PART 1*

# A THEORETICAL SURVEY

*CHAPTER ONE*

# Daniel Stern's model of self-development

*Astri Johnsen, Rolf Sundet, Vigdis Wie Torsteinsson*

Developmental psychology has been a rapidly expanding area of research in recent years. There have been great changes in the traditional thinking around child development, and for this reason it poses a considerable challenge to clinical work. It is our contention that developmental theory is present—either explicitly or implicitly—in the totality of theory on which our work is based. All such theory is about interaction between people—about being together with one person or with several others. This is also the main focus of developmental theories.

The great gap between clinical everyday life and academic research is often pointed to, as are the difficulties encountered by clinicians when making use of research in their practices. Several of the great theoretical innovations have been made possible by an extremely active use of technology. By using video in the study of interaction, it has been possible to focus—in a totally different way from before—on the details in the interaction between the infant and the adult. It has thus become possible—in a totally different sense from previously—to take one's point of departure both as the clinical infant, which emerges retrospectively in the therapeutic context, and as the observed infant, where knowledge is based on solid empirical research (Boalt Böethius & Berggren, 1998).

The psychoanalyst and infant researcher Daniel Stern has in many respects been a pioneer in these areas. Stern's main concern was to attempt to turn research-based knowledge into a resource also for clinical practice. By integrating these two perspectives—the observed infant and the clinical infant—he puts forward what he terms a working hypothesis about the subjectively experiencing infant. With his developmental model he wishes to contribute to a greater understanding of the infant and how it experiences the world—both itself and others.

His two major works are characterized by these two perspectives: research and clinical studies. In *The Interpersonal World of the Infant,* the main focus is on the relation between the individual and the relationship (Stern, 1985). Earlier developmental theories have been greatly intrigued by the issue concerning the extent to which the infant experiences itself as separated from, or as totally engulfed by, a larger entity. All developmental theory has taken this issue into account in one way or the other, albeit in very different ways. The very first period has been described using such opposite concepts as "autistic" and "symbiotic". Daniel Stern's focus on empirical research in this domain has given him a starting point in "both/and" thinking. He says that, from the very beginning, the infant has its own perspective, its own slant on the world, based on its own point of departure. This he almost gives the status of an instinct (Stern, 1985, p. 8), with the consequence that in all understanding of relationships one needs to incorporate in one way or another the individual's organizing and initiating activity as a key element. On the other hand, it is the relationship and the forms of companionship that make the senses of self (see Stern, 1985, pp. 22 ff.) appear as activity on the part of the child.

The same question about symbiosis and separateness is also relevant to the infant's general experience of its surroundings. Does the infant live in the "blooming, buzzing confusion" proclaimed by William James, which enables it only gradually to organize its perceptions as patterns and coherence? Research has shown how the perceptual world of infants is organized—to a far greater extent than previously assumed—in cohesive perceptual patterns and entities. Thus their preconditions for entering into coordinated activity are not, as we have believed, so very different from those of adults. And Stern uses this knowledge to point to the infant's active participation in the forming of its early relationships. This active participation is, for example, reflected in the fact that the concept of turn-taking becomes crucial for understanding exchange processes in general.

In *The Motherhood Constellation* (1995), Stern also advocates a both/and viewpoint in his understanding of representations and how these are formed. Representations are formed from within, though from the subjective experience of being-together-with-another. This is discussed later in the chapter.

A both/and model naturally implies that while thinking "self", one must also think "relationship". Just as we need two legs in order to stand firmly, or two eyes in order to have depth vision, so developmental psychology needs two basic concepts in order to grasp the complexity in all developmental processes. Stern describes the concept of self mostly as capacities for entering into exchanges with others—in other words, capacities for gaining experiences of being-with-others. The different senses of self have thus parallel domains of relationships or forms of being together.

This may also stand as a gateway to another of Stern's important concepts: intersubjectivity. For him, this is a key concept for concretizing how relationship and individuality constitute each other. Intersubjectivity is discussed in chapter 3 in connection with the understanding of relationship in the field of family therapy. It is precisely in this connection that attempts have been made to find formulations and ways of thinking that indicate that the whole is more than the sum of its parts. However, family therapists have been more interested in finding a conceptual apparatus that will go beyond the individual perspective. With a few exceptions, it was not defined as a goal in itself to include individual or subject and relationship within the same theoretical frame. Helm Stierlin's concept of "related individuation" is an example of such an exception (Stierlin, Rucker-Embden, Wetzel, & Wirsching, 1980). Individuation always takes place in a relationship, and the degree of individuation must be evaluated according to the relationship in which it takes place. In his book *Ich und die Anderen* (1994), Stierlin also discusses different ways of conceptualizing the self from a systemic perspective (see also Johnsen, 1996).

Another special topic elucidated by Stern, based on new viewpoints, is the relation between affects/emotions and cognition and language. Here there are many traditional research areas taking part in complicating attempts at integration. Stern emphasizes among other things that the basis for being-with-others experiences is feelings, and not primarily individual reactions. In this connection, the distinction between vitality affects and categorical affects is, for example, described as an important condition for inter-affectivity or shared emotional experiences. In chapter 4, we discuss the use of Stern's understanding of affects for clinical practice in particular. Other important topics are to what degree and in which sense this emotional being-with-others also has consequences for our choice of words and for the stories we can tell about ourselves.

Before presenting the five different senses of self as described by Daniel Stern, we briefly sum up some postulates that he uses as starting points:

- The infant is an active participant in constructing its own world. Already from the very beginning, there is communication where the infant is an active partner in the interaction. This does not reduce the adult's significance.
- The constitution of the self will always be based on interaction with others. The different senses of self have parallel domains of relatedness. The development of the self and the development of relationships are in all respects two sides of the same coin.
- The senses of self are not perceived as successive phases replacing each other. Every sense of self will continue to function and remain active throughout life after first having been established. They will all continue to grow and exist together.
- Self-development is not characterized by phase-specific themes. Clinical themes such as dependency, trust, autonomy, control, and so forth are not linked to age-specific phases, but are conceived as important themes from the very beginning. They will

be worked through and repeated in each developmental phase and are formed and expressed according to developmental competence.

- Capacity and ability are the basis for defining developmental phases. New behaviour and new capacities imply new ways of organizing subjective experience with oneself and others. This is the point of departure for the five different senses of self.

Stern's developmental model is thus characterized by developmental lines, not by developmental phases. He calls this model a continuous-construction model, as distinct from a fixation-regression model. Each new sense of self is added to the preceding one. It does not replace the preceding self-domains or push them aside. This means that they remain important ways of being in relationships, throughout the life span. In all significant relationships the crucial themes are those concerning dependency and autonomy, control and trust. These are not phase-specific themes, but life themes.

In the next section we give a presentation of Stern's self-developmental model (Stern, 1985, 1990). We also discuss his account of how representations are formed (Stern, 1992, 1995). Special attention is drawn to the aspects of his model that have been significant for our clinical practice. We have read him in our own way and let ourselves be inspired by what we considered useful for us. A different reader would most likely have selected other things and understood the material differently.

Stern's model has also met with criticism, and this criticism is discussed later in this chapter. Criticism is naturally coloured by the critic's own theoretical standpoint, whether based on object-relations theory, on traditional self-psychology, or on social constructionism. We discuss particularly the criticism that has come from social constructionism.

Stern's theory has been a source of inspiration to us in our work as therapists with individuals, couples, and families precisely because of the questions he poses. What is it like to be together with another? What is it that makes other people know that you are feeling something that is similar to what they are feeling? How can I know that you understand me?

## *The five senses of self and domains of relatedness*

The five senses of self with their domains of relatedness are:

1. the sense of an *emergent self;*
2. the sense of a *core self;*
3. the sense of a *subjective self;*
4. the sense of a *verbal self;*
5. the sense of a *narrative self.*

These are the key concepts in Stern's theories. But they may just as well be regarded as a point of departure for discussing topics in general developmental psychology—for example, regulation, imitation, or affect attunement. In this presentation, the concepts are used as headings in order to acquire new ideas about how to understand the phenomena that we are often confronted with in clinical practice.

## *The sense of an emergent self (0–2 months): the world of feelings*

In Stern's opinion, the infant is capable of experiencing a sense of an emergent self right from the very beginning, and it is active in forming an emergent sense of self in the course of the first two months. This sense of self will be present for the rest of its life. New experiences, transitions, or changes can give us a dawning or growing sense of something emerging. Falling in love can serve as an example. Women who have experienced pregnancy will also recognize the sense of something novel emerging in their experience of what is happening with them and inside them. This emergent sense of self is also characteristic of the years of youth (see chapter 7, where Stern's model of the senses of self is used as a metaphor for understanding youth).

The newborn infant has sensory capacities that enable it to perceive its surroundings through all sensory modalities (vision, hearing, smell, touch, kinetics). From its global experiential world, the infant creates active organization, coherence, and meaning. It is this sense of organizing processes that Stern describes as the sense of an emergent self. Stern makes a general point of the importance of being interested in the process; this, as a comment to developmental theory, has had a tendency to call more attention to the product.

In the description of the sense of an emergent self, we can recognize the inspiration from dynamic systems theory.

*Amodal perception* and what Stern terms *vitality affects* are two characteristics of the sense of an emergent self that we find interesting in our context.

*Amodal perception* enables the infant to sensually perceive wholeness and coherence. It deals with the ability to translate impressions from one sense to the other, as well as storing impressions across the senses. This means that the infant is capable of experiencing a connection between what it can smell, see, hear, and feel.

Stern mentions that certain types of learning difficulties can be due to deficiencies in amodal perception. Several types of therapy—for example, hypnosis—also aim at ascertaining one's preferred sense modality. Both pedagogy and therapy make use of amodal perception in their concern to activate and communicate via several sense modalities.

*Vitality affects* refer to mobilization, activity, and the quality of the feelings. The infant's experiential world is coloured by the feelings it awakens. The feelings help the infant to find its bearings in its surroundings. Each experience has its own emotional nuance, and the infant—as well as the adult—is influenced all the time by vitality affects. They do not refer to a biological pattern, but to an internal information system. Vitality affect is based on intensity and contour, and not on affect categories such as anger, joy, surprise, and so forth. Vitality affects concern the subjective quality and the quantity of feelings following an experience. Vitality affects are best described via metaphors of motion: explosive . . . decrescendo . . . effusive . . . boisterous . . . emerge . . . undulate . . . fading away . . . quiet.

In *The Motherhood Constellation* (1995), Stern discusses the ways in which affects and experiences are represented. He suggests the concept of temporal feeling shape and says that feelings are represented in the same temporal form as narratives. This is discussed later in the presentation of his understanding of representations.

*Regulation.* The care person's interaction during this period is mostly connected with regulation. The early interaction is about modulating vitality affects. It is about communication concerning the regulation of the child's state (sleep–awake, hungry–satiated, crying–quiet). Comforting and soothing are central aspects in the early interaction.

Thus the focal point of the interaction is to help the child achieve transitions between the different states.

### *The sense of a core self (2–6 months): the close social world*

While the sense of an emergent self makes possible a sense of wholeness, the sense of a core self is based on the idea that the infant gives an impression of having an integrated sense of self, of being distinctly and physically separate from others, with its own actions and feelings.

This is perhaps the most complicated of Stern's senses of self, with the development of memory or episodic recall. Here he also describes a model for the way in which interaction is represented (see Stern, 1985, pp. 97, 112).

Both academic and clinical developmental theories describe an infant where the development of a differentiated and separate sense of self first takes place towards the end of the first year of life. Stern believes that the ability to merge is secondary and is dependent on an already existing sense of self and others. Thus the sequence of one's view on development is reversed: first comes the formation of a sense of self and others, and only then will an experience of merger become possible (see chapter 3 on intersubjectivity).

The sense of a core self is a physical self with meaning and coherence connected to action and experience. Four experiences form the basis of the sense of a core self: self-agency, self-coherence, self-affectivity, and self-history. Stern calls them self-invariants—something remains the same in all that is changed. Pattern and entity are created from experience with variation and repetition of experience. The interplay is characterized by themes-with-variation. In the repetition of a theme—for example, comforting—the adult introduces a variation in the comforting behaviour, which will thus represent something new in what is already known. The repetitions with variation will prevent the infant from habituating, which means that an adaptation or perfunctory reaction takes place. At the same time, it will learn about what remains the same within a world of variation and difference.

With the term "self-agency", Stern means that the infant itself experiences that it is capable of having an influence, of making things happen in relation both to people and to the physical world. The difference between one's own actions and those of others is that one has volition and is in control of actions generated by oneself (your arm moves when you want it to; when you close your eyes, it becomes dark). Self-coherence describes the experience of physical wholeness and coherence. Self-affectivity implies experiencing the affects as established patterns belonging to the sense of self.

The sense of a core self would be impossible without a sense of continuity in time. This presupposes a capacity to remember. It is this that is implied in the self-history, one of the four invariants. For the infant, this means remembering motor function, perception, and affectivity. It is an experience of being in a constantly changeable world. Chapter 7 contains a description of how these concepts may be helpful in understanding certain behavioural forms in adolescents.

In the period 2–6 months, the infant gains sufficient experience with these four self-invariants so that an organized subjective perspective—termed "the sense of a core-self"—can emerge. The child is very sociable during this period. Stern calls this period "the close social world". Smiling, prattling, and eye contact are important, as is the meaning of the face. Close social interplay is the typical feature of communication.

The infant discovers that regulation of affect is greatly dependent on others (a self-regulating other), while self-with-others experiences belong to the child itself. The child is also itself able to regulate interplay and feelings.

The infant begins to internalize experiences of interaction. Internal representations are memory structures, which represent experience (see later discussion about representations). Stern speaks of an episodic memory: a special memory of experiences that facilitate an integration of coherence, being the agent in one's own life, affectivity, and continuity to an organizing subjective whole. The abstraction of many specific memories creates a generalized memory structure, an average experience or prototype. On the basis of different concrete interplay episodes—with mother, for example—the infant will construct an abstraction or a type of average of these experiences. This average experience is an internal representation. Working models are then created that offer a starting point for relational expectations and actions. In Stern's terminology, these are representations of interactions that have been generalized (RIGs). When these representations of generalized interactions are activated, the infant will re-experience different forms of being together with a historic self-regulating other—in other words, one with whom the infant shares a history. Stern uses the concept of evoked companion for the subjective experience of being together with a (historic) self-regulating other.

In this period, imitation is an important way of regulating the interplay. By copying each other's bodily expressions with small variations, the mutual regulation of affects is especially taken care of. Imitation is therefore an important source of being-with-others experiences during this period.

In some of the criticism levelled at Stern, the concept of the sense of a core self has been made synonymous with the Western concept of self: an autonomous, independent self. We think this has been done at the expense of his descriptions of how relational experiences develop. We shall return to this point at the end of the chapter.

### *The sense of a subjective self (7–15 months): the world of the mental landscape*

The next leap in the sense of self happens when the infant feels that it has an internal world itself, an internal life, with feelings, motives, and intentions, and that others also have it. Stern says that the infant has now acquired a theory of separate forms of consciousness. New forms of being-together-with-another are developed. The infant experiences that other people have an internal psychic world similar to its own. Internal experiences are possible to share with others. The infant now has a new organizing perspective on its social life. Sense of self and others includes internal and subjective experiences in addition to open behaviour and direct sensation, which characterize the sense of a core self and others.

Stern points to three states that can be shared within this nonverbal self-domain: sharing of mutual attention, sharing of intentions, and sharing of affective states. This is what is meant by intersubjectivity. Stern points to a number of experiments showing that infants around the age of 6 months are able to share focus or attention with the care person. At this age the infant also starts pointing. This happens parallel with looking at mother in order to check whether she is sharing the infant's direction of attention. Stern (1985) maintains that the infant can experience having a special focus of attention, that the care person also can have her/his focus, and that these two mental states can be alike or different. If they are not alike, they can be brought together and shared. Interattention is a reality.

Stern places sharing of intentions in connection with research on the infant's language development. Gestures, postures, and nonverbal vocalization have been looked upon as such types of original acts of communication. There seems to be a consensus in this research that the infant shows intentions to communicate during this period. This kind of intention differs from an intention simply to influence another person.

The sharing of affective states is clinically the most relevant feature of intersubjective relatedness. How does this happen, and what is included here? What are the actions and processes that let other persons know that you feel something of the same as they are feeling? How can you, without using words, "penetrate to the inside" of the subjective experiences of others and then let them know that you have got there? Stern points out and maintains that imitation does not suffice here. He emphasizes that before one can speak of an intersubjective sharing of affect, the following processes must be present: (1) The parents must be able to read the child's feeling states from its external behaviour. (2) The parents must carry out a behaviour that is not strict imitation, but yet corresponds in some way or another with the child's external behaviour. (3) The infant must be able to read this corresponding parental response as something that has to do with the infant's own original emotional experience, and not just be imitation. It is only in the presence of these three conditions that feeling states in a person can be recognizable for another, and that both—without using words—can experience that a joint action has taken place. This is what Stern calls *affect attunement*. In chapter 4, we have demonstrated the clinical significance of this concept.

Interpersonal interdependence, as created by attunement, will play a crucial role for the infant. The discovery that internal feeling states are forms of human experiences that can be shared is of extreme importance. The reverse is also true: feeling states, which are never attuned, are experienced alone, isolated from the interpersonal context of experiences that can be shared. At stake is nothing less, according to Stern, than the form and the degree of the internal world that can be shared.

### *The sense of a verbal self (15–18 months): the world of words*

The sense of a verbal self is connected to linguistic meaning and context. When acquiring language, a new organizing, subjective perspective is developed that evolves, and this opens up a new way of being together with others. The sense of a verbal self implies the possibility and ability to reflect about oneself and to communicate about oneself to others. The child is now capable of symbolic play and the use of metaphors.

In Stern's perspective, meaning is an interpersonal and socially created phenomenon. Meaning linked to language implies a negotiation about what one can agree upon. Linguistic meaning is based on a shared experiential world. Linguistic development is therefore rooted in dialogue and interpersonal experience. Words are given their significance through a concrete interactional negotiation. This negotiation does not, of course, start anew every time a child is born. We are born into the language and into the meanings dictated by culture. Stern maintains that the word-and-language culture has more than a one-to-one relation to things and occurrences. Words have an existence, a life of their own. In this way, language permits transgressing lived experience.

The sense of a verbal self can also be called a symbolic self. The ability for symbolization facilitates self-reflection, and the child is now able to use symbols in its thinking and communicating. This also gives the child an opportunity to create a private internal world, but in a way different from that in the subjective self-domain. Language is only one particular aspect of the ability to symbolize. Other examples are play and dreams. Stern emphasizes the dual nature of language. It implies new opportunities for communication, interplay, and intimacy. But at same time language entails possibilities of alienation and splitting. It may also become a tool for manipulating and distorting experiences and may lead to a heightened sense of loneliness. According to Stern, language is a double-edged sword. It also makes part of our experiences less accessible to ourselves and to others. It creates a division between two forms of interpersonal experience—the one that is lived, and the one that is represented verbally. Experiences in the sense of an emergent self, the sense of a core self, and the sense of a subjective self will continue independent of language and can only be partly grasped in the area of verbal relatedness.

Language is a new form of relatedness. Language also poses a problem for the integration of the senses of self and the sense of self-with-others.

### *The sense of a narrative self (3–3½ years): the world of stories*

The sense of a narrative self is about creating meaning and coherence by telling one's own stories, and talking about oneself in one's own words. The appearance of language brings about the ability to tell one's own life history, with all the potentials this implies for being able to change the way one sees oneself. The child now has the ability to think about its own experiences, to find meaning in them, and to create an autobiography, a history that the child can tell to someone else.

The construction of histories is based on a number of elements from the other self-domains. This autobiography is also based on the way in which the parents communicate their own reality. The child sees itself in the parents' perspective, as it is now, as it was, and as it will be. Parents and others compile a kind of biography of the child. The primary function of the narrative history is to organize experiences, including those that in themselves can be incoherent and chaotic. To make up a story implies seeing and interpreting connections in human actions. The stories are about performers with wishes, motives, and feelings, taking place in a physical, historical, and interpersonal context.

At a seminar in Oslo in January 1996, Daniel Stern was asked to comment on his 1985 model of the senses of self. In the 1985 model he did not distinguish between the sense of a narrative and the sense of a verbal self, as he does in *Diary of a Baby* from 1990. He replied that today he would have placed greater emphasis on the narrative, not merely as a special sense of self, which was formed around the age of 3. The significance of the narrative and the narrative structure can be found as a recurrent theme quite early in development—in any case, after the formation the core self. He believes that already at an early stage the infant has the ability to create an overall, coherent, and meaningful experience of the world, of how it is to be with another. In *The Motherhood Constellation* (1995), he uses the concept of proto-narrative envelope to describe how the infant creates meaning and coherence in its experiences, and how these experiences are represented. The understanding of an early narrative structure is in line with the ideas of cognitive psychologists such as Jerome Bruner (Bruner, 1990a).

The senses of self, which are formed during the first years of life, function continuously and simultaneously. None of them is dominant at any given point of time in development, or is linked to different clinical topics. Once formed, they continue to be active and offer opportunities for experience and development while at the same time also being vulnerable and exposed to stress and trauma in later periods.

The emergent self deals with the process as the organization emerges. The sense of an emergent self is created through concrete processes with amodal perception and vitality affects. This gives us the potential for experiences of wholeness, creativity, and learning (Havnesköld & Mothander, 1995). The emergent self and its focus on organizing processes opens the way, at the next level, to the experience of a sense of a core self. The experience of being the agent of one's own actions, of being a physical whole, of having affects, and of existing over time will illustrate this sense of self as a comprehensive perspective. In the encounter with others, this perspective will remain, even though one also wishes to experience interdependence. Physical and sensory distinctions between the self and others are established. At the same time the experiences are regulated in this encounter. A new dimension is added with the experience of a sense of a subjective self: a feeling that, what I am experiencing and feeling, others too can experience and feel: "I can experience that I experience that the other experiences." In the first two senses of self, it is most important to experience action. In the sense of a subjective self, an experience of an internal world in oneself and in the other is created. The senses of a verbal and narrative self increase the possibilities to grasp a common world. Language is also a condition for self-reflection and thus also for being able to formulate one's own history.

## *Stern's view on representations*

Stern's project is to study the infant's subjective experience of its own world. This project also includes the question of how these experiences are represented mentally.

Stern addresses this issue in several places. Here we take as our point of departure his view on the formation of representations, in line with his discussions in his two main works (1985, 1995) and in an article from 1992. The point of departure in his book *The Interpersonal World of the Infant* is the question of how the infant develops a coherent representation of itself.

We have described this earlier in this chapter when presenting the sense of a core self. Stern links the formation of representations to memory structures representing experiences of being-together-with-another. He calls this the representations of interactions

(RIGs), which are internalized. Stern emphasizes over and over again that representations are about real experiences as distinct from fantasies.

In his article from 1992, Stern polemicizes against the psychoanalytic understanding of unconscious fantasies as a fundamental entity for psychic experience in the infant. Unconscious phantasies—a concept introduced by Melanie Klein—refer to innate, inherited scenarios that contain an object, the means, and a goal.

These scenarios are internal correlates or the psychic content of instincts. They exist independent of experiences and show a content that is innate. According to Stern, this type of understanding is difficult to explain. There is no space for thinking and representation of ego-functions, and, in this way of understanding, the surroundings are accorded no significance.

Stern believes that a fundamental entity aiming at explaining the infant's total experience has to contain a theory of thinking and a perspective on observable interaction. In narrative thinking, both motive and goal have been found to be crucial aspects. Purposefulness is also important in the study of affects and motor actions. Goal and motive include external and internal states of need, thinking, social attachment, and affects. He calls this purposeful entity that can explain and predict human behaviour a "pre-narrative envelope", because it comes into being prior to the development of language. It is this entity from which narratives are evolved. What distinguishes it from unconscious fantasies is that it is the result of the infant's own mental construction, though being connected to real relational experiences. This construction is evolved from the infant's own experience of instincts, which are handled in an interpersonal context. The constellation of constant elements required to compose such a entity is sensing, perception, affect, motivation, thinking, and so forth (Stern, 1995, p. 81).

In his article about the pre-narrative envelope, Stern leads a theoretical discussion about which basic concept is most useful for the understanding of the infant's early mental representation, while at the same time fitting into a developmental perspective. In his book *The Motherhood Constellation* (1995), the material is again both empirical data and theory. Representations are defined on the basis of his descriptions of interactions and his understanding of relationships. An interaction consists of observable behaviour, an act between two persons. In his understanding, relationship is the remembered history of earlier interactions. The relationship becomes tinted according to how the interaction is perceived and interpreted by the participants in the interaction.

In his thinking about representations, Stern has let himself be influenced by theories of cognitive development, those of Piaget in particular. Even though Stern also uses the concept of schema, he does not maintain the usual distinction used in developmental psychology between schema and representations. He believes that this distinction is scarcely relevant clinically and that modern infant research, especially with its emphasis on interpersonal and affective events, makes this distinction superfluous. The understanding of representations as procedures or processes for re-experiencing, rather than as mental products and structures, also tends to obscure this distinction (Stern, 1995, p. 80).

In his conception of representations, Stern emphasizes the interactive experience. The representations are formed from within, from the subjective experience of being together with someone. The infant starts forming a representation of how it feels inside itself while being together with someone. Fantasies are possibly later formulations of these experiences.

There is a difference between the representation of physical events and things, and subjective interpersonal events. Mental events are usually not isomorphous with events in external reality—they are affect-loaded. Piaget and others have described perceptual schemas, conceptual schemas, and sensorimotor schemas to describe how elements of experiences are represented. A fourth basic schema has also been added: a simple script, scenario, or sequence of events (event representation). Even though the two last-mentioned schemas (sensorimotor and sequence of events) connect elements of experiences to a certain degree, Stern is of the opinion that these concepts are inadequate for explaining person-related subjective experiences, which can also be of clinical interest.

Two other forms of representation are necessary: one entity for representing feelings—temporal feeling shape—and one entity for representing the whole experience as a meaningful event—a proto-narrative envelope, earlier termed "pre-narrative envelope".

Earlier in this chapter we described how Stern distinguishes between categorical affects and vitality affects. In *Motherhood*

*Constellation* he uses the expression "free-floating feeling" to describe the subjective qualitative and quantitative characteristics of feelings that accompany every experience. Since he here chooses to use this expression in preference to vitality affects, he does it in order to stress both the subjective character of the experience and the fact that it has a time dimension. The stream of thoughts, perceptions, and motor patterns creates feelings without reference to classical emotions. He also wishes to avoid arguments on the topic of feelings being secondary in relation to cognition. Feelings are represented in a temporal form, and they are experiences in time—hence the term "temporal feeling shape" (Stern, 1995, p. 85). The time shape makes the representation of feelings possible. Vitality affects, as he described them earlier, are also characterized by intensity, duration, and shape (Stern, 1985). The temporal shape depends on the type of feelings and motivations that are involved. There will be a beginning and an end of the period, which is subjectively structured time. In chapter 4 we discuss in detail how Stern's views on feelings and the way in which they are represented can be useful in therapy.

The display of a motive together with the affect that is triggered lead us to the concept of the proto-narrative envelope. The idea that certain interactive events are directly perceived and understood as meaningful can also be found in Bruner's writings—for example, in his expression "acts of meaning" (Bruner, 1990a). These meanings do not have to be constructed from different separate parts; they arise as a global intensive experience.

The main characteristic of a proto-narrative or pre-narrative envelope can be summed up as follows: it is a purposeful envelope. Motive and goal orientation are important aspects and include internal and external aspects of relationships, affective states, and so forth. It is a subjective experience, which unfolds in time. The temporal shape, too, creates coherence and meaning. It contains a dramatic line and the fundamental characteristics of a proto-plot. It arises before the development of language and constitutes the envelope from which narratives are evolved. It is not an innate structure, but the result of the infant's own mental construction. This construction is developed by the infant's subjective experience with instincts, which are handled in an interpersonal context. Instincts create patterns for events, while thinking gives them subjective coherence and meaning.

Stern's views on how representations are formed would merit a chapter of its own. There are many challenges here regarding the relation between representations, family script, myths, legends, paradigms, and premises. Stern calls these "representational entities", which are generalizations and abstractions of interactional events (Stern, 1995, p. 31). He refers to systems theory and cooperation with family therapists. It would also have been interesting to make a further study of the relation between interactive experiences, representations, and narratives.

## *Therapeutic consequences*

In the Introduction, we argued in favour of the notion that family therapy can benefit from acquiring knowledge and inspiration from current developmental theory. We have been especially interested in Stern's understanding of the senses of self as the organizing principle in development, and that these senses are always connected to domains of relatedness. The continuous-construction model also provides other opportunities for understanding problems and symptoms and will consequently have therapeutic consequences. In his book *The Interpersonal World of the Infant* (1985), Stern himself expresses a wish that his theory will have clinical relevance; the book also contains a chapter about how to use thinking in therapies with adult patients (chap. 11). He uses here, among other things, the concept of the key therapeutic metaphor when working with an understanding of the link between symptoms and senses of self. Bjørg Røed Hansen, a Norwegian psychologist, has made use of Stern's thinking for a number of years in her therapeutic work with children, and she has especially focused on the relation between nonverbal/affective and verbal/narrative forms of communication (Hansen, 1996a, 1996b).

In *The Motherhood Constellation* (1995), Stern draws concrete therapeutic consequences of his thinking on representations for the work with the mother–child unity and partly also the parent–child unity. In the present chapter, we have limited ourselves to his presentation of the infant's representations and have not discussed the significance of the parents' own representations—for example, the mother's representation of herself as a mother. Since we, as family therapists, aim at understanding feelings, we consider that his concept of temporal feeling shape deepens the understanding of feelings, as does that of vitality affects. Another issue with great relevance for family therapists is how interactive and relational experiences are felt and represented. Stern's concept of proto-narrative envelope describes the conditions for the development of narratives. His emphasis on the importance of experiences for the formation of representations cannot be without significance for our field, where discussions about the utility and validity of narratives are most relevant.

## *Critical remarks on Stern*

One way of approaching Stern's work is to take one's point of departure as the fact that human behaviour is ambiguous or ambivalent. It can be given different meanings or different significance, depending on one's own point of view. Stern's theory is one possible interpretation. As we have seen, he is preoccupied with the senses of self and speaks about the "infant"—that is to say, the picture of the clinical and the observed infant as a construction.

Senses of self and interaction are the principal elements in his interpretation. These are given a special content. Keywords are, for example, regulation, theme with variations, evoked companion, self-with-others experience, social referring, affect attunement, negotiation about meaning, and joint construction of histories. In these key words lie potentials for idealizing the interaction between infant and care person based on the idea that the infant is "perfect" from the beginning and, furthermore, that it can be destroyed from the outside through interaction partners who are not up to standard. What is excluded from this conception of the infant—according to some—is sadness, frustration, aggression, and violence. These elements are introduced from the outside world via those who have caring functions—often it is the mothers.

This type of interpretation is risky because it may blame the mothers for possible problems, or prepare the ground for blaming the fathers when they start taking an active part as caregivers.

Stern's perspective shows explicitly that being-with-others contains an element of mutual understanding in the sense that the infant "knows" or experiences the other's internal state. This is what Stern speaks of as the experience of the sense of a subjective self. Again, there is the possibility of perceiving the interaction as a kind of idyll where understanding is a normal state. Bradley (1989) stresses that this can be interpreted differently. It is not a matter of understanding on the part of the child, but that it uses others to expand or overcome its own internal state. The child participates with the other in order to be regulated. The danger with Stern and this type of developmental psychology is that it creates a new idealization of the infant, and that the "not-social" experiences or feelings are easily turned into something secondary and a result of negativity in the interplay from the other, meaning the caregiver. Another comment here is that hatred, violence, anger, obstinacy, and greed can be looked upon as social behaviour, since they are directed at others and are "pulling" others into the interaction. The effect of the behaviour is often negative for others, but that is not the same as saying that the behaviour does not "invite to interaction". On the contrary, a number of negative behaviours are only negative because one cannot get away from them. They are persistently "social".

These critical comments on Stern's work are included in the criticism from social-constructionist quarters. We therefore wish to explore this further in line with Philip Cushman's (1991) criticism. His point of departure is that the self is not a universal phenomenon, but can be viewed as being dependent on history, culture, and context. A description of the self is therefore a report on how society is shaping it, while also being a report on the values and preferences of society in regard to its inhabitants. He emphasizes, for example, that the description of the self-invariants linked to the sense of a core self is strangely in conformity with the emphasis placed on the dominant views on the self in America. He therefore maintains that Stern's work is not so much a matter of discovering universal aspects of the self, but more the fact that it represents an active participation in the shaping and specifying of the self as a historical, cultural, and contextual product. Cushman sees this infant as a virtual product of social conditions. This infant does "exist", but not as a universal infant. At the same time, he is critical of the conclusions drawn by Stern from his own observations. Cushman has no doubts about the infant being able to carry out the actual acts and skills that are described, but he believes that Stern is over-interpreting these observations. The topics of identity that are brought forward by Stern belong—in Cushman's opinion—to the world of adults. To speak of the experience of mastering or of being the agent in one's own life is to transport a theme from the adult world over into the infant's world. One might say that Stern's theories imply a new type of adultomorphization (Peterfreund, 1978), which was precisely Stern's own critical point of departure in regard to developmental psychology. Cushman replies that this is so and that Stern is under the influence of a cultural description or pre-understanding where the self is concerned. Again, Stern is criticized for confirming a culturally conditioned description of the self, rather than revealing a universal self. Cushman perseveres in this criticism of all the self-invariants described by Stern. Self-coherence is preferred to a description where the infant might just as well be described through the experience of being part of a group. Self-affectivity is preferred to descriptions emphasizing the collective or socially oriented affective experience. The same applies to self-history. Why is this brought to the fore, and not the experience of having a common, social history with relational partners? Again, Cushman poses the question, did Stern discover a mastering, delimited, feeling, and continuous infant in his data because it is in this way that infants are conceived in our culture?

Cushman continues this type of criticism of the concept of affect attunement. Again, Stern's alleged claim about its universal aspect is attacked. Cushman's response is that it concerns not universal qualities in the self, but a special tool that the child learns to use in our culture. Looked at from this viewpoint, it exemplifies how the social constructionist's arguments come true. The processes described in affect attunement offer an excellent description of how a special type of self is constructed. Other selves can be constructed on the basis of other interactional processes.

In conclusion, we wish to refer briefly to Cushman's criticism of Stern's views on language. This criticism has many aspects. Our point of departure in what we wish to emphasize is that Stern's view on language is a double-edged sword. It renders possible a division of meaning, while at the same time—as he points out—distancing the child (and us) from the direct experience. This is in many ways Stern's version of the story about Adam and Eve and the first fall of man. Their apple-pinching can be interpreted like this: by eating from the tree of knowledge, they acquired knowledge in the sense of language, and, at the same time, they (we) were also evicted from paradise. Cushman's version of this criticism is that it represents what he terms the "noble-savage" viewpoint (Cushman, 1991, p. 216) on infant development. The preverbal child is in direct and unbroken connection or community with nature. Language takes it out of this state; it is fragmented, split, and becomes dependent on communication, on abstractions. What is close and belonging is exchanged for the distant and superficial. This perspective can easily lead to a continuation of the ancient dualism between nature and culture. Nature becomes the original. Culture—through language—pollutes and destroys the original idyll. We are back to our starting point with mothers (parents) who are always potentially "guilty" where it concerns their children's problems and pathology. A criticism in line with Cushman would therefore be that, of course, parents are potential "sinners". The problem with presentations such as Stern's is that they can easily lead to a marginalization of all the other societal and biologically possible factors that can create problems and pathology.

We look upon Cushman's criticism as an important corrective to take along with us, while his criticism in many ways also confirms Stern's description of the Euro-American infant. Stern's presentation can be seen as a feasible and important description of a historically and culturally produced infant. It is this infant that we primarily work with, and it is in this Euro-American context that we are positioned. In this book we choose to take Stern as our point of departure as a description and a model produced by our culture. Where this infant is concerned, we see no reason to argue for universality.

What we are sceptical about, however, in Cushman's criticism is the fact that he, in our opinion, underestimates the relational perspective in Stern. When reading Cushman's article, one can get the impression that culture is something the individual is submerged into or enveloped by. This perspective on culture turns it into a macro-phenomenon limiting and controlling the individual person and the relationship of which he/she is a part. In our opinion, this is only one aspect of the phenomenon of culture. Culture is not only something we are enveloped by, or something that is superior to individual persons and their relationships. The individual persons and their relationships are culture too. Culture is also a local micro-phenomenon. That is to say, culture is something that is brought about by individual persons and their relationships as much as by something superior. We believe that Stern offers—as also pointed out by Cushman—good and useful descriptions and models of interaction between individual persons which exemplify how cultural values and phenomena are produced.

Cushman's main point is that Stern's model has obvious political implications. Stern's concept of the self can be looked upon as an argument for a special perspective on the individual that draws attention to certain power relationships and marginalizes others. We recognize that every theory and model has these implications, Cushman's as well. Cushman's views on culture marginalize, in our opinion, important local, close interactional relationships as the supporting elements in every culture. He can be understood along the lines of drawing attention to the macro-perspective and marginalizing the micro-perspective. In this dichotomy, one part is brought to light while the other is concealed. Paradoxically, this makes Cushman a worthy member of the Euro-American culture and science of which he seems to be so critical. To us, this means that both he and we belong to the same cultural community. We consider it useful to become acquainted with this community because it is also from there that our clients are coming. Both Stern and Cushman are helpers in this work.

CHAPTER TWO

# Perspectives on the concept of self

*Vigdis Wie Torsteinsson*

Some children are brown
like newly baked bread,
some children are yellow,
some nearly red,
some children are white
from top to toe,
much is different
it is merely on the outside.

Some children are from Finland
some from Sudan
some children are Norwegian
some from Japan.
Yes, there are children
in every land and realm,
much is different
but inside they are alike.

Some children say "yes"
and some say "ja"
some say "oui"
and some say "da"

some say "si"
and some say "hi",
much is different
but it is on the outside.

Think if we could play
together all of us,
we would have a row
from Africa to Drammen.
Some would laugh
and some would scream,
much became different
but inside they were alike.

Jo Tenfjord/Johan Øyan

This children's song has for a long time been a source of speculation to me. I believe that I always understood the author's intention as an attempt to bridge the gradually increasing and far-too-wide gap between individuals in our culture and to counteract differences on the grounds of different external characteristics. And on this level, she has my total approval. But, as a child, I never completely understood what made her claim that we were so alike inside. I thought it might have something to do with the fact that we all needed food, as well as mummies and daddies, and a bed to sleep in at night. Otherwise, I thought that there were plenty of differences inside too. Some always wanted to fight, some talked all the time, some thought it boring to read books, some were shy. Nor could I understand that all differences could be connected to what was "outside", as it says in the song. But how do we understand these differences, and what would it be meaningful to call them? And which conceptual frame do we need so that this diversity can also be useful in a therapy that primarily has our common point of departure in view—namely, the relationships? These are the main issues raised in this chapter.

The concept of "self" is used in the literature in a large number of ways that are partly conflicting (McCall, 1990). Different concepts such as subject, subjectivity, identity, and person are linked to the concept of self, with all the different associations implied in these concepts. Often it is also connected to a particular theoretical school—namely, the self-psychological tradition after Kohut (Karterud & Monsen, 1997). Daniel Stern has a more explicit phenomenological point of departure. He uses the concept of self mostly as a basic category for commenting on what it feels like to be a human being in the world, and as something inextricably connected to all our experiences. In this chapter the concept is basically given a broad meaning, as a way of describing ourselves as individual persons with a perspective, and with a position in the world. The chapter presents a number of ideas on how to use the concept of "self" in ways that are inspired by the research on developmental psychology. The underlying statement is that if we vary the ways in which we use the concept, it may significantly expand our thinking on the relationships and contexts of which we always are a part.

In many contexts, the concept of self is precisely one of the concepts used to characterize difference or delimitation. And using it as a key concept for therapy understanding has largely depended on whether individual- or relationship-focused thinking has been used as the basis for one's approach. Traditionally, the theory of therapy has focused on the individual in different ways. Even if an understanding of the background has implied one or the other form of interaction with the environment, the approaches have always been concentrated on the individual and his/her sense of self or his/her self-understanding. The individual has come with relational experiences as his/her personal property and has carried them around in new contexts. These possessions have therefore also influenced new relationships, like old furniture brought into new houses. In an individual approach, one establishes a new relationship through the therapeutic dialogues, as a basis for new experiences or as a re-telling and a re-interpretation of former ones. The common point of departure for most individual approaches is an understanding that in therapeutic work, the sense of self or self-understanding is an essential element. The understanding of pathology is also linked to an individual focus. In this connection, the concept of self can best be understood as an understanding of *identity*: who am I, and what is it that prevents me from being the one I *really* am.

The last decades have brought about a recognition of the fact that the present moment is not only an arena for displaying old experiences, but also a point of departure for gaining new ones—and hence also experiences that will be different. The starting point of family therapy was the assertion that problems could not be seen solely as sediments of problematic experiences in the individual. Problems *belonged to* the relational contexts in such a way that every effort to change individual problems had to be directed at the relationships. It was only by being focused on the relationship that one could change individual functioning. The traditional concept of self was looked upon as a cultural prejudice, which created more problems than it solved because it disengaged the individual from his/her relational context. But the relational context is the precondition for understanding or interpreting experiences or individual characteristics as problematic (Hoffman, 1992, p. 10). To put it plainly: to treat human problems as something isolated from a relational context, and as solely connected to individual persons in an individual therapeutic context, was looked upon by family therapists as having no effect at best and being harmful at worst. A family therapeutic classic, Mara Selvini-Palazzoli's *Self-Starvation* (1974), gives a description of a project for treating severe anorexia within a psychodynamic frame. Selvini's conclusion was that the results were in no way proportionate to the amount of work that was invested. A further conclusion was that one needed totally new therapeutic theories in order to understand and treat psychic problems, because problems originated in the reality created by relationships.

Family therapy theory detached itself from individual, psychological concepts. "Early family therapists were sceptical about the idea of the self", says Lynn Hoffman (1992, p. 10). The preoccupation with the self was connected to fundamental ideas in the psychological literature, as a concept that was used to describe the private internal world and not what happens between people. In this respect, Batesons's article "Cybernetics of Self" (1972a) was an important milestone. Even though he continued to use the concept of "self", he provided it with an alternative theoretical frame. The focal point in this frame was the understanding of the self as a cybernetic concept. This demanded reference to an ongoing communication between the individual and his or her surroundings in order to create meaning. The self could only be understood as a relational phenomenon. At any point in time, the current context created the self and gave meaning to it. The link between the "self" and an "internal being" was dissolved. The concept of self can here perhaps best be understood as a way of understanding and also as an indication of how important it is to transcend our culture's conception of individuality. Our culture's definition of the self as something internal that is able to transcend its surroundings, and is thus also able to control them, was defined as an "epistemological error" contributing to the development of pathology. Inevitably, the focus of the therapy would therefore also have to be directed at relationships, including that part of the client's self-understanding that indicated that "the part could become more than the whole". Individual therapy had to be seen as a kind of illusion. The individual was his/herself unable to change, independent of his or her context. Nor could the individual be in unilateral control of his or her relationships—the relationship was on another logical level, hence demanding other ways of approach.

In family therapy literature, the discussion concerning individual versus relationship is often presented in an either/or form. Family therapists engage in polemics against what is termed an "essentialistic" concept of self, which includes the notion about the self existing as a kind of core inside us that we are more or less given the opportunity to realize through our relationships. The criticism is therefore aimed at a self-sufficient concept of self. The main grievance is associated with the idea that it is the private, individual self that creates and maintains relationships—not the other way round. The basic thesis in "essentialistic" thinking is that each one of us is unique, and that it is this uniqueness that is to be communicated by an authentic expression. I have a kind of core that is me. It can be suppressed or honed, but in one way or another it should be expressed in whatever I am doing. The alternative—or the other extreme often represented by family therapy literature—is the totally relativized self, one that always changes according to the context of which we are a part.

The basic thesis is that without the context or the relationships there would not be a self to relate to. In a family therapeutic context, the essentialist is seen primarily as the counterpart—the one who is referred to when one wishes to create a contrast to one's own standpoint. In the eyes of family therapists, everyone is, in one way or another, preoccupied with relational experiences, even though the significance and the content of these experiences may vary. However, to which extent and in which sense is it necessary to continue the debate with Descartes? Is the fact of having a theory about the subject or about the self hopelessly outdated and reactionary in the sense that we now conceive ourselves in every possible way as created by relationships and belonging to relationships? Is thinking in relation to a concept of self the same as saying that each one of us has an identity that exists from the very outset to the end, in one or the other unchangeable form? Bateson continued using the concept, even though he gave it a different theoretical context. This is also Harlene Anderson's position: to use the concept, but with roots in an understanding of the relationship as the fundamental category (Anderson, 1997, p. 234). A central issue will therefore be: which of our theories and experiences give meaning to the subject in a form that still takes into account that we have a basis in relationships and interpersonal contexts? Perhaps we need to look at this topic with new eyes, and perhaps we are prevented—by a dichotomy like the one described here—from grasping the complexity of the phenomena we are trying to understand.

In many ways our everyday conception of the subject or the self is a light mixture of essentialism and relativism. We encounter one or the other form of essentialism in very many different contexts. All thinking that in one way or the other has understanding human *nature* as its starting point is a form of essentialism. When one says that within the modern school system all children are entitled to teaching programmes that are adjusted to their individual requirements, then this is also a form of essentialism.

But the opposite—the relativistic way of thinking—can also be easily illustrated. We express it when we experience ourselves or others as extremely different, dependent on the context. "I felt like a completely different person" or "I almost did not recognize him, he was so different" are expressions that capture the vicissitudes of the sense of self. "From the moment he sees her again until the moment when he recognizes her again in the way he loves her, there is a certain road to travel", says Milan Kundera (1998, p. 32).

### *An example from the therapy-room*

The point of departure for the issues raised in this chapter can also be illustrated by a concrete therapeutic example. Signe became a client in child and adolescent therapy after increasingly long absences from school, ending with her not showing up at all. She had physical ailments now and then that, she felt, were good enough reasons for staying away from school. She suffered especially from headaches and pains in her joints. Signe was therefore examined by her doctor in every way he considered advisable. No somatic problems were discovered. But her parents became gradually convinced that this did not only have to do with her body and with physical pain. For this reason, her family had an ongoing discussion about her adjustment and well-being at school and about her friends and social adjustment in general. In spite of lengthy discussions, none of them believed that the emerging themes could give a clear explanation or understanding of Signe's physical symptoms or of her refusal to go to school. Some of the discussions also ended with Signe becoming despondent because her pains and discomfort were defined as unreal, as though they did not exist. What became most important to her was the question of who could say something about how she felt "inside herself", and how the words and her subjective experience were connected.

Another topic of major concern to Signe, and which is connected to the experience of being one's own person, were questions about who she was and what she could call her own self. When asked to say how she felt, she formulated it thus:

> "I feel that I am walking on a kind of edge—and I *have to* stay up there. I could very easily fall down—am scared that it will happen. The edge has long, steep downhill slopes on both sides. I am walking on the top. It is a long way down—I just *cannot* fall. It is difficult to stay on top of that edge—others are walking on broader edges, I have one that is a little narrower. I feel that I am losing my balance or my control, and then I may fall down. There is nothing which I *mustn't* do, just have to be careful. Down there—then I might be lost for ever—then there is nothing more—*then I won't be myself again.*"

The picture of the edge was about knowing who one was and being able to be oneself. But how do you find this out? The narrow edge was, for Signe, a metaphor for how she experienced being uncertain about who she was, who she wanted to be, and partly also about how others saw her. Signe felt a need for authenticity—she did not want to be one who only copied "the cool ones". Neither did she want to do the opposite—for it would not make her feel, either, that she was doing exactly what she wanted. Nor did it help her very much that other people offered concrete feedback as to how she was seen by others and told her what impression she made. She cites her teacher: "She says to me—to everyone—sort of what everyone is like—you are a good girl at home, she says to me—she sort of *affirms* what the person *is like*—so then one almost tries to prove the contrary a little. . . ." For her this was a serious and difficult issue, and she spent hours brooding over how she could solve it. In a way, she imagined that she could take on different roles, choose different ways of behaving, depending on which impression she wanted to make, or in which context she found herself. But on the other hand, she regarded this position as a form of falseness, which she did not wish to have in her life. Something had to be there, something that was more real and more her own than everything else. Thus Signe's question became similar to ours: to what extent can we speak in a way that will give Signe a feeling of being herself, and how can it be possible to find out when and how she feels at home in her own life? One way of looking at this is seeing Signe as also enmeshed in a set of either/or problems, in the terms of social-constructionist thinking. Either she has a core, an identity independent of interactions with others, or else she is a social chameleon turning the way the wind is blowing and shifting identity according to her surroundings. Signe felt that none of these alternatives was good enough. She problematized this dichotomy in a way that made it necessary to search for other modes of concretizing the concept of self, with a different conception of the relation between the self and relationships.

In our culture we are used to seeing these problems partly as a phenomenon of adolescence. Erik H. Erikson (1994) calls this phase the identity/confusion phase, where finding one's identity is a presupposition for and also presupposes a type of autonomy that is held in very high regard. Ever since the age of Romanticism, we have believed that the answer to the question of who we are would be found inside us—as a core of uniqueness in each one of us. Only a few decades ago, the motto was "finding oneself". Most of us are probably familiar with the fact that when adolescents are referred to treatment, "low self-esteem" is the recurrent theme.

Signe's dilemma can therefore serve to illustrate an extensive theoretical debate. These sets of problems have obvious historical roots that can be usefully concretized. Can we now discard the debate with Descartes and, rather, focus on an understanding of the subject which does not have the same implications about individuality and autonomy as postulated by an essentialistic way of thinking? Is the only alternative the social-constructionist relativism that says that I am at all times being created by the linguistic context in which I find myself?

In relation to therapeutic practice, this also concerns ideas about how working with a relational-based sense of self can become significant in a family therapy context. How can one work with problems centring around the sense of self as expressed by Signe and based on significant relationships?

## *The debate about the concept of the self*

The common starting point for all those interested in the social self has been the criticism levelled against the Cartesian concept of the self (Bakhurst & Sypnowich, 1995). They are united in their negative attitude towards a concept of the individual that was clearly formulated at the beginning of the Age of Enlightenment and has had a profound impact on Western culture. Descartes' formulation "Cogito, ergo sum" postulates that what characterizes the individual is thinking, or consciousness. Originally, Descartes formulated this statement as a kind of response to the question of how we could acquire true and certain knowledge. There may be good reasons for doubting everything that is outside us and of which we gain knowledge through our senses. Just think of, says Descartes, how an oar appears to be bent when you see it halfway in the water. What has been handed down by tradition can also be questioned. The sole facts that can always be ascertained with certainty are doubts—or thinking and consciousness. In Signe's case, one might think that all the hours she spent alone in her room, thinking about what she could really call herself, what she was, and what she could be, would have yielded results in the sense that the process of reflection in itself would have given her an experience of being a self. But it did not. On the other hand, it is difficult to reject it as just useless, unessential, or harmful. At least it made her a most interesting person to talk to and to be with.

Implicit in a Cartesian understanding is a theory about the relation between consciousness and the world. Every single one of us can only know the content of our own consciousness. Our knowledge of the external world is always indirect and communicated by mental representations. And mental representations can only be compared with other mental representations, and not with the world around us. The psychological world becomes a self-sufficient world, but directly transparent to itself. Introspection enables us to discover who we are and what characterizes us as individuals. Meditation by a tranquil mountain lake without distracting social relationships should therefore provide a more favourable context for "knowing oneself".

However, within these confines the self becomes a profoundly asocial phenomenon—the self is my private relationship to my own thoughts and ideas and is an introspective phenomenon of consciousness. Thus mental life also has content and structure prior to and independent of my interactions with other people. Other people are a part of the external world, and the external world is only known to us as a derivation from our own private ideas.

Family therapy theory also had a period with focus on the internal structure. In many ways, Maturana's constructivism expresses a similar line of thought. The inner logic of the nervous system is decisive for what we conceive. It is not the world in itself that creates the impressions; it is the internal logic in the perceiving organism that determines what can be perceived. And Descartes' assertion that "one representation can only be compared to another representation" has an affinity to the current postmodern assertion that the meaning of a word is only given by other words. It is not the connection of words with "something else"—in today's terminology, often called the external world—that gives them meaning. It is the inner logic in language as an independent system of signs which creates and maintains meaning, just as structure did for Descartes in the system of mental representations. The difference between them is nevertheless conspicuous regarding the outer/inner dimension: to focus on the language places the structure *outside* the individual, or *between* individuals.

In a sense, Descartes has remained the symbol of atomistic individualism and is opposed by the adherents to the idea of a social self. If one takes as one's starting point the notion that the self is a socially constituted phenomenon, the idea that the self is a concrete, empirical manifestation of a not-concrete internal essence is of no value, or even interest. Today, the motto is that my self is constituted in the social dialogue. My identity is a result of my social existence. The importance of language for the sense of self is especially emphasized. We return to this later. The social-constructionist critique against the concept of the self is explicitly directed at this type of Cartesian interpretation (Anderson, 1997; Gergen, 1994).

Signe's experiences are marked by the inadequacies of the Cartesian perspective. Something is missing in this way of thinking, something that makes her more withdrawn and gives her a feeling of first having to find out something before she presents herself to the world. In this sense, this type of reasoning creates problems, just as Bateson (1972b) pointed out. We must therefore continue to ask ourselves whether the question of the singular person, the individual self, thereby is superfluous. Or, expressed differently: which alternative formulations make more allowances for the importance of the context for our experience of having our own view or conception of the sense of the world, of being a self?

## *Two different approaches to the social self*

However, the argument that the self is social is certainly not an unambiguous or uncomplicated point of departure (Bakhurst & Sypnowich, 1995). What we may call a weak invariant is based on the notion that we are socially constituted beings since our individuality is formed to a great extent by social or cultural influences from the outside world. Growing up in London makes Signe a different person from who she would have been growing up in Scotland or in Vienna. Socialization is a key concept in this tradition and implies the internalization of experiences and values as basic premises. The self is more or less pure plasticity; it is malleable, but it nevertheless has a kind of existence prior to any influence. Signe is onto the same thoughts when she reproaches her parents for having given her an excessively "girlish" upbringing which made her more unassuming and less aggressive than she could have been. She is thinking of herself in this connection as a girl who—with influences of a different kind—would have had possibilities to present herself differently, although even then she would not have been a totally different person. These premises would then have constituted this malleability as a kind of "essential" self. It is possible to speak of a type of self as an ever-present substance that is not given a concrete form before we have a world to relate to. "We instinctively process our experiences in such a way that they appear to belong to some kind of unique subjective organization that we commonly call the sense of self" (Stern, 1985, p. 6). With Stern in mind, we must also expand the context by turning it around. The relationship both creates and is created by this subjective organization. And it is not shaped if we exclude the subjective perspective or what Stern calls the "sense of self".

The radical or strong argumentation assumes that the self is not only social in the sense that what we believe in—and the way in which we conceive ourselves—is profoundly influenced by the social circumstances in which we are living; the basic assumption here is that the very capacity to think and act, and to conceive ourselves as delimited individuals, is socially constituted. In all these arguments, the dialogue or the social experiences are not the form in which a pre-existing self is moulded; the dialogue is what brings the self into existence. "Social constructionism is not only saying that our cultural milieu has an influence on our psychology, or that our nature is a product of milieu (including social) factors rather than biological factors. *Both* of these perspectives are essentialist" (Burr, 1995, p. 6). The very idea of the self is a social and cultural product. We could just as well have thought about ourselves in different ways. In a different linguistic context, we would have been preoccupied with quite different matters and experienced ourselves in completely different ways. The professional focusing on the topic creates and maintains this cultural tendency to look upon the experience of the self as a central human phenomenon (Gergen, 1994, p. 128).

Consequently the social-constructionist concept of the self has been developed as an alternative to a concept of the self that, in a certain sense, is defined as an individual property, as something inherent in the individual that—facilitated by the surroundings—can be more or less developed or expressed. Kenneth Gergen says that it is this form of essentialism that is under attack by constructionism. We have no inner essence—the self is constructed in the exchange between people. "If one feels split between several selves, torn between competing tendencies, capable of multiple personalities . . . the literature suggests that a state like this can become an emerging cultural form. And this we should not grieve over" (Gergen, quoted in Hoyt, 1998, p. 357). It is not difficult to agree that ideas about the self that do not include the relational contexts that are always part of our lives are not appropriate for an understanding in most contexts, and perhaps especially not as a philosophy of therapy. The problem with Gergen, and the point of departure in social constructionism, is that all other possible ways of using the concept are traced back to Descartes and thus represent the same essentialism expressed in his thinking.

## *Experience of self—identity or subjectivity*

The alternative to a social-constructionist understanding is consequently characterized as a subject that is "separate, self-sufficient, independent, uniform and private" (Wetherell & Maybin, 1996, p. 221).

The current discussion is, however, primarily a discussion between what we have here called a weak and a strong understanding of a relational point of departure, regardless of the attempts made to confirm that Descartes is still alive and kicking. What Sommer (1997, p. 189) calls the "extremely dogmatic argumentation" of social constructionism makes it difficult to discuss many of the topics without ending up in an either/or discussion. One of the paradoxes in the current discussion, to give an example of how intricate these questions are, is that even with interaction-based perspectives on the processes of self-construction, the emphasis is stronger than ever on the subjective aspect of the reflective process. As an example: even if your self is created in a dialogue with me, and it is inextricably connected to this dialogue, then your self will in principle be unrecognizable to me—I cannot know anything about your standpoint or your perspective. This is formulated in the spirit of hermeneutics. "Hermeneutics maintains that all is interpretation", says Harlene Anderson (1997). "If . . . all understanding is interpretation, then one can never reach a true understanding, another's opinion cannot be fully understood . . ." (p. 39). Everyone has to speak for himself/herself. The very idea of ambiguity or diversity in descriptions of reality in family therapy is, in my opinion, a way of emphasizing the unique quality in the individual's perspective. Subjectivity is alive and kicking, even though the subject is outdated. "The entire dialogue is based on the idea that an understanding is possible even if we know that it may be impossible," says Steve de Shazer (1994, p. 55). And he continues: "Of course the client knows what she means ... but we cannot know it." To understand the sense of self will thus imply understanding the unique perspective—what the context alone cannot clarify. Subjectivity is therefore a more accurate alternative concept of the self than identity.

Another central point is the question of the degree to which language is the sole source of the sense of self. According to Harlene Anderson (1997, p. 219), "Whom we regard ourselves to be, is a linguistic construction." Vivian Burr (1995, p. 39) states: "The person you are, your experience, your identity, your 'personality', is all an effect of language." With this kind of starting point, one might think that Signe's lacking experience of an authentic self was a consequence of the fact that she seldom participated in conversations where the use of pronouns was an essential part, or that these conversations gave exaggerated emphasis to the importance of an unambiguous and consistent use of the same pronouns. This would be the consequence of understanding Signe's problematization of her sense of self solely in relation to her as one who uses language. However, the significance of language is sometimes treated in a confusing manner. In a fundamental sense, language creates the world. However, sometimes language is subordinated to a further concept of interaction or practice, as, for example, in Kenneth Gergen. This is discussed later.

Dion Sommer (1999) criticizes social constructionism for its lacking possibilities to say something about the ever-present sense that there is a "me", in spite of shifting contexts. This is also Signe's problem in relation to the relativism implied by a purely context-based, chameleon concept of the self. She wanted a third alternative that would embrace the relationships, but where she would not be reduced to a product of them. While being a part of something, she also wanted to understand herself as one who was able to make a contribution, as one who made a difference in the contexts in which she took part.

### *A developmental psychological understanding of the self*

One of the basic assumptions in developmental psychological theory is that a sense of self, in the form of an experience of one's own position in relation to the other, *also* is a precondition for participation in a dialogue.

Daniel Stern chooses—as he himself formulates it—to place the self at the centre of his reflections about developmental psychology. He does this explicitly in order to convey the infant's *subjective experience of its social relationships* (Stern, 1985, p. 5). He therefore takes it for granted that the relationship is the point of departure, but that everyone who is a part of this relationship has her/his own gateway to or experience of relatedness. "How we experience ourselves in relation to others provides a basic organizing perspective for all interpersonal events", says Stern (1985, p. 6).

He also stresses that even though the self is a difficult concept to grasp in a scientific context, its impact is so crucial in all our everyday experiences that for this reason it is necessary to dwell upon it. It appears in all our experiences—for instance, in the experience of being an integrated bodily whole, of having volition and intentions, and in the experience of reflecting on and communicating experiences that are fundamentally one's own. Stern sees the social-constructionist definition of the experience of reality being exclusively created by the linguistic context to which we belong—and which therefore could have been completely different in a different linguistic context—as important, but lacking in several aspects. A sense of self permeates every human experience in one way or another (see chapter 1 for a discussion of the criticism against the tendency in developmental psychology to universalize its understanding). By focusing on the concept of "self", Stern is often associated with the tradition after Kohut (Boalt Böethius & Berggren, 1998; Karterud & Monsen, 1997). Basically, Stern does not make this conceptual connection himself. Rather, he gives the impression that he wished to grasp the phenomenological core of the experience of being present in the world. For Stern, this implies the experience of always being present as *someone*. A "sense of self" is an ever-present phenomenon in all interactional contexts. With this statement he argues against two opposite alternative positions for a conception of the infant's world. First and foremost, he argues against the notion that it is born into an autistic position, enclosed in its own world. In this view, the child opens itself to the world through the socialization inherent in experiences with others. Gradually the child is shaped into a social being and thus becomes able to participate in an intersubjective world. The alternative is to see the small child in a symbiosis where its subjective world, its own perspective, gradually is separated from the common world. According to Stern, none of these perspectives covers what a theory should include in the way of recapitulation of the early interaction, as we understand it today.

## *A preverbal self?*

An important difference in the understanding of the self in family therapy and in developmental psychology is the question of conceiving the self as a not exclusively language-based construction. Stern uses the term "senses of self". His explicitly states that some senses of self exist long before language and self-awareness become a part of the child's potential modes of expression. The three first domains of the self in Stern's model are based on affective forms of exchange, where regulation, imitation, and affect attunement are the typical forms of being-together (see chapter 1).

Assuming this to be a continuous-construction model, it means that these are forms of togetherness that are present as part of all significant relationships throughout life. It is Stern's main point that within the frames of these modes of togetherness, the infant organizes its own perspective all the time, as a precondition for being able to participate in a coordinated way of togetherness. Senses of self are defined as "invariant patterns of awareness" (Stern, 1985, p. 7), which again is a form of organization.

There are two crucial implications here. First, Stern uses the concept of "sense of self" as something more fundamental than subjectivity. He links the concept of subjectivity to the subjective domain of the self. His use of subjectivity implies a difference between the child and others, based on a distinction between internal and external. Others have an internal world, which is potentially but not necessarily accessible to me. In a way, all senses of self therefore do not imply an internal world. In the domain of the core self—where imitation and themes with variations are the most important forms of togetherness—the sense of self is represented by the production and reproduction of bodily expressions. These forms of togetherness are a condition for coordinated bodily action with others. Or, in the words of the social anthropologist Henrietta Moore (1994): "What is at issue is the embodied nature of identities and experience . . . a mode of knowledge that draws on an understanding of experience as a form of embodied intersubjectivity" (p. 3). Stern therefore distinguishes between having one's own internal (and hence potentially inaccessible) world and being a singular self on the basis of one's own bodily expression. Bodily expression is personal, but it is always created in coordinated interaction with others.

For Stern, this coordination of action is also a requirement for transforming experiences into language and narratives. In Stern's theory, a concept is created on the basis of pre-narrative experiences. These experiences exist prior to verbalization. The main characteristic of the infant's representations is that they deal with interactive experiences (RIGs). These are experiences of being with particular others who are internalized, and not of external events or persons (Stern, 1995, p. 81). These experiences are affective and unfold in time in an irreversible way—in other words, they have a beginning and an end.

How, then, does the infant represent these experiences? One of the forms accessible to the infant is what is called "event representation", which is defined as "an invariant sequence of events which is represented as a coherent scenario" (Nelson, 1996, pp. 84–85). Being together with an other is a sequential event. Moreover, in this context the infant's capacity for representing feelings is important. Affectivity (used here both for vitality affects and categorical affects: see chapter 1) is crucial because their representations structure the subjective *experience of time*. This experience is created by the changes unfolding in time. According to Stern, these temporal contours make it possible to represent affective experience. Feelings are represented as "temporal feeling shapes"—that is to say, lived patterns of change. The infant's ability to evaluate time is very much like ours. This capacity is an important condition for the coordination of action which is developed in the earliest interactions. All turn-taking is based on coordination of one's own and others' initiative in the interaction, also in relation to a time-axis.

This also implies that the child sees the world and the events in it as intentional (Bruner, 1990a; Stern, 1985). The other's actions contain an "in-order-to"—there is an intent in what one is doing. The concept of coordination of action therefore also includes a claim that even if we function as an entity on one level, the difference between my point of departure and yours is important for the understanding of the relational structure that coordinates action. We have different positions in the world and yet are inextricably connected to the common structures we create.

In Stern's understanding, the coordination of action and the representations of events are linked to narratives in the following way: a narrative always contains a plot or an intrigue that is played out as a line of dramatic tension. This tension curve corresponds to the affective curve and gives Stern a reason for stating that the infant recognizes narrative structures that exist before they can be told (Stern, seminar in Oslo in 1999). Like very many other modern authors, Stern says that the narrative structure provides the frame for the possibility of understanding and relating to interpersonal events. It is this format we all use in order to comprehend human action.

In order to describe this linkage of affects, events, and narratives, Stern uses the concept of "proto-narrative envelope". It comprises both time and event, thus connecting the feeling schema with a narrative schema. A central point is, therefore, that language is given a double task: it can express an experience already existing in another experiential modus, but it can also create new experiences or transform earlier experiences (Stern, 1985, p. 6). This leads Stern to take a clear stand on the idea that, in a certain sense, language has a relation to an experienced world, and that it thus may refer to something different from other linguistic expressions. Consequently he separates himself from an understanding of language that a great number of family therapists are representing today.

The French philosopher Paul Ricoeur emphasizes a point that, in my opinion, is essential in this connection. In his book *Oneself as Another* (1992), he makes the following comments on the relation between language and action: "The implicit axiom that 'everything is language' has often led to a closed semanticism, incapable of accounting for human actions as actually *happening* in the world, as though linguistic analyses condemned us to jumping from one language game to another, without thought ever being able to meet up with *actual* action" (p. 301). A semantic analysis deals only with utterance as a statement and not with the changes occurring in a subject that is capable of making decisions of its own by assigning significance to the world, including the relational contexts of which the subject is a part. In this sense, the use of language is a process that exceeds boundaries, where the *use* of language contains something that cannot be understand on the basis of an analysis of the specific internal structure of language. Social-constructionist family therapy, on the other hand, has been interested in the opposite phenomenon—that language exceeds each linguistic utterance. When using language, we always speak from a wider context of relations and possible meanings (Schrag, 1997, p. 111). With Stern in our hip pocket, we can get other ideas about the linkage between the individual's action, the coordinated interaction (the common, interactional reality), and the stories we tell about ourselves and our lives, and the relation between action and narration.

Robyn Fivush (1993, 1994) has underlined another point in connection with the significance of narratives. By studying how families interact in creating narratives around events in the history of the child, she shows that there are different cultures in different families in regard to these topics. She divides them roughly into two groups: those who are "fact-oriented" and attach importance to naming the actual events, and those who also include an evaluating aspect. This evaluating aspect emerges in the sense that the experiences are related to the importance they have had for each person, and the feelings these events included. This comes about with the help of emotional exchanges, words, and descriptions referring to these.

A concrete example from a family therapy session with Signe's family may illustrate this point:

> Mother: You were so worried about Signe in that period—you were so afraid that she would break down that I had to comfort you too—I remember that very well.
>
> Father: It was more like it was bad if she isn't feeling good. It was more like that, well, that she is in a situation she doesn't enjoy at all, I don't like that. Perhaps I was afraid that we wouldn't manage to help her either.
>
> T[herapist] (to Signe): Did you notice that he was thinking of you?
>
> S: I noticed that someone was worried. I'm also worried. But I didn't know it actually. Something or other that Mummy said . . .

Signe expresses that she both knows and does not know. All of them are aware that they are relating and organizing themselves around a form of worry. But Signe does not know this in the sense that it is an experience she can take hold of as words or with words. In one way, they all both live and speak about sequences of coordinated action.

Seen from Signe's perspective she is participating in these sequences, but she does not relate to them as events that can have different meanings for the persons included in them. When we use this as a starting point in our talks, she can recognize the experience of knowing but not knowing, from many different contexts—also in relation to friends and classmates. This often makes her feel insecure. She participates in these exchanges but does not know how to act intentionally in the sense that she can choose between alternative actions. She feels drawn into exchanges, but not in such a way that she can contribute with her own perspective.

Another episode, but with a different point of departure, can be described as follows: mother turns to Signe and, while they are talking to each other, starts fingering Signe's scarf, which is lying across the armrest of the chair. Signe immediately straightens up and puts the scarf properly across her own shoulders. Mother turns slightly away from Signe while they continue talking to each other; she straightens her own clothes. This short interaction is just one of the innumerable small sequences in the course of one hour. What makes it special is that Signe uses it a little later to put into words an example of how mother is always "picking at" her. Considered as a statement, this is a very ambiguous formulation. It can be about taking the initiative, responding, closeness, distance, approach, or criticism.

One way of understanding this is, of course, to say that the entire family is worried or is struggling with the difference between closeness and distance, criticism and recognition. On the level of coordinated interaction, this may be an adequate description. However, this coordination of action is also a condition for being able to formulate one's own perspective, one's own history, about, for example, being worried. Words give their experience of coordinated action new dimensions. When we address the significance of "picking at" in our talks, this common starting point will become meaningful as a source of both similarity and diversity—as something that binds them together and also separates them from each other. They perceive this differently, and yet they feel that they have something in common.

## *Language as the world—or language in the world?*

Let us for a moment return to the philosophical roots. It is important to point to the fact that a great deal of the origin of a language-based perspective is derived from Nietzsche. He criticized the philosophy of subject (i.e. those who believed the subject to be a kind of essence prior to all experience) by saying that it had ignored the role of language in the constitution of the self. In his opinion, the *"I"* expresses a grammatical phenomenon and not an independently existing essence.

This notion is the point of departure for the French philosophy of language, which has had great inspirational impact on the field of family therapy. Roland Barthes says in his famous quotation: "Do I not know that *in the field of the subject, there is no referent*" (quoted in Eakin, 1992). When using words like "I" or "self", there is no substance, or no phenomenon we refer to, that has its own existence independent of our linguistic expressions. The fact that we generally refer to something which we call a subject is, in every respect, a linguistic construction.

In his book *The Singular Self* (1998), Rom Harré discusses possible ways of understanding a language-based concept of the self. He outlines the primary problems thus: in all contexts where we engage ourselves in the issue of human behaviour, the "personal singularity" will sooner or later become a central topic. Wetherell and Maybin (1996) are also onto this in their reference to the social anthropologist Marcel Mauss. They quote his assertion that "there has never existed a human being who has not been aware, not only of his body, but also at the same time of his individuality, both spiritual and physical (Mauss, 1990, p. 3, cited from Wetherell & Maybin, 1996, p. 230). According to Harré, however, this is also a topic that can be discussed in various ways. First, this is about individuality—namely, that Signe is different from all others. Second, it is about the fact that Signe is unique, that she is not like anyone else. This may look like an ingenious difference—completely in line with what one may expect from philosophical quarters. But for Signe, too, this is a crucial issue—because Signe knows that she is a separate person, that she is not someone else. Her question does not only concern her wish to know that she is separate from others, even though this is also an important concern for her. She would also like to have a content of her own, be unique, be able to know herself in a way that when she speaks, the words are rooted in her experience in a way that makes her feel genuinely present in her own expressions. To say it in theoretically controversial terms: that she has a kind of substance.

Harré's main assertion is that the self is not a thing, but a *place*, a place from which one understands the world, a place to act from. Having a sense of self is therefore the same as having a sense of one's position, one's point of view in relating to other people. The fact that we conceive of the self as a thing or a separate entity is, according to Harré, a consequence of the way we speak about it. The "reification" is due to the fact that we describe the self with nouns. It is the grammatical form in which we use "the self" in our talks that creates the reification—it is not a characteristic of singularity. This results in subjectivity being looked upon as something different from being a subject, which for Harré is a purely linguistic construction. The self as a *position* therefore becomes crucial for Harré. Compared to Ricoeur's idea that the *use of language* in a certain sense transcends the *language*, we can say that each person's contribution to the talk both confirms and expresses a context that transcends the individual but cannot give a complete picture of the subjective perspective. Again, it is the distinction between subject and subjectivity that can get us out of an either/or position. The self as a *position* also reminds us of Stern's representation of the self as a fundamental process of organization, which is a part of and also a condition for mutual coordination of action.

Jerome Bruner (1990a) emphasizes the same point: "We speak as though the self had an essence which preceded our attempts at describing it, as though all we had to do was to inspect it in order to reveal its nature" (p. 99). Since all human action is *situated*—that is, rooted in a historical and cultural reality—it is important to underline that the process of formation takes place going from the outside and in.

However, human actions cannot, in his opinion, be explained by a one-sided "from-the-outside-in" viewpoint. For Bruner, our reflexive capacities and our possibilities of imagining alternatives indicate that in a certain sense we have to be regarded as autonomous or self-regulated. A perspective therefore goes also from within and out. We find the same way of thinking in Stern when he refers to the infant's way of representing experiences. When children are given drawings of fifteen different faces to look at, they will at the end prefer the sixteenth face—the one that represents the best summary of the fifteen faces already seen. This preference therefore expresses an inner processing of the impressions the child has been subjected to, a process of organization and generalization that in an important way transcends the concrete sense impressions. This process moves from the inside and out, even if the premises for it come from the outside and in. In regard to Signe, the same processes are operative: a processing of the impressions she receives is taking place inside her. But the basis for this processing are her experiences and her participation in an experienced relatedness.

In today's theories, the self is viewed as a linguistic construction in the sense that it is the cultural traditions of narrative history that supply the setting for its existence. The idea of subject is today linked to the space the self occupies in a narrative, in a coherent story. In this way, one attempts to connect it even more firmly to a purely linguistic context, while at the same time reinstating the subject, the intentionality, and the development in time in the form of a plot. However, the ideas of developmental psychology about a connection between affective and narrative exchanges can provide other possibilities. From this viewpoint, a sense of self is rooted in coordinated action and concrete interactional sequences with others. Without a focus on Signe's sense of belonging in different interactional sequences, it became impossible for her to experience the "authentic" expression that she desired.

What gave Signe a sense of herself was having her own experience of patterns of action that she shared with others, that could also be verbalized and become a part of a—for her—coherent narrative. This made her feel that she was someone who had come further than one who just "went along with the crowd", someone with a form of integrity, which she explicitly yearned for. Focusing on shared experiences made it possible for her to find words, but the words needed to be rooted in the shared reality that constitutes coordinated action. Focusing on shared or coordinated experiences enabled her to find "her very own words", which in a significant way had their roots in relatedness, a kind of common reality.

Even if one focuses on language as the common source of meaning, it does not follow that either the nonverbal interaction or each single perspective has become meaningless—on the contrary. Developmental psychology focuses on the relation of language to a lived, common reality and on the relation of every statement and its significance to the totality. As emphasized by Jerome Bruner in "Autobiographies of Self" (1990b), the recognition of my own position is something other than a recognition of the other's perspective on me. The latter presupposes reflexivity, and the possibilities for this are both reinforced and changed by using language.

## *Concluding remarks*

In the literature of the French philosophers of language and of the most prominent social constructionists, it is possible to point to formulations indicating the same contradiction or ambivalence as expressed by Signe. On the one hand, the self is a linguistic phenomenon, an effect of discourses or modes of using language. On the other hand, it is easy to find formulations stating that we as subjects have an existence beyond language, an existence that language quite simply cannot express. In his book *Realities and Relationships* (1994), Kenneth Gergen goes so far as to say that the important concept is practice or coordination of action: "This emphasis on practice must also move beyond the boundaries of the language" (p. 112). Here there are patterns of mutual action going beyond the framework created by language that suddenly become the focus of attention. This is clearly a marginalized interpretation in today's social constructionism.

The concept of practice is also included in the current philosophical debate. It is used first and foremost in contexts where one wishes to describe how the acting subject takes into account or includes the actions of others in its projects. In a certain sense, the actions of others are included in my actions because we take part in a practice—they are included in a common pattern that gives meaning to our individual actions. The concept of practice thus becomes a concept for conveying coherence between the actions of individual subjects in a meaningful way.

We find one example of this type of reasoning in Charles Taylor's book, *Sources of the Self* (1989). Taylor introduces the concept of practice in order to indicate that it is our physical patterns of action, adapted to the relational context in which they appear, that are our primary source for understanding the world in which we live. He calls this the "pattern of appropriate actions" and defines it as stable configurations of shared activity. A concretization that one can obviously refer to is the favourite metaphor of all social-constructionists family therapists: the dialogue between the therapist and the client as a *dance*. Anyone who has tried to dance—and perhaps especially if one has not been successful—knows, of course, that it is difficult to find a better example of the importance of action coordination. The concrete forms of dance are examples of what is meant by practice. Another example of such practice is what Signe refers to when she tries to teach her mother how to approach Signe's girlfriends. Mother tries to be friendly and interested based on her own assumptions, asking them if they have had a good time when she fetches the girls after training. Signe's rejection of this strategy has one simple explanation: "We don't do it like that." Signe knows that the youth culture she is trying to take part in has its own rules and directions for how to act, but this is difficult to articulate on the basis of general, logical premises. It is just that they have their own ways of doing things that is different from the rules and regulations applying to the world of her parents. Ideas, or linguistic utterances of opinion, are developed as an attempt to formulate the underlying rationale behind these patterns.

Perhaps we can say that this emphasis on practice as a basic concept substantiates the idea that it is precisely coordination of action or coordination of interaction which should stand more in the centre of our efforts to understand these complicated connections. And perhaps this is also the important aspect of all the central modes of exchange—in Stern's vocabulary, regulation, imitation, affect attunement, verbality, and narrativity. However, the coordination of action implies an understanding of subjectivity that goes beyond what an understanding by us as linguistic constructions can offer. Language is *also* an important source of coordination of action, but in this context it is not the only one.

The consequences for the concept of self are that it also becomes a both/and concept: it presumes relational totalities but without the subjective perspective becoming irrelevant or destructive. It helps us to understand a dimension in the picture of our common existence that places it at the centre, even when the focus is on the relationship.

CHAPTER THREE

# Intersubjectivity as a philosophical and psychological concept

*Vigdis Wie Torsteinsson*

> When Peter Fortune was ten years old, grown-up people sometimes used to tell him he was a "difficult" child. He never understood what they meant. . . . It was not until he had been a grown-up himself for many years that Peter finally understood. They thought he was difficult because he was so silent. That seemed to bother people. The other problem was he liked being by himself. Not all the time, of course. . . . Now, grown-ups like to think they know what is going on inside a ten-year-old's head. And it is impossible to know what someone is thinking if they keep quiet about it. People would see Peter lying on his back on a summer's afternoon chewing a piece of grass and staring at the sky.—Peter! Peter! What are you thinking about? they would call to him. . . . Grown-ups knew that something was going on inside that head, but they couldn't hear it or see it or feel it. They couldn't tell Peter to stop it, because they did not know what it was he was doing in there. He could have been setting his school on fire or feeding his sister to an alligator and escaping in a hot air balloon, but all they saw was a boy staring at the blue sky without blinking, a boy who did not hear you when you called his name.

> As for being on his own, well, grown-ups didn't much like that either. They don't even like other grown-ups being on their own. When you join in, people can see what you're up to. You have to join in or you'll spoil it for everyone else.
>
> Ian McEwan, *The Daydreamer*

The epigraph above can serve as a heading for an important therapeutic approach to problems, as can the following excerpt from a family talk with Yngvild, her older sister, and her parents. Yngvild is a 13-year-old girl with severe compulsion problems and anorexia that disturb most of her life. In many of the talks we have with the family, both jointly and separately, the problems emerging are those concerning the topic of shared or separate experiences. The following brief dialogue is a typical example.

> Y (to mother): You can't know how I feel! No one can know it. You say that you understand, but I know that you don't!
>
> T: Do you notice when your mother feels alright, when she enjoys being with you?
>
> Y: No, I don't! I can't know that . . .

Under other circumstances, however, she describes her mother as the only one who can understand her and who knows how she is feeling and what attitude she should take towards her own experiences.

Both these quotations illustrate situations where the unitive, central topic is what we can have together—what cannot be shared, what is mine, and what is common to us. They are taken from two separate contexts—one fiction; the other, case notes from a therapy session. The issues each raises are, to a great extent, identical. They are expressed by two children who in many ways describe the same thing: in what sense, and to what degree, is it possible—and necessary—to experience something as a common or shared experience? And what do we mean when we say that we are sharing an experience? One may also query whether these children give voice to something that we, as therapists, ought to worry about. Or do they find words for a universal human experience—the certainty that each one of us has a world inside us that is not immediately accessible to the other? Because in the statements of these children, there is also the idea of an internal world—the idea that, in a certain sense, all of us are alone, in spite of belonging to different communities.

One difference can be pointed to in these two descriptions. The fictitious child expresses an almost tranquil happiness about this private, secret world. Yngvild's statements are far more characterized by a conviction that the impossibility of being understood is a logical impossibility, and that the realization of this is bitter and painful.

From a perspective of the history of ideas, our culture has over the last 2,000 years moved continuously in the direction of more individualization. This is described as a process where what is happening inside each of us becomes constantly more important, constantly more of what is real (Taylor, 1989, 1992). This is a development many wish to counteract, and which—in our professional milieu—has its strongest opponents among the American social constructionists. These, in turn, have had a strong impact on the field of family therapy. And it may not be difficult to imagine that the strongest resistance comes from them, in a context where a European may easily feel that a word is of no consequence unless it begins with the prefix "self". The ideal became to stand on one's own feet, to be independent, and the hero was the lonely horseman riding into the sunset.

We would not do justice to this development without emphasizing its positive aspects. A great deal of our ethical thinking is organized around an understanding of autonomy as a basic concept. This applies, for example, to all ethical guidelines for health professionals (see chapter 13). Respect for the integrity of the individual and the right to take part in deciding one's own fate in all contexts, from democratic elections to informed consent in therapy contexts, are established values that most of us unreservedly consider justified. However, in many areas this strong focus on the individual has limited our understanding of how we belong to the world we are living in. This has been the credo of family therapy for the last twenty-five years: to underscore the significance of context and relationship for everything we are and all we undertake.

Psychology as a professional field has been firmly grounded on the idea of the "inside"—the individual psyche as a point of departure for an understanding of the forms of existence of both individuals and of relationships. "It is the long tradition of psychological essentialism, supported by important institutions and justified by a century of social sciences which constitutes the basis of the everyday processes which we conceive as self-understanding and self-realization—and for the ways in which we pose questions, evaluate and explore the self" (Gergen, 1994, p. 128). This is clearly demonstrated by the central position held by Freud and psychoanalysis during the first part of the last century. Actually, one of the chief assertions of psychoanalysis was that we are not even comprehensible to ourselves. Thus the relationship between what we knew and what we did not know about ourselves became a more interesting angle than the relationship between ourselves and the social context of which we were a part.

Behaviouristic ideas created for a period a climate that made the thought of sharing an internal world irrelevant. The internal, psychological world—if it was there—was unnecessary for the understanding of actions and statements. The development into cognitive theory changed this, but even now the psychological mind was conceived as rules or schemata for processing information. Intersubjective understanding was only possible if one had identical schemata or models for understanding.

The popularity of the concept of intersubjectivity often causes it to be used for a variety of purposes. Often we see it used as a collective term for everything we share, for being social beings relating to each other. But in many ways this is a complicated concept that contains many miscellaneous guidelines for understanding how we share experiences. Another important question is whether, and in what manner, it tells us something else about relationships other than what has been supplied by the relational concepts used in family therapeutic literature.

## *Concepts of community in family therapy*

Family therapy has evolved as an attempt to build an understanding of human life on the understanding of relationships. The first "catch-phrase" was "the whole is more than the sum of its parts", which precisely expressed the idea that in order to understand individuals, one had to focus on the relational totalities of which we are all a part. And in order to substantiate the notion that the individual could not transcend the relational context, Russell and Whitehead's theory about logical types was used as a theoretical basis. Since the relationship was on a different level from that of the individual, it became logically wrong to explain relationships with concepts from individual psychology.

The history of family therapy can therefore be described as the history of a search for concepts that would capture these totalities. At first, theories of communication (Haley, 1977; Watzlawick, Beavin, & Jackson, 1967) held a central position. The basic idea is that separate statements become meaningless without reference to the communicative context in which they arise. A statement is always a reply to another statement. It is the logic in the interaction as a totality that is crucial, not each separate statement. Minuchin's (1977) understanding of relational structure also set a trend. The relational structure as a totality gave meaning to the individual's action. The individual acted from his/her position in the totality.

Gradually family therapy turned its attention more to *meaning* than to action. The analyses of structure and communication presumed a perspective on the therapist as the one who analyses families and relationships from the outside, and who through her/his observations could give an unbiased description of how the family *really was*. The Milan group (Boscolo, Cecchin, Hoffman, & Penn, 1987) adopted Bateson's formulations (1972b) of the relationship between the map and the terrain. The map—as expressing meaning—was what the therapeutic system should and could work with. With its emphasis on meaning and the therapist as a fellow originator of this new meaning, the focus gradually shifted from action to language. It is through language that meaning is created, thereby expressing this totality to which we are all subjected, and which we are dependent on to create meaning (Anderson & Goolishian, 1988; Gergen, 1994). Therapists wanted to abandon the understanding of words as something that has reference to something or other in "reality" and say, in the words of Wittgenstein (1958), that "the meaning of a word is its use in language" (p. 20). Feelings of loneliness and of a sense of community thus become a consequence of the stories we tell about our lives—for the alternative is that there is something prior to or between the words that we try to convey with words as the means at our disposal. Words have reference to something in the world. Wittgenstein himself was not as categorical as this in regard to this topic. As he says: "For a large class of cases—*though not for all*—in which we employ the word 'meaning', it can be defined thus: the meaning of a word is its use in language" (p. 20, emphasis added).

Consequently, family therapy theory created an alternative to the existing theories, with its focus on something common—a common context or frame that we all refer to or are referred to in order to create meaning or connections. At the same time, it seems as though we have to renounce having an internal world as one way to understand our experience of ourselves and one another. At the least, we have to raise the question: do we want to reject the whole set of problems concerning sharing and having different experiences, on the grounds that it is a consequence of erroneous philosophical theories? If it concerns themes arising from elements in the human experiential world, a necessary focus for understanding what goes on between people, it might make us better therapists to include reflections on them in our theories. The mere fact that we use the concepts of communication and dialogue implies a recognition of distance, in the sense that my perspective is different from yours. If my perspective were not different from yours, it would not be meaningful to speak about communication. This means that communication implies a difference between dissimilar perspectives and, in a sense, a possibility for building bridges across this difference. And if we recognize this difference, then we are left with three different phenomena: having something in common, sharing something, and having something completely to oneself. The concepts of family therapy have mostly focused on what is common, on what—in a certain sense—constitutes the frame and the context for understanding the individual family member. The subjective perspective has to a large extent been the domain of individual therapy.

As already mentioned, intersubjectivity has lately been given the position of yet another word that in one way or another tries to take care of what we *share*, or have in common. In a certain sense, it differs from the conceptual world of family therapy in that it describes the relationship as something *in between*—and not as a level *above* the individual participant. In this way it may provide new approaches to an understanding of relationships.

## *Intersubjectivity in a philosophical context*

In philosophy, the concept has primarily been a response to solipsism, which means that the only thing I can know anything about in this world is the content of my own consciousness. This way of thinking has created a distinction between myself and others that one may attempt to bridge but in principle is insurmountable for a solipsist. There will always remain an "irreparable loneliness of the soul". The concept of intersubjectivity is an attempt to understand human behaviour *both* as a common project and as an individual project.

In philosophy, however, the concept has not been used in an unambiguous form. There have been several suggestions as to how we should understand this twofold human behaviour. In philosophy, Husserl, Buber, and Merleau-Ponty are well-known exponents of different ways of understanding this problem (Hansen, 1991b). In this chapter, I attempt to give a brief summary of the guidelines provided by the different philosophical positions and of which alternative formulations we have to deal with.

## *The limited concept of intersubjectivity —or, "it takes one to know one"*

Husserl may hold his place as the exponent for a way of thinking about intersubjectivity with an individually oriented point of departure. Husserl is basically a phenomenologist, interested in how the world is represented in consciousness. According to him, we are ourselves active contributors to the construction of the world as meaningful. It is my consciousness that constitutes the way in which my world will appear to me.

This immediately raises a potential criticism. So what about other people? Are they to be merely reduced to my constructions of them? Husserl himself answers this question with a no and indicates, among other things, that there are ethical and epistemological reasons for this (see Crossley, 1998).

How, then, does one establish a concept of intersubjectivity on a phenomenological foundation? At first, Husserl examines, through a phenomenological reduction, how other people are represented in one's consciousness in ordinary contexts. He believes that at first we experience others as objects, as separate others, who are psychologically controlled by their own motives, reasons, ideas, and so forth. So far, Yngvild would agree with him. She is perfectly aware of the fact that others conceive the world in their own way, which is different from hers. But Husserl also says that we conceive others as subjects who experience and know the world, and who experience and know us as part of this world. In addition, we experience the world as a common world, an intersubjective world. These three elements add up to what Husserl terms an "empathic intentionality". Yngvil will not recognize the existence of the last two elements—because she does not believe in the experience of sharing with someone, of living in a common world in which she also becomes understandable to others and not only to herself.

Husserl emphasizes the importance of the point that, with the help of empathic intentionality, we are able to transcend the particularity of our own perspective and actually share the experiences of others, or that we can experience ourselves and our own world just as we are experienced by others.

According to Husserl, however, this knowledge about others is nevertheless significantly based on my own knowledge about myself. His analysis takes us through yet another reduction, where all traces of difference will be put in parentheses. His conclusion is that the psyche is basically monadic, and that the knowledge I have of my own mind is the fundament for understanding subjectivity and consciousness in others. What we know about ourselves therefore helps us to understand others, to construct knowledge of other minds.

How, then, do we carry out this transition? Husserl describes it with the concept of analogous apperception. He believes that in all perception we see more than we are actually seeing. We add to it our earlier experiences, our expectations, and our understanding. Since we have no concrete experience of forms of consciousness other than our own, but resemble each other, we undertake an analogous transference of our own experiences onto others. In addition to this, we are different, at least in the sense that we are in different places in the world—you are "there", and I am "here". Therefore, we have to recognize *both* that others have their particular point of observation in relation to the world *and* that the world can be recognized from different viewpoints. Analogous apperception is therefore our opportunity to transcend our own limited standpoint and experience empathy with others. Maybe, says Yngvild, someone who has experienced similar problems will be able to understand some of her experiences. But she is not certain, because the similarities can never be complete. With this she emphasizes the limitations in Husserl's way of thinking. If the experiences of others are too different from mine, she says, then this gap will become too wide. It is not possible for anyone to understand what this kind of experience embodies who has not experienced the elements of compulsion in "having to do something".

But regarding empathy: phenomenology retains a form of solipsism because it turns the construction of the individual's consciousness of his/her own reality into the decisive element in understanding others. Meeting another means meeting someone we do not know, one who is not ourselves. And yet we only have our own experiential world to refer to when we try to understand the other person. There are two limitations in this line of thought that are crucial to what follows. First, the theory is based on observation of others, and not on interaction with others. Second, the relation between language and meaning is not discussed. The important point in this presentation is the fact that in this perspective, subjectivity is a premise for intersubjectivity.

### *The radical intersubjectivity— or, "in the beginning was the relationship"*

With this point of departure one goes all the way and turns the relationship into the primary phenomenon. Martin Buber and Maurice Merleau-Ponty, for example, are the central figures in this understanding of intersubjectivity. In Buber's *I and Thou* (1958), a book familiar to many therapists, he describes the infant as a communicative being who communicates with gestures. The communication constitutes a level of its own—both the self and others are secondary phenomena that are constructed on the basis of these interactional experiences. "There is no sharp sense of distinction in this case, no reflective awareness of either self or other" (Crossley, 1998, p. 11). In Buber's (1974) words: "Man can become whole not in virtue of a relation to himself but only in virtue of a relation to another self. . . . in being together the unlimited and the unconditioned is experienced" (p. 204). With this Buber wishes to demonstrate that he does not reduce the encounter and the relationship to whatever conscious thoughts or reflections each of us has about what is going on. Self and others are relational topics and elements of a common structure.

Intersubjectivity, according to Buber, will therefore imply living in a common space where self and otherness have not yet been separated as experiential modes. He adopts the opposite position to Husserl: here, intersubjectivity is a condition for subjectivity. Both I and the other as a subject are inseparable from an analysis of the interaction as a whole. What may be difficult to understand in Buber is how an encounter between two, where the other is conceived as being-different, can *also* be an intersubjective encounter.

Merleau-Ponty elucidates intersubjectivity from a totally different perspective. He starts with analyses of perception. From an individual point of departure, this is the way in which we win access to the outside world, our channels from the outside in. He criticizes all research on perception for being based on a lack of understanding of the fact that perception is what he calls an "activity". If perception is a part of the area "in-between", says Merleau-Ponty, then in perception the one who senses has to transcend himself, open up to what is not himself. A glance *questions* more than it receives. "Perception is an opening out onto and an engagement with otherness, which neither reduces it nor is reduced to it. It is an active interrogation in search of form" (Crossley, 1998, p. 27). "Perception is not . . . an experience of objects. . . . It is an enjoinment and an involvement with them. It is a 'communion' with otherness" (p. 28). The analysis of perception therefore also shows this "world-in-between". In this way perception becomes an active involvement between two parties. When I see another person, I do not see a physical object, but I am touched by meaning. This meaning touches me in the direction of giving an answer.

It is also important for Merleau-Ponty that all perception implies a perspective. The body exists in space and is the *place* from which we perceive. But coordination in *time* is just as important in the establishing of this world-in-between. The meaning of our actions is not immediately obvious. They unfold in time, with a rhythmical structure. Interaction is not possible if the time-horizons do not melt together and become a shared horizon. This common rhythm is important for all coordination of action and therefore also for communication.

In this way Merleau-Ponty can state that an "intersubjective system" is formed between physical subjects that are irreducible to each participant but bring about actions by the participants. This description resembles Buber's I–Thou relationship: the actions are motivated and coordinated by an orientation towards the other, but without conscious positioning or reflexive attention, towards neither the other nor oneself. The "conversation" thus becomes a primary unit, a system that is more fundamental than the participants. The dialogue becomes a communicative system that is immediate and is always something different from the sum of its parts. Based on an analysis of the contributions of one or both participants, we cannot predict what each person will say, or how the conversation will end. It is the *conversation* that creates all contributions. In the moment of conversation, all statements belong to the system of interaction that is formed between the partners in the conversation.

Previously I have used the concept of conversation in a broad sense, to include gestures or other nonverbal expressions. Merleau-Ponty's basic assumption is that on this level of interaction, too, we act in meaningful ways—ways that we can describe as containing a form of understanding. But the understanding is reflected merely in a limited sense. All perception contains an element of reflection, because in a certain sense the process of perception is reversible (Madison, 1981). When I am touching, I am also touched by what I am touching. Linguistic communication, however, contains several elements of reflexivity that do not exist in other forms of communication. Language does not only refer to internal states. It also makes it possible to create transcending transformations of the individual's behaviour. Language facilitates this transformation into a reflecting and reflexive subject (Madison, 1981; Priest, 1998).

This brief review of some fundamental philosophical positions demonstrates a number of general dilemmas when one attempts to see the relationship as an intersubjective space. For Husserl, subjectivity is fundamental. Our understanding of others is essentially based on analogous inferences. Both Buber and Merleau-Ponty raise this debate to a new level with their basic notion that, in a sense, we are living in a shared world. In Buber's conception, there is a problem as regards understanding the world either as shared, in the sense that we are two separate people experiencing the same, *or* as common, in the sense that what we experience only has meaning to the extent that it is related to the same linguistic, meaning-creating dialogue. This latter topic is at the core of social-constructionist family therapy. It is the language-based community that is in focus here—it is only through the use of language that experiences have meaning. This does not imply a common meaning in the strict sense of the word, but it is the same dialogue, the same linguistic system, that gives meaning to each one of us, as well as giving an experience of limits. The relationship between what is similar and what is different between us has therefore not, to the same extent, been put on the agenda of family therapy. Merleau-Ponty's point of departure is simultaneity: the subject and the other are constituted in a relational movement; relationship and subject mutually imply each other. Merleau-Ponty is thus closest to the point of departure of today's developmental psychological thinking on this concept.

## *"She says a little more"— an extract from a therapy session*

So, when it comes to the crunch, what is this all about? How can we recognize these topics as something relevant and important in the therapeutic context? Perhaps an extract from an individual session with Yngvild will be useful to illustrate these points. For, through the course of therapy, Yngvild gradually becomes able to give examples of short sequences of shared experience. A written account does not do justice to this girl—all the episodes of thoughtfulness, smiles, eagerness, and hesitation remain hidden in a written rendering of an exchange. But her thematizing is still important.

T: If you were to give a description of what it is that makes you and Camilla [a girlfriend] have a good relationship—what would you say? Which words would you use?

Y: Oh . . . We're fine together. We respect each other for who we are. . . . It doesn't matter that I like handball and she likes snowboard. . . . That's only one example—it might just as well be something completely different—something deeper. . . . We don't agree with each other, but we are not mad at each other.

T: Could one say that you both tolerate being different?

Y: Yes . . . but I have this special thing. . . . I can't stand it when people don't understand. This is really so stupid, but I get mad inside me.

T: How do you notice that someone understands . . . how do you find it out?

Y: They say things—it isn't enough to say "I understand"—that's what so many are doing . . . well, I don't know . . .

T: Are you able to remember a situation where you and Camilla were together, where you really had this feeling that she understood you?

Y: When she said that there were things she had to do as well . . . "well, otherwise it won't be right", I said . . . "yes, right," she said . . . and with this she meant that I said it correctly . . .

T: Does that mean that when you feel that you are being understood, the one you are talking to will also find an example of what you are both talking about?

Y: Mm.

T: Are there other things that are important?

Y: It shouldn't be like they actually don't want to be together with me—then it's all wrong. When I have to leave, for example—like when I had to go to come and see you, then she says: "Oh, are you leaving . . . so then I'll be all alone"—and then she pretends to cry. Then I know that she likes being with me. I don't believe that she is lying. . . . I can sort of feel . . . that she doesn't fool around . . . that it's actually true.

T: How do you realize what it is that she wants to say?

Y: Don't know, I . . . She says a bit more, not just "Oh, what a shame" . . . don't know—I can just feel it. It can happen that I'm wrong . . . no, that can't happen.

T: What happens with you then?

Y: I feel happy . . . I understand her a bit. . . .

Many of the sessions with Yngvild alone or with all her family or a part of it are influenced by these topics. Yngvild herself is perfectly aware of the fact that her peers often look upon her as a strange bird. This impels her to sometimes try to convey something to them of her own world, her own experiences. As a rule, the response she gets is, "Oh well" or "I understand". Even though her girlfriends use words that should indicate that they have understood, these situations are extremely frustrating for Yngvild. After these attempts at conveying something about herself, more often than not this leaves her with an even stronger experience of loneliness and despair—even though she does understand that it is difficult for others to understand what she is talking about. She has a lot of experiences that others have no concrete experiences of, and she therefore feels that it is difficult for her to rely on recognition as the only point of departure for intersubjective or shared experiences.

And yet there are exceptions—and this is thematized in the extract from the session. There is this "something more" that

Camilla and Yngvild experience together, and which Yngvild otherwise thinks she rarely experiences. Even though, when summing up her feelings, Yngvild does not have any experience of being understood, she is able to give examples of shared experiences in her descriptions of small interactional sequences.

Basically, Yngvild is a most eloquent girl. She has a well-developed ability to convey her experiences in words, and she also conveys that she is interested in doing this in a way that will make her understandable to those listening to her. She thinks it important to try to be as precise as possible—she samples her words and, if the first attempt does not feel right, often reformulates them. Her stories are also told with a good portion of humour. In this sense, she is a stimulating girl to talk with.

However, what Yngvild is mostly concerned with is what is "more than" or between the words. She tries to describe what cannot be described, and yet she passed on a feeling of harmony and warmth in this reciprocal meeting. For Yngvild, this is about the feeling of sharing something or being a part of something.

If we return to the philosophical positions, we see that, in terms of this example, thinking in analogue is a too-limited concept of intersubjectivity. The feeling of harmony is certainly not only part of a picture where Camilla understands how Yngvild is feeling, or the other way round, even though this is also part of it. The crux of the matter is that they experience something together that basically does not belong to either of them.

Yngvild also emphasizes, as we can see, that this is happening because they are different, and because they organize themselves and their empathic reactions on the basis of two different perspectives. "For a real event does not only consist of someone getting up to speak and addressing a conversation partner; it also consists of the person's wish to express and share a new experience which takes place in a situation with an other" (Kemp, 1999, p. 53). However, it is also easy to point to the necessity of being able to establish an understanding in spite of great differences in what is experienced. Yngvild often expresses dreams about one day having experiences of relatedness without dependence on similarity. This is a possibility she wants for her own sake: to be able to share something of herself with someone who is totally different from her.

## *Intersubjectivity as a developmental psychological concept*

Most of the phenomena described in the theory of developmental psychology are exemplified in the brief excerpt from the conversation with Yngvild. Sharing feelings, sharing focus of attention, sharing intention—all this can be found in Yngvild's descriptions of her encounter. But the most important point in this connection is her description of how they are connected, and how the meaningful conversation is built across a mutual, affective resonance in each of the two girls.

The topic of intersubjectivity has gradually become one of the most central topics in the current research in developmental psychology. Developmental psychology has aimed in many ways and almost to the same degree as family therapy to transcend the thinking about the separate subject that in a way becomes "socialized" into interaction with other people. It has been important to find concepts that point to the infant as a social being from the very first moment—for example, by spontaneously reacting differently to people than to things in its surroundings. Colvyn Trevarthen was the first to use the concept of intersubjectivity in connection with infant research (Havnesköld & Mothander, 1995; Stern, 1985, p. 134). He says, when reflecting on the history of modern infant research, that the intention is not to say that the infant does not learn, or that it does not need care, but that it immediately enters into conversation-resembling negotiations with others about aims and intentions (Trevarthen, in Bråten, 1999, p. 16).

Bjørg Røed Hansen describes this development in her article from 1991 on the concept of intersubjectivity in developmental psychology (1991b). In order to underscore the unfair deal given to the concept of intersubjectivity by earlier developmental psychological research, she refers to Bruner's descriptions of the basic premises of developmental psychological theory and research (Bruner, 1990a). These are obviously both empirically and theoretically justified. However, the most important factor in this connection is perhaps the fact that psychology as a subject has mostly been an individual-based project, where the understanding of the individual psyche has been the central issue. Some have put it so strongly as to say that psychological research has had a tendency to "ignore the contexts which have produced the behaviour about to be studied, and to re-attribute it as a quality in individuals—in isolation" (Danziger, 1990, p. 186). From this viewpoint, the intense focus on this concept represents an attempt to play down the solipsistic angle in psychology, in line with the basic ideas of family therapy.

Defining the contents of this concept, Hansen formulates herself as follows: she says that it is firstly "a relational concept which describes something that takes place *between* people, something that people *share*. However, the concept specifies even more by emphasizing the *subjective* or *experiential* aspect of what is shared" (Hansen, 1991b, p. 568). Affective attunement is used as a concept for describing the form of exchange in an intersubjective exchange. Affective attunement is characterized as a process where two people somehow share an internal state but express this state in different ways (Stern, 1985). It is therefore the mode of expression that constitutes the "little extra" and tells us that we are dealing with two different subjective experiential worlds (see chapter 1).

Stern outlines three concepts that can be used to characterize the space *"in between"*—in other words, what we can share. These concepts are inter-affectivity, inter-intentionality, and inter-attentionality. What we can share, in other words, are feelings, intentions, and attention. The sharing itself, however, is not an expression of intersubjectivity. Only when an experience belongs to the subject—in Stern's conceptual world, inside the subject— is it possible to use the concept of intersubjectivity.

In this sense, Stern develops a specific way of using the concept of intersubjectivity. He reserves it for what he calls "the subjective self-domain". His explicit intention is to say that intersubjectivity is about seeing the other as *subject—in other words, that the other has an inside.* In this way a distinction is also created between the outer behaviour and the inner state. Therefore, it only becomes intersubjectivity when one experiences the same in a certain sense, but expresses it differently. This also leads to another important element in Stern's conceptual world: the distinction between "self" and "subject". This distinction is difficult to maintain because these concepts are often used synonymously.

However, the concept of intersubjectivity is employed in different ways in today's research and development of theory. Bråten (1999) distinguishes between three main types of application. The first describes an immediate experience of intersubjective relatedness in and between persons who together are interested and involved in this relatedness. The resemblance with Martin Buber's I–Thou relationship is obvious. Bråten also refers here to Trevarthen's "primary intersubjectivity" as an example of this type of immediate subject–subject relationship. "I called this expression an individual consciousness and intentionality *subjectivity*, and concluded by saying that in order to be able to communicate, the infant must also be able to adapt this subjective control to the subjectivity of others; they too must be able to demonstrate *intersubjectivity*" (Trevarthen, 1999, p. 27).

The second mode of application is—still according to Bråten—an external reference as a common attention towards an external object. Here, intersubjectivity is a three-part relationship having something in common outside the dyad, which nevertheless constitutes the relationship as a community. What is common is the focus of attention, but what one directs one's attention to is not basically a part of the relationship. Stern's use of the concept of intersubjectivity coincides with "the child's ability to share the focus of attention" (Hansen, 1991b, p. 572).

Third, this concept also deals with a reflexive form of intersubjectivity. Here the conceptual application implies a communicative understanding where symbols and the uses of symbols are crucial (Bråten, 1999, pp. 1–2). This type of application can also be linked to Husserl's understanding of intersubjectivity. By processing our own experiences, we can become open to descriptions of reality that differ greatly from our own.

In certain contexts, these distinctions are not used in an explicit way. Haldor Øvreeide and Reidun Hafstad (1996, p. 216n) make use of the concept as follows: "By intersubjectivity one understands . . . an experience of reciprocity, a similarity in the experience of emotionality and cognition, or experiencing that the other is capable of entering into the quality of one's own experience." Included here are both common (shared), similar, and different experiences as the basis for intersubjectivity. The question we must continue to explore is, therefore, whether they represent different aspects of experiences of intersubjectivity, thus complementing each other without competing.

## *Intersubjectivity— but which subjectivity?*

Stern's understanding of a subjective experience implies, as we have seen, a different experience from the emotional relatedness that is established through imitation. Therefore, intersubjectivity as a phenomenon does not exist in the infant before the age of 7 to 9 months. Stern differs here, as already mentioned, from Trevarthen, who uses the concept of intersubjectivity about the child's behaviour right from its birth. Trevarthen justifies his standpoint by saying that the child is born as a social being—in other words, that it "is born with motives for finding and using other people's motives in 'conversation'-negotiations about objectives, emotions, experiences and meaning" (Trevarthen, 1999, p. 16). Trevarthen focuses on a congenital communicative competence and sensitivity for other people that is different from the way we relate to physical objects in our surroundings. He terms this an "intuitive sympathy". Proto-conversation, a concept he borrows from Mary Bateson, is a mutual rhythm or pattern in the use of voice and gestures. The infant shows sensitivity for and identification with the expressive form of others. A 2-month-old infant will show signs of anxiety if mother's responses—however friendly—are not synchronized with the child's own actions. Here, Trevarthen also refers to Bråten's "virtual other". Bråten defines the mind as being dialogical. One acts with the other's actions in what Bråten terms "a sympathetic sense of felt immediacy".

Trevarthen therefore uses the concept of primary intersubjectivity in order to characterize the infant's actions from the beginning. He does this because he interprets the infant's actions in terms of an interest for and assumptions about the other person having motives and intentions. They read into the other's action not only an expression, but an expression *of something*. Secondary intersubjectivity deals with having a common focus towards an external object and entering into an interaction about it.

In order to clarify the difference between Stern's and Trevarthen's use of the concept of intersubjectivity, it may be useful to illustrate it with an indication of how they understand imitation.

The concept of imitation has a central position in current developmental psychology. For Stern, imitation is the point of departure for the experience of a community of feeling in what he calls the core self (see chapter 1). Many researchers have demonstrated the infant's ability to imitate bodily expression right from the very start (Meltzoff & Moore, 1995). And the most important implication in this context is probably the fact that imitation as a relational phenomenon supplies us with arguments for assuming a form of self–other dualism from the first moment. Forceful statements have been made to the effect that "both logically and psychologically, an initial dualism is a precondition for human imitation at birth" (Kugiumetziakis, 1999, p. 78). Imitation implies an experience of a distinction between oneself and others as two separate persons, but who are *together as an interactional whole*. In the very earliest studies, one demonstrates the infant's ability to copy facial expressions. This implies that the infant translates the visible facial expressions of another person into expressions in its own face, which it *cannot* see. The infant understands the equivalence between the visible bodily changes in another person and the non-visible changes in its own body, changes that the infant takes in with its proprioceptive senses. An immediate coupling takes place between oneself and the other through a common "code" for understanding one's own and others' bodily expressions. It implies that there is no basis for thinking a phase of confusion around the relationship between oneself and the other, or an original symbiosis where the child is gradually separated as a separate person. The bodily being-together is a coordinated being-together, where the simultaneous similarity and the difference between one's own body and the other's body and the forms of expression are crucial for an understanding of what is taking place.

In a different context, we pointed to the fact that imitation as a form of exchange can have problematic consequences when it remains without the supplementation and variation given by other forms of affective exchange (see chapter 4). The experience of this may vary according to the emotional content of the exchange. Yngvild describes an episode with Camilla in this way:

> "We were just sitting there next to each other, in exactly the same way, with our arms around our knees [she demonstrates] looking out across the town. . . . I almost think we wore the same clothes too . . . it's quite possible that she was thinking of something completely different and not of me . . . and yet we were sort of together . . . sometimes we looked at each other . . . it was just like I became someone, too."

The two girls had climbed onto the roof of a house and were looking out across the town. They shared an experience, and being in the same position created this feeling of togetherness.

For Stern, intersubjectivity in the sense of developmental psychology is mostly about affective sharing and exchange. In the domain of the core self, imitation is the source of a feeling relatedness. When the child uses its voice, then the mother responds by using her voice. Small variations in the established exchange patterns can nevertheless create enough differences to exclude a symbiotic state—on one level, these two are separate individuals. However, according to Stern, this is not sufficient for calling the exchange *intersubjective.* To justify this concept one has to refer to the said difference in expression. Therefore, Stern distinguishes between experiences of relatedness (which can also comprise regulation and imitation) and intersubjective experiences. With Yngvild's brief story in mind, it is difficult to see that the distinction between the external and the internal can have the importance accorded to it by Stern. Yngvild feels at least that she "becomes someone" within the frame of the brief experience of relatedness through imitation that she describes.

As mentioned before, Stern distinguishes between the concepts of "self" and "subject". He also uses the concept of self in relation to the earliest experiences of sharing: regulation and imitation.

Trevarthen also introduces a distinction, but he defines it as a distinction between primary and secondary intersubjectivity.

In addition to the numerous discussions brought about by this difference, I would like to point to yet another possibility, taking my point of departure in Yngvild's many reflections around this topic, and the differences introduced by the philosophical distinctions in the use of this concept. Perhaps intersubjectivity can also be understood as a dimension from an immediate to a conveyed intersubjectivity. The immediate intersubjectivity is expressed in Buber's I–Thou and in Trevarthen's primary intersubjectivity, as well as in Stern's concepts of the "emergent self" and the "core self". Secondary intersubjectivity and the subjective-self domain already contain an element of conveyed presence: both because the relationship is conveyed to a greater extent via a common attention to an external focus, and also because it is expressed and conveyed to a large extent as analogies (Hansen, 1991b). In Merleau-Ponty's linguistic usage, this is expressed as degrees of reflexivity. Gradually also, the symbols and the language will offer opportunities for intersubjective experiences via words and narratives. Conveying language opens the way for an experience of relatedness in spite of great concrete differences between us.

According to Stern's use of concepts, this implies that differences between the internal and the external will become less important than the degree of mediation in what is communicated, and the degree of symbolization in regard to experience and expression. This will also imply that we need different formulations of intersubjectivity. The formulations already mentioned are connected to each other, but they cannot be reduced to each other. This is, among other things, what we are reminded of by Yngvild's different experiences.

### *Two understandings of relation—two different worlds?*

The question that nevertheless remains is whether the subjective experience constitutes the essence, or at least the most important part, of our relationship to others. The social-constructionist scepticism about the concept is based on the issue of whether one should count on the individual, or on the individual consciousness, as being the source of meaning. If meaning arises and is formulated in the individual consciousness, withdrawn from all relational contexts, how can we then bridge the differences and understand each other? If the individual consciousness is the source of meaningful action, how am I to know then what your world looks like, what your intention is? What we need with this type of starting point is what Gergen (1994, p. 245) has termed the "intersubjective transparency". Understanding an other is the same as gaining access to that other's inner being and understanding what action and statement represents as the other's intentional expression. Gergen says explicitly that he is extremely sceptical about this, because the assumption that meaning is the same as individual significance will necessarily lead to the conclusion that intersubjective understanding becomes impossible (Gergen, 1994, p. 256). Understanding is only achievable as a consequence of the fact that we have the same meaningful structures—language as well as all other forms of cultural expression—to deal with. However, with this point of departure it becomes difficult to understand Yngvild's different interpretations of the "I understand". For her, those are two different experiences, dependent on *other* characteristics of the relational context in which she finds herself. It is the affective exchange in *addition* to the exchange of words that is essential and that turns this into two different contexts. For her, the meaning of the words is also a consequence of the emotionally regulated social interaction.

Yet this is not the same as saying that words are *without* importance. Through words and the use of metaphors and narratives; the scope of significance is both formed, developed, and expanded. One example is the way in which Yngvild verbalizes that she and Camilla are different. She could have chosen many other words to describe the differences. For example, she could have chosen words that limited the importance of what was common, because the difference between them was also obvious. But in our conversation that day, the difference turned into a bonus, a confirmation of the significance of what she had experienced as something they had in common.

Once more, one criticizes Gergen because he creates an insurmountable chasm between the individual consciousness and the relational context. When ruling out the possibility of sharing experiences in this way, he is also deprived of the possibility, in the first place, to be able to recognize the different meaning of two completely similar formulations, and, in the second, to recognize that also the possibilities of viewing the productivity of words in relation to experience are limited. Language can, *with* this connection between words and experience, expand and re-create the possibilities of intersubjective experiences, of experiences of relatedness.

## *Concluding remarks*

Today's therapy theories—both family therapy and developmental—have gradually and in various ways attempted to create concepts that, literally speaking, will reduce the difference between me and others. A part of this endeavour is also the attention given to language as a meta-individual phenomenon that we all use and need in order to create and express meaning. The perspective of developmental psychology is strongly directed at the notion that shared experience, with a different point of departure, is a precondition for all developmental processes. In therapy contexts, it is meaningful to concretize experiences of this as part of the relationship between the persons who are in a dialogue regarding a problem, including the therapist. It is possible that in some contexts it may be a productive hypothesis that linguistic competence presupposes a communicative competence as the basis for using language. A part of this can be covered by what the concept of intersubjectivity attempts to describe.

When working with families, it seems that the concept of intersubjectivity can expand the scope of our understanding in a constructive way. It covers or focuses on different phenomena, different experiences, from the relational concepts of family therapy. One important difference is that to understand the phenomenon of intersubjectivity, you have to include an explicit understanding of how bodily expression and feeling operate in human relationships. In addition, if one wishes to focus on the question of the elements in the interaction that create and maintain an experience of sharing something with someone, the concept of intersubjectivity will supply ideas and gateways to meaningful exchanges. But still it cannot replace the family therapeutic concepts. These largely describe the context that supplies the framework for the micro-exchanges that constitute the experiences of intersubjectivity. In our efforts to organize the diversity of experiences that constitutes therapeutic work with relationships, we can perhaps make use of concepts on different levels—that is to say, concepts that have a bearing on both self-experiences in dyads *and* on contexts that include larger structures of stable relationships, which to a greater extent are mediated through symbolization. And perhaps the concept of intersubjectivity will prove to be most useful in the descriptions of concrete dyadic experiences of relatedness—which need words transcending the fact that we are formed in and by the same context.

*PART II*

# RELATION-ORIENTED THERAPY AND MODERN DEVELOPMENTAL PSYCHOLOGY: CLINICAL IMPLICATIONS

CHAPTER FOUR

# Understanding each other—what does that mean? On emotional exchange, self-experience, and interplay

*Astri Johnsen, Vigdis Wie Torsteinsson*

The importance of feelings for the relationship between people will hardly be contested by anyone. Feelings intensify one's attention towards the internal world as well as the surrounding world. Affects and feelings can be understood as intuitive evaluations of the individual's attitude to his or her surroundings. At the same time they are also bodily expressions. They have profound roots in our history, but they are also influenced by cultural and social conditions. Many schools of psychotherapy have attached great importance to feelings, although in different ways. Psychoanalysis emphasized the importance of feelings for development and for the occurrence of psychic illness. The abreaction and ventilation of feelings was one way of freeing oneself from connections to traumatic events and other repressed experiences. We also find this way of thinking in the historically oriented family therapy (Hoffman, 1981). Ivan Boszormenyi-Nagy and, among others, Helm Stierlin in his early days, have demonstrated the significance of speaking out about repressed, prohibited, and taboo feelings in a family context. In his subsequent work, Stierlin showed that this did not always have a healing effect, and he made a distinction between what he called "healing through encounter" and "healing through systemic change". The degree of usefulness of affective confrontations and working through depended—in his opinion—on the system's or the relationships' degree of deadlock (Johnsen, Tømmerås, Hundevadt, & Haavardsholm, 1987).

Systemic family therapy had the work with deadlocked systems as its point of departure. This may be one of the reasons why feelings were given such an unfair position in this area of therapy. Doubtlessly the ambiguity of concepts such as affects, feelings, emotions, and the mixing up of theories of instinct and affect have all contributed to this attitude.

But the main reason is probably that the focus of individual psychology which embraced all the traditional approaches to feelings has been difficult to combine with a consistent focus on what lies "between". This is Lynn Hoffman's primary concern when she says that "social constructionists look upon them (feelings) as just one more part of the complex web of communication between people, and do not give them special status as interior states" (Hoffman, 1992, p. 12).

Studies of affects have been given a new theoretical angle these last ten to twenty years. Modern theory of affect has combined theories from different fields, such as psychoanalysis, cognitive theory, systems theory (Tomkins), and also knowledge gained from infant research (Lichtenberg). Modern affect theory deals with what goes on not only inside the individual, but also between the individual and others—that is to say, it deals with both the intrapsychic and the interpersonal developmental processes (Havnesköld & Mothander, 1995). The relation between modern psychoanalytic self-psychology and modern affect theory has been an issue in psychotherapy research. Jon Monsen has done special work using Tomkins's affect theory in clinical practice (Monsen, 1997).

Within family therapy, the social-constructionist understanding of feelings has aroused more interest (Gergen, 1994; Harré & Parrott, 1996). Social constructionism stresses the role played by culture and socialization in the development of feelings. Traditional psychological studies of emotions have, according to the evaluation of social constructionists, neglected the significance of context. Feelings are part of a context, feelings *are* evaluations and interpretations, and this presupposes information about the situation (Harré & Parrott, 1996). Gergen states explicitly that we do not *have* feelings—we *make* them. Feelings are not inner, biological or experiential states; rather, they acquire their meaning through being part of cultural patterns for interaction (Gergen, 1994, p. 222). And precisely for this reason they are given a status different from any other bodily mode of reaction. The disagreement concerning different affect theories concerns—among other things—the issue of whether feelings represent a mode of experience that is, or can be, preverbal, or whether feelings are exclusively linguistically constituted, through the names we give them and the discourses they enter into as a result of this. As far as we can see, the latest contributions within affect theory have only had a minor impact in the field of family therapy. One exception in Norway is Anne Johnsen's and Terje Tilden Nordby's utilization of Monsen's feeling-consciousness interview in their work with couples (Johnsen, 1998; Nordby, 1998). In our own work with families, we have also used Stern's distinction between categorical affects and vitality affects, as well as his concept of affect attunement and affect matching (Johnsen & Torsteinsson, 1997).

In this chapter we intend to take as the starting point Stern's understanding and description of the affects and the importance of feelings for development, since his model is both inspired by modern affect theory (cf. Karterud & Monsen, 1997) and also supplements it. One question we would naturally ask in this connection is to what extent all significant relational exchanges can be incorporated into an understanding that first and foremost is founded on linguistically constituted and conveyed experience. And if affective exchanges are an important part of our common life—does it mean that experiencing an emotional sense of relatedness is a condition for creating our narratives? What does it mean that, according to Stern (1995), feelings have the same temporal form as narratives? We wish to assert that this is a central issue in regard to the narrative wave that characterized family therapy in the 1990s.

Inspired by Daniel Stern's theory, Bjørg Røed Hansen has made a clarifying distinction between what she calls affective and narrative dialogue, and she has used this distinction in psychotherapy with children (Hansen, 1996a).

Individuals, couples, and families often come to therapy because they feel that neither are they understood nor do they understand each other. Sometimes this experience is confirmed in the therapy—they do not feel understood by the therapist and they do not understand each other. We would here like to share a number of experiences about how the therapist can deal with this situation, and how the therapeutic encounter can promote an understanding between the participants. We believe that knowledge about affective exchanges, or a lack of these, can be of use.

## *"A pet child has many names"— about different words for feelings*

Affects, feelings, and emotions are concepts that are used differently and interchangeably, depending on which theoretical tradition one refers to.

*Affects* are today seen as a fundamental biological system that successively evolves towards a higher complexity through human contact. Instincts and affects are conceived as separate, inherited biological systems. Affects are connected to biological patterns, while *feelings* refer to the subjective quality and quantity of the experiences. Feeling-consciousness is defined as a subjective experience of an affect being triggered, and it presupposes, therefore, both a subjective experience and self-reflection. *Emotions* can be linked to biographical narratives and episodic memories. An emotion can be defined as a complex combination of memories of earlier experiences and the affects that are triggered by them. To put it simply, we can say that affects are biology, whereas feelings are self-reflection and emotions are biography (Havnesköld & Mothander, 1995). In everyday speech, we mostly use the word "feeling", which refers to our subjective experiences. This is also in line with Stern, although affects, according to Stern (1995), refer to both the subjective and the objective aspects of certain congenitally organized experiences.

## Vitality affects and categorical affects

As mentioned before (see chapter 1), Stern makes an important subtle distinction between two different types of feelings or affects. One of these types is what we usually call feelings, and what Darwin (1872) at first classified as *categorical affects* (joy, anger, etc.). In addition, Stern defines something that he terms *vitality affects*, which follow any kind of experience. For example, the flow of thoughts, perceptions, motor patterns, and acts can also create moods with or without any connection to the classical affects—the categorical affects (Stern, 1995, pp. 53–58). The vitality affects can therefore come together with or without a categorical affect. Stern calls this a different form of "expressiveness", and the concepts he uses to elaborate on the phenomena are, for example, activation contours, dynamic shifts, or patterned changes in ourselves. Contour and pattern are the words he uses to tell us that this is something different from the activation level. He attempts to describe the very rhythm in the experience, that it starts slowly, continues with a sudden escalation, which is followed by just as sudden a reduction in intensity. Stern describes the vitality affects as a form of comprehensive experiences. Activation is only *one* aspect of the vitality affects. These activation contours accompany all experiences and can therefore easily be transposed to an amodal form that can be re-created in a different form of action or mental activity. This is the underlying quality in every form of vitality affect. It is precisely this amodal form of presence that causes Stern to believe that feelings are one of the fundamental sources of interpersonal experiences. This we can return to later. And in addition to the fact that they are important forms of communication—that is to say, important signals to others—they also constitute the basis of several of Stern's self-domains. These are crucial for an understanding of the developmental patterns of both individuals and relationships. In order to explain how feelings are represented, he subsequently introduces the concept of temporal feeling shape (Stern, 1995, pp. 82–88). The feelings are represented in a narrative form. They have—similarly to his description of the vitality affects—a beginning, an escalation, a reduction, and a termination. The vitality affects take care of the experience of wholeness. They continuously influence the individual and emerge as background music or hedonic tone. In the infant as well as in the adult, each experience is followed by a special hedonic tone (Stern, 1990).

### *Regulation, imitation, and affect attunement*

The central issue in the treatment of feelings in developmental psychological contexts is the fact that they are basically experiences of relatedness. They give us experiences of sharing while at the same time shaping us as delimited subjects with our own perspective on the contexts of which we are a part. And even though they are, first and foremost, described as being significant in the first dialogues that the infant is a part of, a continuous-construction model implies that these are central topics in all the significant relationships we enter into or are a part of, regardless of the time of life when this occurs.

The description of the vitality affects takes its point of departure in the infant and its experience and form of expression. The *regulation* of states is important in the early interaction. It has to do with communication linked to the child's state-regulation, where comforting and calming or stimulation are central aspects of the interaction. But regulation is mostly about influencing another's rhythm and letting oneself be influenced by it.

*Imitation* is another important concept used by Stern to characterize emotional sharing. He characterizes imitation as a re-creation of the same overt behavioural expression. In the domain of the core sense of a self, imitation is an important source of experiences dealing with relatedness, equality, and intimacy. The interactional sequences that are primarily directed at state regulation are complementary to those of the child (Stern, 1985, p. 108).

The concept of *affect attunement* is linked to the domain of the sense of a subjective self (see chapter 1). The sharing of subjective states—intersubjectivity—presupposes the experience that others are separate from oneself, according to Stern. Affect attunement points to one aspect of intersubjectivity—namely, the sharing of affective states. The affects are both the medium and the subject for communication. The affective exchange governs the mother–child relationship during this period. Stern discusses affect attunement in relation to concepts such as imitation, mirroring, and empathy and concludes that it is a concept that covers similar, and yet different, phenomena.

*Affect attunement* implies that one refers to a similar inner state with the help of different overt expressions. Attunement has the following characteristics: it reminds one of imitation, yet without being a complete rendering of the child's behaviour, but a different kind of matching. This matching is first and foremost cross-modal, which is to say that the adult uses a different modality for expression, but the experiential pattern remains the same. Therefore, says Stern, what matches is not the behaviour of the other, but an aspect of this behaviour that refers to the person's feeling state. In this way, an experience of relatedness is established that simultaneously delimits those who are involved as separate persons. Somewhat simplified, we can say that imitation reproduces form, whereas attunement reproduces feeling.

Mirroring is a concept that comes closest to affect attunement. Mirroring can be understood as imitation developing into a theme with synchronized variation. Stern thinks that the way, clinically, in which this concept has been used points more to a communication of feeling (from mother to child) than to a reproduction.

Affect attunement resembles *empathy* in that both phenomena presuppose a form of emotional resonance. Attunement takes place automatically, beyond consciousness. The original emotional resonance takes place automatically in another expression, and it is this transformed re-creation that turns affect attunement into a separate phenomenon. Empathy, on the other hand, implies conveying a cognitive process. It implies being able to understand, share, and verbally express the feeling state of another person. Empathy means listening from the inside of a person's perspective and, at the same time, communicating this cognitively (Karterud & Monsen, 1997).

One example of an imitation response is when a mother's eyes fill with tears immediately after observing these in her daughter, who experiences that no one can understand how she feels. The mother experiences the tears as a kind of "contagion" that is good neither for her nor for her daughter. In a sense, she regrets not being able to transform the empathic matching in a way that would give the daughter a possibility of "owning" her own feeling, while at the same time having a feeling of sharing it with someone. An example of empathic response is the use of introspection ("how does it feel to be scared or sad?"), empathy, and at the same time a cognitive processing of the experience ("I understand that . . ."). In affect attunement, one shows that one knows and understands the feeling through a different channel or modality.

Stern emphasizes *inter-affectivity* as being perhaps the most central part of intersubjectivity. In his opinion, feelings—and especially the vitality affects—are ideal for shaping a sense of an intersubjective self: first, because they accompany every experience and thus function as a source of background information that continuously specifies an interpersonal self; second, because mutual regulation of feelings is a unique trait characterizing human social interaction. The vitality affects are central precisely to affect attunement. They are important for registering or understanding the hedonic tone, the mood, the experience. The amodal quality of the vitality affects enables the other (the mother, the therapist, etc.) to communicate an understanding of the subjective experience, although through a different modality.

## *Some therapeutic implications*

When confronted with individuals who are grappling with the problem of understanding each other, we have found that Stern's concept of affect attunement is of value. Perhaps we can say that the concept of empathy has been particularly useful or widely held within a psychoanalytic/psychodynamic tradition, where the main emphasis has been on the relationship between the therapist and the patient. In the field of family therapy, different concepts have been used to describe the therapeutic relationship, such as neutrality, respect, an anthropological attitude, curiosity, "multipartiality" (attention, participation directed towards everyone), "joining", and a not-knowing attitude. These concepts have been rather inadequate for grasping the emotional interaction. The family therapist is required to take care of his/her therapeutic relationship to everyone in the family while at the same time directing his/her attention to the relationships existing between the different members of the family, expressed verbally and nonverbally. In the last decade a number of articles have been published dealing with the importance of being understood, the therapist's involvement, and a systemic understanding of the concept of empathy (Flaskas, 1997; Pocock, 1997; Wilkinson, 1992). These concepts have been introduced precisely in order to take more notice of the importance of feelings in family talks. In addition to this, affect attunement also draws attention to the nonverbal communication of feelings.

Stern underlines that the vitality affects accompany every experience—in children as well as in adults—with or without connection to the categorical affects. But how can we make use of this distinction in our clinical work? In our opinion, the vitality affects are useful for capturing and understanding the interaction between people. It is just as important to grasp the tone in the experience—the quality, the intensity, and the subjective experience—as it is to grasp the content, whether the person is angry, unhappy, pleased, and so forth. An example of this can be found in chapter 9: by focusing on form instead of on content, we were given a different understanding of the interaction between Line and her sister and mother, and also a different understanding of her participation in the therapy.

In our experience, it can be useful to focus on vitality affects when working with eating disorders. Eating disorders are often classified as a disorder in the ability to express feelings or a lack in the ability to do so. The only experience or feeling such patients describe is being anxious. The therapist may sometimes become eager and try to find or draw out the "real" feelings, such as anger or joy, disappointment or anxiety. Our experiences are often depressing, and we are confirmed in our belief that these persons do not have access to their feelings.

## *Moving out of the fog*

Hanne, who is 32 years old, has been living with eating problems for the last fifteen years. In the last twelve years, this has resulted in severe bulimia. She goes to work every day from 9 a.m. to 4 p.m.

The remaining hours of the day and all the weekends she spends overeating, with subsequent vomiting. She vomits one to three times a day. It is her sister who has arranged for her to come to therapy and who has nagged her about doing something about her own situation. Hanne has previously made some half-hearted attempts, but she does not believe that she can get herself out of her situation. In a way, it is only a matter of lacking willpower, of pulling herself together. The therapy is an example of the both/and approach that this book wishes to convey (see especially chapter 9). The point of departure for Hanne is individual sessions. The family—sometimes all the family members, sometimes the mother or the sister—is involved whenever it is necessary in relation to the topics we are working with. These couple or joint talks are also limited by geographical factors since Hanne lives by herself, far away from her parents. Her life consists of work, overeating, and vomiting.

The idea that problems are caused by a lack of ability to pull oneself together is something that is shared by all, especially by Hanne and her father. Self-reproach and self-criticism can explain one's own inadequacy, and the problems of others are also caused by oneself. The daughters feel responsible and guilty about their parents' bad marriage, and the parents feel guilt about their daughters' problems (the sister also suffered from eating problems for a while). In this way, one becomes guilty and responsible both in relation to one's own and others' illness and problems. They understand each other, but this understanding leads to apathy, to an inability to act. Everything becomes grey, opaque, foggy. They become opaque for each other and for themselves. Is it possible that therapy will help Hanne to become more distinct to herself and others—that is to say, will it contribute to a different understanding of herself and others? Further on in this chapter, we show how Stern's concept of affect attunement can usefully promote understanding. In the present example, we want to show how the attention given to vitality affects helped to create distinctiveness and enabled Hanne slowly to emerge as a person.

During the sessions, Hanne is charming and pleasant; she willingly rambles on, seemingly open, but everything is like a steady stream. It is impossible to grasp what is essential and what is not. What I [A.J.] am saying as a therapist makes no difference to her, gives no meaning to her. The encounter with the family makes the therapist understand that it is no use ending up in self-reproaches. The important thing here is to be distinct as a therapist. Gradually I notice that there are two things that seem to have an effect, that give meaning to her. One of them is the therapist's involvement. I tell her what I think of her and her situation, and what I think I am seeing. It is the variation, the intensity, and the rhythm in what I am saying that catches her attention. My involvement usually begins somewhat slowly. Little by little, I become eager, my intensity increases, and then towards the end of the comment or "statement" it quietens down again. This characterizes the vitality affects as described by us earlier.

The other factor that gives meaning to her is my use of images or metaphors. This is interesting and in line with the importance attributed by Stern to metaphors as a connecting link or a transition between the nonverbal affective exchange and the development of language, or as a transitional form between analog and digital language (Røer, 1996).

I describe to Hanne that it seems as though the bulimia is enveloping her in a fog, making her indistinct to herself and to others. This makes others indistinct or invisible to her as well. The fog image is meaningful to her; she can recognize it. I also state that I disagree with her explanation that the bulimia expresses a lack of willpower to pull herself together. On the contrary, both she and the others in her family carry the burden of a tyrannical perfectionist on their backs, which constantly sends out the message that nothing is good enough. Through the therapist's active engagement, certain contours are emerging. She too becomes involved and eager, declaring her agreement or her disagreement. The therapist becomes aware of the small variations, of the differences in her involvement in the sessions and of what she is telling. She is gaining experience and is learning; it is not a matter of great experiences or deep feelings, but of small, everyday experiences. The therapist is also interested in the minor details, in the variation in her experiences. What happened before an incident, how did it start, how did it develop, did the experience or the feeling become more intense or did it diminish? At first her experiences were connected to her bulimic episodes and her feelings of anxiety. How did the anxiety start, how could she identify it, how did it increase, and what could diminish it? Registration exercises—a commonly used method in cognitive behaviour therapy for bulimia—were used, and here the variations and the intensity of the experiences were especially discussed. Little by little other experiences were emerging. She started remembering; she came to the sessions with new experiences, eager, curious, hopeless at times, depressed, back in a haze but now in order to emerge again with new experiences.

In my therapy with Hanne, Stern's concept of vitality affects became important for me and helped me to understand my own potentials as a therapist, both in relation to myself and in relation to her. When moving into a foggy landscape, it is important to mobilize activity, engagement, and curiosity. The foggy landscape needs to be actively explored in order to discover what it may conceal.

This active exploration followed a rhythm with varying intensity and variation. In this way the rhythm, the intensity, and the variation in the experiences of the therapist, as well as in Hanne's own experiences, became important ingredients in the therapeutic dialogue. It was only against this background that the verbal dialogue became meaningful. At first, her words did not have meaning for me. In her verbal stream, it was impossible to distinguish between what was important and what was not. Nor did my words have meaning for her. We can formulate it like this: it was only when the words acquired a melody that life and movement entered into the therapy. What we said to each other gave meaning, and we could start sharing an understanding of her problems and her life. She tried out these experiences, at first in relation to her parents and siblings, and later in relation to a boyfriend. The use of metaphors linked the affective and the verbal, as has also been demonstrated by Stern and others.

As mentioned before, the vitality affects are one of the fundamental sources in interpersonal experience due to their amodal or cross-modal quality. For what did actually take place between Hanne and the therapist/me?

Is it an empathic exchange, a mirroring, or a form of imitation? Or is it even more about what takes place prior to both the affect attunement and the imitation—namely, a regulation or modulation of the affects? Can we describe what happened in the therapy like this: through regulation, Hanne is given the opportunity to organize and experience an emergent sense of self and an emergent other?

### *Loving each other is not the same as understanding each other*

The meeting with the K. family can illustrate the problems connected to what it means to understand each other. It can also illustrate some of the differences around imitation, affect regulation, and affect attunement. The problems were anxiety, diffuse eating problems, and the sleeping problems of one of the daughters, Dina, who is 20 years old.

Her problems have increased in the last twelve months and have now become severe. The physician who referred her believes that the social pattern in her family will retard and inhibit Dina's personal development.

*The family.* The father has had a drinking problem for many years. He has now admitted to this abuse, but it still remains a problem in the family. He is described as two persons: kind and caring when he is sober, unpredictable, critical, and hurting others when he has been drinking. The mother is presented—by herself and the others—as the emotionally most stable person in the family. The sister, Siri, is 23 years old, and a few years ago she tried to take her own life at a time when she was extremely depressed. She functions well now but would not like the story about her suicidal attempt to be broadcast outside the family. The youngest in the family, Lars, who is 15 years old, has no special problems. All five live together. Neither Dina nor Siri have many social contacts outside the family.

The family presents itself as being very closely knit, where everything is talked about and all are very fond of each other. Mother's special preoccupation is how the closeness within the family can compensate for difficulties with persons outside the family. At the same time, closeness and security also become a dilemma. Does it promote or inhibit the process of separation, which, especially in the eyes of her mother, is Dina's problem?

They presented themselves as a family who were experts in terms of each other's feelings and thoughts, a family who would be described in the family literature as an *ego-mass family* (Bowen, 1978), a *centrifugal family* (Stierlin, 1974), *enmeshed* (Minuchin, Rosman, & Baker, 1978), or a family with rigid or deadlocked *family premises* (Boscolo et al., 1987). An example of this is Siri, who used to involve herself so deeply in the feelings of others that they became her own (e.g. her involvement in her parents' conflicts regarding her father's drinking problem). Another example is Dina, who feels the same as others are feeling and who has total empathy with the feelings of the others and may then create feelings that are not there (e.g. believing that mother is under stress, and becoming more stressed herself). The father, who feels what others are feeling, becomes anxious when he believes that Dina is anxious, and happy when she is happy.

They are engaged in reading each others' feelings, with the result that they "over-read" each others' feelings. Mother becomes infected by Dina's sadness, "goes down" with her—in other words, she becomes just as sad and powerless. Mother experiences that when she becomes like Dina, matches her feeling or experience, it will still not give Dina any possibilities of developing. At the back of her mind is her experience with Siri—the fact that sharing her worries and anxiety about her husband's alcoholism on an equal basis had merely overburdened her. Mother is afraid that, as long she only provides the security that Dina's anxiety requires from her, she does not challenge Dina enough. Dina experiences that she is dependent on her mother feeling the same as herself. But she also realizes that this can be a strain on her mother and that it is necessary to keep a distance. Either they experience the same, which is a problem for both the mother and Dina, or else they have two totally different experiences, which both will then find unsatisfactory.

Taking as our starting point the concepts of developmental psychology dealing with emotional exchange, one can say that this family is characterized by *imitation* as their emotional response. In the sessions, too, they "copy" each other's reactions, which, according to Stern, is an important source of the experience of feeling-relatedness but is not yet a relatedness delimiting the involved parties as separate subjects.

"Understanding each other—what is that?" This question became the focal point already in the first session. It first emerged as a question about what can and what should be shared. Where are the dividing lines between what is mutually experienced and what is individual? Are my feelings necessarily the same as yours?

We approached this issue at first using our standard family therapeutic methods: circular questions and intervening exercises. These proved to be inadequate for capturing certain experiential aspects in the relationship to oneself and each other.

We began by exploring differences and boundaries between the family members. We used circular questions such as: "How do you (father) look upon Dina's situation? Do you think it is similar to or different from the way Dina looks upon the situation?" To Dina: "When you become anxious, who do you think notices this first? How do you see that your mother understands that you become anxious or unhappy?"

In order to explore the boundaries between their own feelings, thoughts, and experiences, we gave them homework after the second session. Dina was asked to register the symptoms: when and how does anxiety (the lump, as she called it) come? She was also asked to make a note of whether she thought that it was noticed by the others in the family. However, she should avoid talking about it, except when she had her sessions (one hour, twice a week). The parents and the sister were asked to write down when they believed that Dina was anxious, but not to talk about it until their own sessions.

This assignment could be seen as a typical structural assignment or a Milan assignment, which was meant to challenge and explore central family premises, or as a typical individuation assignment inspired by Helm Stierlin's model (1974). On our part, the purpose of the assignment was to discover the family premises that were crucial for understanding the family's deadlock. This type of assignment will, in any case, lead to new information.

The parents, especially the mother, experienced the assignment as the beginning of a breakaway, but for Dina it did not lead to an experience of mastery, but only of want and loneliness. For Siri, the difference between herself and her sister became clearer. Solutions were more important to her than understanding—a difference between the sisters that gradually became more obvious. For Siri, it would have been important to share what she had experienced during her own depressive episode with the family, but not outside it. She was also more interested in mastery than in understanding connections. For Dina, it was different—in fact, almost the opposite. Previously she had been the person in the family who perhaps most wanted to contact others when problems arose in the home. The taboos and the secrecy about central and frightening experiences that can be characterized as more or less shocking made her gradually invisible and incomprehensible to her friends and also to herself and to her own problems. The significance of having a narrative that is comprehensible, coherent, and meaningful for oneself, and which one can share with others, gradually became a focal point.

## *Regulation and exchange of feelings as therapeutic challenges in the family*

The reactions to the assignment raised a number of questions. What is the difference between sharing experiences, thoughts and feelings, and being infected by each other? Is imitating each other's experiences sufficient for making one feel understood? Does involvement convey understanding? What kind of relationship is there between regulating feelings and understanding? And, above all, what does it actually mean to understand each other? What does it imply in terms of similarities and differences, the sense of belonging, relatedness, and separateness? These reflections brought up new therapeutic issues and interventions. For instance: in spite of the family's frankness, the therapist got the impression that Dina did not feel herself understood—"Was that correct?" ... "Yes" "What would it take to be understood?" ... "Don't think anyone can understand without oneself having experienced the same."

Dina makes it clear that the others cannot understand her, and that she does not feel understood by seeing that others feel the same. "The understanding has to come from within." This also raises the question about the extent to which affect attunement is a specific phenomenon in the early mother–child relationship, or whether it is a more general phenomenon. In terms of what has already been said about affect attunement, these phenomena characterize all human coordinated interaction and especially the closest relationships. For this reason, these forms of exchange are operative at any point in time, even though the forms may vary in significance and frequency. The one most frequently found in the period from age 2 to 9 months (sense of a core self) is imitation, while affect attunement reaches its highest frequency from 9 to 15 months (sense of a subjective self).

Stern's concepts of regulation, imitation, and affect attunement were useful to us as therapists in our understanding of the interaction in this family. They wished to share each others' feelings. Instead of leading to an understanding, it increased the anxiety, not only in Dina, but also in the others, especially the mother. As mentioned before, affective exchange is characterized by imitation. This means that none of them can experience a shared internal world. Can we as therapists contribute to this?

### *The prerequisite and significance for Dina and her family to create their own narrative*

Dina asks especially for her mother's understanding, and not just for her empathy. For this reason we chose to invite mother and daughter together to a couple of sessions. In this context, with only two of them present, the atmosphere was calmer and offered more opportunities for exploring the topic of understanding. What was the mother's story in terms of being understood? She had experienced losing her own mother in a most dramatic manner when she was 18 years old. It had been a shock and grief. What had helped her was to talk to others—first and foremost to her boyfriend, to her friends, and also to her family. Is it possible that Dina's anxiety, which comes in the shape of an incomprehensible lump in her chest, also has a story—which proved to be about her insecurity in connection with her father's drinking and the taboos surrounding her sister's depression? A number of questions made it clearer that the anxiety/lump was caused by an experience of loneliness. She had been unable to share with anyone what she had experienced during the episodes concerning her father and sister. This is an example of what Stern calls selective attunement: feeling states that are never attuned will be experienced as loneliness. When Dina's anxiety was linked to concrete episodes and understandable experiences and feelings, they became less frightening and more understandable for the mother. In the sessions alone with her daughter, and relieved from the burden of loyalty towards her husband and oldest daughter, she was also more relaxed when listening to her. Through the affective exchanges that were a part of the mother's and Dina's responses to questions, it became possible for them to maintain a common emotional basis and yet be different. The anxiety was given a narrative, a narrative embracing small and big experiences of shock and insecurity connected to the father and the sister. The anxiety is given a personal meaning; it becomes understandable to Dina, and thus also understandable to the mother as well.

We can say that, so far, Dina has not had a coherent narrative about her own life. She has blended in with the others. She has swallowed her experiences of shock and insecurity, and these experiences have then grown into a large and painful lump in her chest. According to Stern, the analogous responses that characterize affect attunement are important learning experiences for developing language. In terms of development, he points to a path from imitation to analogies (affect attunement), symbols, and language. If imitation continues to be the most important form of communication in relation to feelings, then important steps towards a symbolization of these experiences, such as language and narratives, will complicate the issue. On the other hand, however, we see that exploring words that give meaning to the family as a whole will open up for the development of an individual narrative, as demonstrated by the mother's and Dina's different narratives about understanding.

This narrative about the K. family shows the importance of understanding and the exchange of feelings for the development of a narrative self, an understanding of oneself that gives coherence and meaning. Stern emphasizes that the representation of feelings—what he terms temporal feeling shape—has the same temporal form as narratives. This temporal feeling shape constitutes a part of a narrative structure that Stern calls a pre-narrative envelope (Stern, 1992). It describes the infant's mode of representing reality and is later organized into what he calls the sense of a narrative self, which is formed at the age of 2 to 3 years. At this point the child creates its own autobiography. Affective and selective attunement function as filters for the experiences and feelings that are accepted and permitted and for those that cannot be shared. We can say that central family premises are in this way conveyed to the child, particularly in the sense of which emotional experiences are understood and permitted. The child soon learns which experiences can be placed within the narrative about itself, and which are not permitted. These experiences and feelings are not given a sense of belonging. They do not find any "home"; they become isolated islands. Both psychoanalysts (Schafer, 1992; Spence, 1982) and family therapists (White & Epston, 1990) have been examining the question of how these experiences create conditions for symptoms. For Dina, the sharing and understanding of these isolated and hidden learning experiences became a condition for her being able to create her own autobiography.

### *Being in each other's glance and reading each other's mind*

Harald and Sissel are a couple seeking help to understand each other better. They have had a severe crisis. She fell in love with another man, was unfaithful, wanted a divorce, and had moved out. It came as a shock to him. He fell into a deep crisis but wanted her back again. They had been married for many years. He had been in psychoanalysis for many years, and the psychoanalyst understood that couple therapy would be necessary if the relationship was to have a chance. She was positively surprised about her husband's reaction, had not thought that he cared about her. He had lived in the world of science for the last twenty-five years and had started in psychoanalysis five years ago, to come into better contact with his feelings. It had taught him a great deal about what was going on inside him, but it had not improved his views about what was happening to them. She looked upon the crisis as a chance to do something about the relationship. His psychoanalyst also realized the necessity of directing the attention to the couple relationship.

We will here give some examples from the sessions showing how we as family therapists helped them to communicate about feelings. All in all, we had five double sessions in the course of ten months.

A typical trait of Harald's is that he speaks in big headlines: "She can't love me when she doesn't want sex" (they had intercourse the night before). He has felt that she despises him. "When I lie in bed on Saturday or Sunday, she thinks I am regressive, she hates that." "He lived in his own world and did not see me," she says. Both have had very strong feelings for each other but have only been able to express the negative ones.

In the first session there is, among other things, talk about a situation that made her feel sad:

T: How do you notice that she becomes sad?

H: Difficult question. Notice more when she becomes angry. I have difficulties seeing when she is sad.

T: Is she too withdrawn?

H: I think so. I had a shock, it changed everything. Haven't been able to put myself in the place of anyone. When Sissel begins to cry—I don't feel it—or I feel it, but don't do anything about it. Can see that she is unhappy, but don't feel it. A need to comfort her is not awakened.

Later in the session, about contempt:

H: . . . We each have our own weak points: her contempt, my self-centredness. When I feel her contempt, I become even more self-centred in order to avoid feeling her contempt.

S: That isn't contempt, but rejection.

In spite of these topics of rejection and contempt, the therapists feel that the tone between them has changed. This is a couple moving in step, at the same pace, and it is good to be with them. However, they are wearing some "glasses" that prevent them from becoming aware of this. We suggest that they try out some other glasses—namely, "confirmatory" glasses.

When they come to the second session, they have been feeling better. There has been more physical closeness, and this is one of the themes of this session. Closeness also triggers longings as well as bitterness about what has happened, and they are afraid of falling back into old patterns. What strikes us in particular is the distance between the verbal language and what is conveyed through their tone of voice, their facial expressions, and their body postures. The topics, and the ways in which these are conveyed stimulate the therapists to use a metaphorical language: "Your story resembles a landscape marked by frugality and barrenness. It is as though you did not know of any springs that might make the landscape more fertile and hospitable."

In the third session, the topic is sexuality, rejection, and expressions of love other than sexuality.

S: Harald is constantly wearing these sexual glasses. It is the measure of everything (*in a sad voice, eyes filling with tears*), how often, how it's done, becomes a token of whether I love him. . . . I have to excuse myself if I don't feel like it, but I do love you (*looks at him*).

T: Do you think it is possible for him to see this differently?

S: Don't know (*sadly*), important for him.

T: What effect does it have on you and your interaction that he is so preoccupied with it?

S (*thinking for a while; he is looking at her*): Important not to reject him (*moved*).

H: I experience something similar to Sissel, we had such a good time together [that weekend], but then comes doubt, placed on sex. . . .

T: When you get a feeling of that she loves you, how do you see that?

H: That she wants me sexually—and in other ways.

T: What are the small signals telling you that she loves you?

H: I personally can only see the big headlines. (*Reflects*). She comes and sits close to me, creates an atmosphere of cosiness and warmth.

T: How do you become aware of it?

H: The way in which she does it.

T: What about the way?

H: There is a good atmosphere, a lot of light and warmth.

T: How does she convey this—by the way in which she talks, moves, her face?

H: I'm not able to see it, . . . only have an idea that it's something good, . . . don't actually see Sissel, just feel, sense that it is something . . . I have more of a radar system for negative things, can describe it more clearly, for example rejection and contempt. . . . But we have become better at touching each other.

T: How do you read Harald when he loves you?

S: By his voice.

T: What about his voice?

S: He speaks differently, becomes softer.

T: Is it mostly the voice?

S: The voice reflects him, his emotions, sadness, anger, kindness.

T: Many couples are sensitive to each other's glances: how is it with you?

S: That's more difficult. Haven't got the channel.

T: Not the channel you are both looking at?

H: Have always been afraid of eye contact. I also register the voice.

T: If you were to look for other channels than the voice—for example, the eyes or glances?

H: It's not there that I get the information.

T: Have both of you never done that?

S: Haven't thought about it.

T: I have read a book about early interaction. The expression of "being in each other's glance" is used there. Some describe being in love like this. Has it been like this for you both?

H: No experience of that, haven't had such meetings [with the glance]. . . . The body, that's the channel we have been using, always been afraid to look people in the eye, have done lipreading.

This session confirms the impression of a couple who greatly differ in the way they show that they love each other, and in the headlines they give out. Their marriage is a narrative about a book with some large headlines—rejection, infidelity, sexuality—and it looks as if they have forgotten to read the small print. Their homework is to practice reading each other's glances and faces, not to look for the painful things, but for the good ones. Sissel's face, for example, is a landscape of sunshine and warmth.

The fourth session is about sharing feelings. They have done their homework with the glance. They speak about a difficult period where previously they would have rejected each other. Now they remained in contact.

H: It has been lovely, seeing her eyes, seeing that she loves me.

S: I've also seen his mouth, I can see anger and sadness there, in his eyes there is joy.

They clearly become more interested in the other's perspective, especially Harald, who has been least interested.

H: Instead of just feeling, I try to put myself in the other's place.

This session is also an example of how Harald's individual therapy has taught him something about the feelings he has inside him, that he has a right to feel anger, disappointment, and longing, but it has also taught him that these feelings have stood in the way of the feelings that are between them. It is not a matter of either/or but of realizing that the feelings he comes in contact with can also keep alive those that are between them.

They come to the fifth session with an experience of being in harmony: "We are well in harmony", says Harald at the beginning of the session. The session elaborates the topic of sharing experiences. One of the questions is how one can share something that is basically experienced differently. Harald's condition for sharing was that they should experience it alike. In this session, it is they who are using a metaphorical language.

We talk about what they mean to each other.

H: Sissel has always been the most important person in my life. . . . She is like an emerald or diamond. Although I have felt love, I haven't been able to express it—neither in words nor in action. . . . The world can't be that fantastic.

T: Are you scared that she might become an ordinary stone?

H: Yes, perhaps.

T: What do you think (*to S*)?

S: Would like it to be like that.

T: Which image would you use?

S: He is my fixed point, my cliff—security, stability.

T: Seen like that, there isn't any imbalance, no different scales of values, masculine and feminine images. How is it for you, Harald, to hear the description Sissel is using?

H: Fabulous for me, never heard it before. And this was the first time that I used the word emerald about her.

This session was the last one. And Harald's parting remark was: "Well, we can't go to therapy all our lives."

This therapy exemplifies how the therapist can stimulate a more affective exchange between two people in a couple relationship. For the therapist, the feeling tone in the interaction was just as important as information as the content of their talk. Stern says that affect attunement is integrated in other behaviour and therefore not so easy to get hold of. There are three behavioural traits that can be matched and adjusted, and which give grounds for attunement: intensity, timing, and form. This type of matching takes place intuitively or unconsciously, but it can still be recognized through introspection, direct observation, or video recording. It is our assertion that this form of attunement characterized the therapeutic interaction with this couple.

## *Conclusion*

In this chapter, three case histories have been used to illustrate the usefulness of Stern's conception of feelings. We can say that they also demonstrate the line of development in Stern's theory about the importance of feelings in relation to oneself and others. The story of Hanne demonstrates the usefulness of directing one's attention towards the vitality affects, in the therapist as well as in the client. Meaning and coherence was created through a communication in which the variation, intensity, and rhythm in Hanne's and the therapist's experiences were underscored. She gradually became more distinct and started to link meaning and coherence to what was happening to her. By being together with an other, she was slowly able to regulate, remember, and give names to her experiences.

Imitation is described by Stern as a necessary experience when it is a question of sharing feelings. Imitation is, however, not adequate for having an experience of being understood; the story of the K. family can serve as an example of this. This story illustrates the differences in imitation and affect attunement as two developmentally different forms of communication and sharing of feelings.

Feelings need to have a form or a schema in order to be remembered (Bruner, 1986; Stern, 1995). They are a key word for leading into the narrative that is to be reconstructed (Havnesköld & Mothander, 1995). This is also evident in the history about Dina. Incomprehensible feelings were linked to the context they belonged to. Since this could be shared and gradually understood, she could also begin to construct her own narrative.

Harald and Sissel grappled with the problem of finding a language to make them read and understand each other's internal world. Through the therapist's attunement, which captured the feeling tone between them with the help of metaphors and detailed questions, they became capable of reading the signs behind their outer behaviour.

Stern describes a development from imitation to affect attunement, symbols, and language. The case history of Harald and Sissel is terminated as they themselves begin to use a metaphorical language for conveying their emotional experiences.

CHAPTER FIVE

# The traces of experiences and the significance of time in narrative therapy

*Astri Johnsen*

The narrative metaphor used in family therapy creates new possibilities, but it also raises a number of questions. In this chapter, I mainly discuss two issues: the relation to experience and the relation to time. The narrative form has a need for wholeness and closure. The dramaturgy in a narrative requires that all the elements are given meaning in a comprehensive interpretation, and that the narrative has a conclusion. A narrative can be coherent and consistent, even credible, but what is its relation to lived experience? The sequential character of narratives marking the course of time also holds some possible limitation. It may also create a certain determinism and lead to linear causal thinking. According to Jerome Bruner (1990a, p. 45), we humans have a readiness or predisposition to organize experiences in a narrative form. Bruner discusses the question of what distinguishes the narrative form from other ways of organizing experiences, and he points especially to its sequential character and special structure. The narrative can be true or fiction without losing its power as a narrative. There is no grammatical or lexical distinction between real and fictive narratives. The meaning in the narrative lies in the relation between the plot and the various events, and not in the relation to the factual events and concrete experiences. This similarity between fictive and real narratives creates an ambiguity as regards the type of experiences they refer to (Bruner, 1990a, pp. 52 ff.). Truth and possibility are entwined with each other. It is difficult to distinguish between a good narrative and an actual event. But within this ambiguity there are also possibilities; narratives open up for human possibilities rather than for rigid truths.

The question of the significance of experience also touches upon ethical issues. The plot and the characters in fictive narratives are created without the author being held accountable to real persons. Therapeutic narratives, on the other hand, involve existing people and their mutual relationships. The therapeutic dialogue requires fidelity to lived experience. Telling a narrative that also involves other people requires an ethical obligation. Who has the right of ownership to the narrative?

In order to elucidate these issues, I shall make use of two cases. One is called "Guilt, parents, and childhood". The other I have called "In search of identity".

In my attempt to understand some of the problems connected to narratives, to time, and to experience, I shall avail myself of aspects in the understanding of narratives set forth by Jerome Bruner, Luigi Boscolo, Paulo Betrando, Donald Spence, and Jim Sheehan. Sheehan's references to Paul Ricoeur and Gary Saul Morson have also been important for me. Daniel Stern's use of the narrative metaphor is illustrated in chapter 6 by his concept of the key therapeutic metaphor and will therefore hardly be touched upon in this chapter.

## *Guilt, parents, and childhood*

I receive a letter. It is from the parents of a young man, Karl. It is Karl himself and his therapist who have wanted family therapy. Karl, who is 30 years old, has been struggling with an anxiety neurosis for the last ten years and has had many different therapies. Now he is asking his parents to find a family therapist. They have had several discussions about the family circumstances and what effect these may have had on him as a child. They write that he had been active and energetic as a child. Now he is anxious and afraid to speak his mind at home. They also say that they spent a great deal of time together with him when he was a child. And they ask: if any of Karl's anxiety is a result of the conditions at home— "Can we, as parents, now contribute to relieving some of his anxiety neurosis?"

Karl is partly unfit for employment and lives at home.

### *The past: the unhappy childhood*

Until he was referred, the parents had considered Karl's problem as his own personal problem. Karl, on the other hand, had begun to think of his problems as having to do with his family and with them as parents. In his present individual therapy he has become preoccupied with his childhood. He thinks that he has had a childhood where he had not been seen. He is anxious, however, that family therapy might be too tough on his parents, and he is afraid of hurting them. The parents find it difficult to recognize Karl's narrative. In their eyes, he was a happy boy until the age of 19. Then he met a girl, and after that things went wrong. However, the parents have also begun to think that something must have happened when Karl was a child. He was an only child. Even though the parents remember Karl's childhood as a happy time, the mother still asks herself: "What have I done wrong? And what is wrong with me as a mother since he is so afraid of women?" In spite of good memories, the father also wonders whether they as parents may have done something wrong. They did not quarrel, they kept their conflicts under control. "Perhaps I've been too kind and indulgent since Karl is afraid and anxious not to show his anger," he says.

The interaction in the family is now marked by mutual consideration and caution. The parents feel that everything is done on Karl's terms. They walk on tiptoe, become impatient, but dare not say anything for fear of increasing his anxiety. The interaction in the family today is seen as proving that the interaction in those days, in Karl's childhood, had been equally unfortunate. This is how unhappy childhoods and difficult parents can be created.

Both parents are, however, preoccupied with the fact that Karl had been an exchange student in the United States, and that this had been a difficult time. Karl has been preoccupied with a wish to return to America in order to confront the family he had been living with there. It was the mother in that family who did not like him. The parents had noticed that Karl was a little more serious after he had come back from America. When asked whether they believed that Karl thought they understood him at that time, or whether he was given sufficient opportunity to tell his narrative, it emerges that the family itself had been in a crisis at the time of Karl's return. The father's business had gone bankrupt, and he was out of work for a period. The mother had to take work outside the home for the first time. It goes without saying that, in a situation like this, Karl may have felt that he was not seen, or that there was not so much room for him to talk about what he himself had experienced. Karl's America narrative turned into a lonely experience. There was no room for sharing his painful experiences with his parents. Could the trace of these experiences, and not his experiences in childhood, give meaning to Karl's narrative?

### *The past: from an unhappy childhood to a difficult adolescence*

In the following session the father began by saying: "I've thought a lot about what you said; even with a good childhood one can experience painful things. I've always believed that if one got through the first six or seven years, one was protected. You [therapist] were quick to mention this about America and also the crisis I went through in connection with my job. I had not thought about this combination before." Karl has thought a great deal about America, but not about the family crisis. He does not remember much about it. But he confirms the lasting impression made on him by his stay in America. "I've been thinking of America and all I endured." There were two things that prevented him from speaking out: "It was difficult, well, scary to say that I couldn't fix this. Of course I could have picked up the phone and told them how it was. But it's been like that at home: preferably one shouldn't say exactly how things were. I can see where that comes from." The other thing that prevented him was his anxiety: "I was so scared of her when I lived with there. She frightened me, she grounded me, she hit and threatened me, I was terrified all the time." He had talked a little about it when he returned, but he does not believe his parents understood the emotional impact it had on him, does not think they were able to empathize. He had thought that he might go back and square things with them. "There are still many feelings connected to it," he says.

The mother says she had noticed that he was more serious than before he went away, and she feels that they as parents had not been there for him when he returned. Karl thinks this is because they all have a way of dealing with each other that is difficult. "Our way is to keep off, it is cowardly." The parents walk on tiptoe because they are uncertain of what he might tolerate. Karl walks on tiptoe because he is uncertain of what his parents might tolerate.

He is also worries that family therapy will make him more dependent on his parents.

### *The time lost*

In the next session it emerges how Karl's life and the family's mutual interaction is controlled by anxiety. And yet the parents feel that they have now become better at being more direct. The mother is intent on speaking her mind, the father is intent on showing more of what he himself feels. Karl has been thinking a great deal about different ways of settling matters, but he is afraid that anxiety will paralyse him and keep him locked up in a cage. His anxiety keeps him totally under control. He misses pleasure and joy. Both Karl and his parents are locked up in time. Only the past and the present exist—the future is non-existent. For this reason the therapist introduces what is called the miracle question: "If a miracle took place tonight and you woke up on Sunday morning without anxiety, how would you notice that? How would others see it on you?" Karl would feel delight; he would see that the sky was blue and that the world had colours. He would feel like getting up, doing something, going shopping, and taking an initiative as regards friends. With girls, he would have waited a little while longer—the last time had been too difficult. The mother weeps about the time that was lost, and all the years her son has lost. Confrontation creates new opportunities, and grief is also a part of the healing process.

### *The present: the desire, the anxiety, and all the demands*

The parents come alone to the following session. Karl does not have the strength to come. The parents are worried about the future. Karl has now cut out all therapy arrangements and has also taken a break from his odd jobs.

They are worried that there may be ten more years of anxiety. They had talked about the previous session. Karl was pleased that the mother had shown feelings. The father would like to be more spontaneous. It emerges that Karl has had less anxiety, fewer pains. He himself has said that he is feeling better. He only tries to do things that he wants to do and is eager to find out what is right for him. The therapist's conclusion is that he has made his own therapy arrangements and taken a break from traditional therapy. The parents themselves would like to continue in family therapy, but they wonder whether this would have any effect on his anxiety. The most important thing, however, is that Karl can become freer and have a better relationship with them. Karl has also shown more initiative at home, and they have dared to require more of him. They have also talked about Karl's right to rehabilitation.

### *Creating a future for oneself*

Karl has continued his "self-therapy" by trying out his own boundaries in terms of what he feels like doing and what he can tolerate. He considers family therapy to be different from the other therapies, and he feels that it is important that the relationship between the three of them should improve. He has also taken the initiative to apply for rehabilitation, which he previously would never have had the energy to do. He has been especially anxious about his father's reaction—that he would be disappointed. He himself believes that half a year of rehabilitation would be sufficient. His parents believe that he will need more time, perhaps one year. They are also afraid that he will never get rid of his anxiety. At the same time, they expect and have faith that he can become well, which is encouraging but can also be experienced as a strain or a demand on him. The family therapist wonders whether this brave and talented young man has made far too great demands on himself, and whether both he and the people around him have overestimated his possibilities in regard to the great and serious problems he is struggling with. He has battled intensely with his anxiety and his physical pains for many years and believes that the pains are connected to his anxiety. That fact that he now takes a break from his own demands and those of others is a positive sign. All three—the parents and Karl—have this in common: they make strict demands on themselves and on each other. It is important that family therapy does not result in new demands. Karl wept on hearing this and said that he felt relieved, and also relieved that he had been seen.

In this session, the contours of a new future are emerging. In spite of his anxiety it is possible to imagine a future where he himself will have more influence.

### *The return to the present and the past: grief and reconciliation*

A great deal happens in Karl's life during the next few months, in regard both to himself and his parents and to his male and female friends.

This is a family where, when regarded as a whole, feeling, action, and thought has been present, but it has been unevenly distributed.

Karl has been the sensitive one in the family, with little energy. Now he has started acting. He has gone to visit friends, he has got himself a girlfriend, and he speaks out and sets limits. The father has been a man of action whose wish it has been to be able to express more feelings. In one of the sessions, he describes the pain he feels because he cannot help his son: "It is like being out at sea in a boat and seeing my son drowning right nearby without being able to help." He cries bitterly.

This image has popped up again during a conversation at home, and Karl has said that the father does not need to do anything, it is sufficient for him to know that he is there. This man of mastery and action has begun to show other sides to himself, that he is in fact a very sensitive person. The mother, who has kept her strong reactions and feelings to herself, has now started speaking out and taking up matters, whether they concern her husband or her son. A better balance has been established.

The theme of the interaction between them emerges in a new way. The focus is no longer on guilt but on curiosity, understanding, and reconciliation. Karl was frightened when he was in America, and his adolescent development was halted. But how is he to understand the fact that he let himself be frightened in this way? What caused him not to speak up? He remembers that his father sometimes suddenly became furious when he was a child, but that was not frightening in the same way. The mother was also angry much of the time, but she tried to talk to him afterwards, explaining why she had been angry. The father had a father whom all were afraid of. Why did the father not develop anxiety? And the mother had a mother who was psychotic at times. Why did he, Karl, get sick and not they? What was the difference between being frightened by a psychopathic "mother" in America, as opposed to the father's experience of an authoritarian and despotic father? Or an unpredictable and sick mother whom mother had had?

The interest in the past veered away from what the parents had done wrong to who they were as persons, and what their different and also similar experiences had been in relation to him. What was their narrative, and what was its significance in terms of understanding all three of them and their mutual relationships?

### *In search of identity*

Again I receive a letter, this time from a young girl, Ingun. She is 18 years old. She writes that she would so much like to get help to improve her relationship to her parents. When she was 14 years old, she reported her father for incest. The whole family was interrogated, the father lost his job, but the case was dismissed owing to lack of evidence. She herself was put into an institution for adolescents, and there was a break-up with her parents and siblings. Later she understood that she had been "infected" by some girlfriends and realized that it had been a lie. She went to the police and gave new evidence and also told her parents that it was wrong. She wishes to re-establish contact with her family. They are sceptical, but have said that they are willing to participate in family talks.

### *The lie*

Ingun and her parents come to the first session. The parents do not want to burden the two younger siblings with a revival of the narrative and the circumstances before being certain that they can trust Ingun again. They are relieved that she has withdrawn her formal complaint and that she understands that it was wrong. Ingun realizes that she has caused them much pain, and she hopes for a reconciliation and forgiveness. The father has given a lot of thought about how Ingun could come up with something like this. In his experience, he was the one closest to her and defended her in her conflicts with the mother or the siblings. Ingun got the idea about incest at a summer camp, where a kind of incest-fever almost raged. The father has been angry with the leaders of the camp, who failed to intervene either at that time or later in connection with the report.

The mother is more reserved. She feels that she has never really understood Ingun, who was adopted when she was about 1 year old. With the other two children, also adopted, she has had quite a different type of contact. Since Ingun has frequented the drug scene in recent years, the mother worries that Ingun may have a bad influence on the other children.

Ingun says that she has never really felt herself understood by her mother. She felt that the contact existing between her mother and her siblings was quite different. She herself felt different and lonely, without understanding what was wrong. It was also difficult for her to hear her father and mother quarrel about her, and she did not understand why she had not been happier about her father's involvement. When she heard about incest and several of the other girls at the camp told her about sexual abuse by the father or step-father, it was as though something fell into place. It gave meaning to her experience that something was wrong, a feeling of guilt about not being good enough, that she did not feel grateful to her parents who had adopted her. At the institution, most people had believed her. But instead of feeling relief, she gradually began to feel uncomfortable. When talking with a psychologist, she began to have doubts. She remembered more good feelings for her father. But her relationship to her mother was more difficult. She was tormented by her bad conscience, started on drugs, and also made a few attempts to take her own life.

In the family therapy, the therapist emphasizes Ingun's attempt to create her own identity, to create meaning in her life. Her accusations of incest, her attempt at suicide, as well as her drug abuse are conceived of as a way of trying to discover who she is, or who she should be.

The father also says that Ingun has always behaved marginally—for instance, in her choice of friends and in relation to her own appearance.

### *A new narrative—*
### *new accusations or reality-based experiences*

The first couple of sessions were used to clarify the old lie and to understand how it could happen and what it had done to Ingun, to the parents, and to the whole family. Both parents were extremely relieved that their daughter had tried to make amends for the damage she had caused. She had also written to relatives and friends of the family apologizing for what had happened and explaining herself.

After the first feeling of relief about having explained herself and understood how it could happened, Ingun again becomes anxious. She is angry with her mother, who she feels is directing the family, keeping her siblings away from her, and must always be in control. She makes another suicide attempt and leaves a farewell letter to her parents in which she again apologizes but also writes that she feels she will never win the parents' trust and can therefore never present the real truth.

The parents become anxious and frightened. They want to do everything to avoid a repetition of something like this and are wondering what Ingun means by the real truth.

Ingun is angry with her mother. She feels that her mother is too inquisitive about her life, while she herself does not really feel that she knows her mother. She knows little about her and her relationship to her own mother.

Their (mother's and Ingun's) homework is to meet a few times. Ingun is to ask questions about what she is wondering about, and mother is to give answers to what she herself feels is reasonable for Ingun to know about.

In the next session, the mother says that she does not trust Ingun. She feels that whatever Ingun finds out, she will use against her. Ingun has also become even more angry with her mother and repeats this in several sessions and then discloses that her mother had beaten her as a child. The mother does not directly deny that she had beaten her, but she says that she was mostly alone with the children, was worn out, and that Ingun had been a child she did not understand. She would lose control and shake her. During the whole first year after she came to them, her mother experienced her as inconsolable: "She was crying and fretting all the time."

Ingun starts in individual therapy at this point, and the family therapist has heard from one of the milieu therapists at the institution where Ingun lives that Ingun has said that she has been exposed to child abuse, and that she considers reporting her mother. As the ties between Ingun and her family are still very fragile, the therapist is somewhat reticent about investigating what has actually happened. There is also some uncertainty as to whether this is a newly fabricated narrative in an attempt to create meaning in a difficult mother–daughter relationship. The topic is left alone. The parents break off the treatment after Ingun has accused her mother of having maltreated her as a child. And the family therapist is left sitting there, wondering what kind of experiences make it necessary for this young woman to tell such extreme stories.

## *The traces of experiences*

How do the various theories of narratives deal with the issue of truth and with real experiences in relation to told stories?

As an illustration of the difference between what Spence (1982) calls the narrative truth and the historical truth, he compares the French and the English titles of Marcel Proust's masterpiece. In the original French title, *A la recherche du temps perdu,* the emphasis is on the author's year-long quest to create a meaning for what occurred at that time. The same event can have different meanings depending on the conditions that are present at the time of remembering. Regaining the past is compared to recognizing a face; vague contours are filled out with special thoughts and feelings from the remembered moment. Spence uses the French title to exemplify what he calls the narrative truth: it is dependent on continuity and closure and on the composition of separate parts being given an aesthetical form. When constructed, narrative truth is as real as any other truth. One problem with this concept of truth is that it puts parentheses around what the narratives refer to.

The English title, *A Remembrance of Things Past,* pays special attention to the memory and to the historical truth. Concrete occurrences from an earlier point in time can be taken along into the present and the dust wiped off them, so to speak. This reflects a belief in reliable recollection that can furnish an accurate image of the past. The analyst as an archaeologist, unearthing layer after layer in the narrative, can serve as an image of therapy being a search for the real and true narrative.

Spence discusses the issue of whether one can differentiate between these two forms of truths. The narrative influence can cover deficiencies and incompleteness in the material and can prevent one from exploring further conditions for the emerging information. And yet Spence becomes vague in his understanding of historical and narrative truth. The validity of a narrative is dependent on whether it fits into the narrative of the patient's life in a way that gives insight and meaning. The incentive is to find a narrative home for incidents lacking a sense of belonging.

The Irish family therapist Jim Sheehan (1998), when applying the narrative metaphor, is interested in exploring the narrative's connection to lived experience, and in this exploration he makes use of Ricoeur's thinking. Ricoeur has said that the past always leave an imprint. For this reason, personal narratives are linked to a real past. When we construct a narrative, we also give life to others. This can constitute a hazard in an individual therapy unless the therapist is conscious of the ethical obligation and responsibility implied herein.

In his individual therapy, Karl told a narrative about an unhappy childhood and about parents who had not seen or understood him. This has made his suffering and his symptoms understandable, but it has not brought about sufficient change. But what are the traces in this narrative, what are the concrete experiences this narrative is based on? The parents cannot recognize it. It does not tally with their own experience, but they are willing to declare themselves guilty if it can help their son. But will this narrative about childhood and guilt be sufficient to create a change? Needless to say, experiences of childhood are felt and interpreted differently by the different persons involved. And children and parents have different perspectives and different premises for interpreting events. And yet it does make a difference if it is here that the pain is buried, or if there are other sources linked to lived experience that are more suited for creating change. Narratives are a way of presenting experience, but they are also a way of dissolving tension and dilemmas. A person telling a narrative does not only report one set of events; he/she also constructs a social identity. The narrative that is told also indicates something about the intention, the identity, and the feelings of the person telling it.

In chapter 4 we have posed the question of whether the fact that a narrative leads to change is conditional on an experience of emotional relatedness. As mentioned before, Stern introduces the concept of a key therapeutic metaphor about a narrative that is sufficiently potent to create understanding and meaning (Stern, 1985, p. 257). He has a narrative approach to therapy that is combined with the self domain that is activated and carries the affect. Feelings are crucial for the personal meaning of a narrative and for the place the narrative is given in the person's sense of self. Karl's time in America can serve as a key therapeutic metaphor. It is a narrative referring both to a self and a relational domain (core self—he became incapable of acting) and to an affect-laden experience. "I became absolutely terrified", he says. He also has strong feelings connected to his desire to revolt. Stern says that it is not necessary to revert to the problem's historical point of origin. The narrative point of origin must, however, according to Stern, find an echo (see chapter 6). Since Stern focuses on the subjective experience, it is somewhat unclear to me what are the criteria on which he bases his evaluation of the narrative's validity, apart from the demands made on the narrative form.

During Karl's stay in the United States, there were also some experiences that left noticeable traces. The parents can confirm these experiences. The ban on correspondence, telephone calls, and visits alerted them to the possibility that something might be wrong. In the family therapy, Karl furnishes concrete examples of these frightening experiences. However, this narrative has gone astray in pursuit of the difficult childhood, the root of all evil. In order to understand his own experiences in terms of the parents' experiences, it was also important for him to return to the parents' background and experiences and to realize how their experiences of anger and anxiety resembled, or differed from, Karl's own experiences. Ricoeur also speaks about the ethical relevance or commitment to recollection. Recollecting is a form of recognition or knowledge. It is a matter of challenging the truth and of distinguishing between real and unreal, true and untrue. Forgiveness and reconciliation presuppose recollection, not oblivion. If we do not remember, we are doomed to reiteration, to repetition.

Sheehan (1998) indicates that the narrative metaphor creates as many problems for the therapist as it creates possibilities. Inspired by Ricoeur, he cautions against the notion that one can be the author in one's own life, an expression used by both White and Epston (White & Epston, 1990). In literary narratives, one differentiates between being the author and being the narrator. The author has control over the characters in the narrative and their actions, and over the way in which their development and their relationships are portrayed by crises, and then finally he will present a conclusion. However, in life there is no such point of departure where one can be in control of persons and events as well as of one's own life and those of others. We also have an ethical responsibility towards the other actors in the narrative. We cannot treat them as we wish. We cannot create an unhappy childhood just like that, or parents who abuse us, without casting an eye at our own experiences. And, as a therapist, one has to be precisely in search of the traces left by these experiences.

A narrative of abuse can give meaning to particular experiences that one has previously not been able to explain—for example, a difficult relationship to mother or father. Yet the narrative does not necessarily have to be true or tally with the experience. When Ingun heard about the incest experiences of her peers, she got the idea that this had also happened to her. It gave meaning to her feeling of being different from her sisters, of lacking a sense of belonging to her family. The piece in the jigsaw puzzle which could give an answer to her question of who she was seemed to fall into place. But she soon began to realize that it was not right. The drug scene gave her a brief feeling of belonging, a kind of identity. Stories about maltreatment were also circulated there. We never found out whether this milieu or her own experiences had given rise to her idea of maltreatment on the part of her mother. Some may have thought, as did the parents, that her ideas about sexual or physical abuse had their roots in an obscure and unknown past prior to her adoption.

Stern discusses the current strong tendency to emphasize language in preference to action (Stern, 1995, p. 77). We find this tendency both in psychoanalysis and in today's family therapy. The language and the narrative decide the meaning we ascribe to our experiences. Stern warns that the interpretation and the narrative may create a psychic reality that is given priority over the action itself. The reconstructed experience will then—as it happened with Ingun—become the real event. She is certainly not the only one who is unable to distinguish between lived experience and a construction of these experiences.

Stern describes how a small child's experience of being together with a depressed mother is very different from the adult's reconstruction of such an experience (Stern, 1995, p. 99). The moral that can be derived from this is how important it is to revert to the traces of experiences and to pose concrete and detailed questions about actions as well as feelings.

Narratives about life cannot be finished products; they are processes undergoing development and change. As mentioned earlier, narratives have a form with a tendency towards closure and a structure that sets limits for alternative paths leading to a credible plot. This urge and tendency towards closure will also confront us in therapy. Spence (1982) describes how both the narrator (patient) and the listener (therapist) depend on the narrative structure to create meaning and cohesion in what is being narrated. This is even the case in the psychoanalytic situation, where the analysand is asked to associate freely and the analyst will listen with free-floating attention. This creates a certain determinism. One attributes to events that are being told a kind of necessity that is deduced from the meaning in the totality.

McLeod (1997) also suggests that the metaphor of therapy as authorship may conceal the unifying and creative nature of narratives, and, I wish to add, the ethical responsibility that lies both with the therapist and with the client. McLeod introduces the word "voice". Therapy means giving voice to experiences that have abated or have become silent in all the implicated parties.

When narratives are regarded more as a process than as a product, then several new possibilities will become available. We introduce here alternative ways of looking at time.

## *Narratives and the many faces of time*

One of the special features of narratives is their sequential character. Events and experiences are organized in terms of a past, a present, and a future. In *Time and Narrative,* Paul Ricoeur distinguishes between three forms of time: cosmological or objective time (calendar time), phenomenological or subjective time, and narrative time. Narrative time is a bridge, a poetic solution, between objective and subjective time. The experience of time is made human through narrative action (Ricoeur, in Sheehan, 1998). The difference between the map metaphor, as introduced by Bateson (1972b), and the narrative metaphor is precisely the fact that the latter includes the time dimension. The map metaphor is static and says nothing about development. The narrative metaphor, on the other hand, guarantees that human action takes place in time.

As a systemic family therapist, one wishes to introduce more possibilities, more options, and greater freedom. What are the limitations and possibilities implied in the sequential presentation of time that characterizes narratives?

Bruner (1986), in the chapter "Two Modes of Thought", discusses the relation between the understanding of causality in the paradigmatic (logical-scientific) mode of thought and the narrative mode of thought. The paradigmatic mode of thought concentrates on generating general causes, on creating fundamental hypotheses that are logical and can be checked against what can be observed. This does not necessarily exclude intuition but implies the ability to see possible formal connections even before one is able to prove this in more formal ways. It is based on abstractions and on the transcendence of the special. Meaning is linked to empirical or logical connections. Narrative thinking is constructed in consideration of human and not logical reasons. It has to confront both action—what Bruner calls the "landscape of action"—and consciousness, the thoughts and feelings of those who are involved in the action ("landscape of consciousness"). It is the interpretation of the events that creates meaning. One mode of thought cannot replace the other. Both are necessary, but each has its own domain; they convince one of different things. Arguments convince one of the truth, stories of their similarity to life. Narratives are about possibilities and not about certainty.

The sequential character of the narratives, the construction around past, present, and future, can easily invite a linear-causality explanation. The past explains the present which then predicts the future. The narrated events take place within an image of time that is dominated by a logic connecting actions and events throughout the entire time of the narrative. But is this conception of time too limited—are we becoming more deterministic in our exploration of stories than is actually necessary?

The narrative form, of course, does not rule out coincidences, options, or surprises, but these are subject to the demand for a comprehensible and meaningful course of events.

Sheehan (1998) raises the issue of how one can introduce more freedom and more options when confronted with these deterministic features in narratives.

*Time casts shadows*

Literary critics and literary theoreticians have also occupied themselves with this question, and Sheehan refers to one of these, Gary Saul Morson. For Morson, the issue about freedom is closely linked to how we think about narrative time. Most narratives leave little room for coincidences, which reduces the idea that every single moment in time calls for many possible options. The way we speak about time casts shadows over the events that are included in the narrative (Morson, 1994). These shadows can reduce or expand a feeling of possibilities that are linked to each narrated moment. This perspective is widened with three concepts:

1. "Foreshadowing", which reminds one of anticipation, which is a well-known narrative technique. An event is used to foretell the future, as a kind of "omen" or prophecy—the future is decreed by fate.
2. "Backshadowing" reminds one of retrospection. An event in the present is explained by way of an event one remembers from the past.

Both these concepts present an image of time moving in a linear, predictable way.

3. "Sideshadow" casts shadows from the side—that is to say, from other possibilities. It is a kind of antithesis to "foreshadow". Two different alternative presents—the real present and the possible present—are simultaneously made visible. Something else had once upon a time been possible, even though it was not actualized.

When, for example, Karl wonders why he did not protest that time in America, there is a possibility to explore other actions. What could have made him protest, report to those who were responsible for the stay, and notify his parents? Instead of looking for other options, he spent his time searching for events or explanations in the past that, so to speak, had predestined his actions that time in America and represented an excuse for not being able to act differently. The literary scholar Bremond is also interested in the fact that a situation can be open to a possibility and then close down on it (Bremond, in Engelstad, 1976). In therapy, one can open up for possibilities that had once been closed down on.

### *The reflexive and non-linear character of time*

Family therapists have also given a great deal of thought to the issue of our relation to time. At one time, the belief that the past influences the present led to a rejection of the importance of the past and to an emphasis on the present, as exemplified by the tradition of the Mental Research Institute (MRI). There are therapeutic schools today focusing especially on the future (de Shazer, 1988) and laying little emphasis on the past and the present.

Boscolo and others introduce time as a new perspective in systemic therapy, as a lens or glasses through which you can study therapy (Boscolo & Bertrando, 1993). Time as a variable in therapy has often been underestimated, especially in the interaction between past, present, and future: "The Reflexive Loop of Past, Present and Future in Systemic Therapy and Consultation", as Boscolo and Bertrando have called an article (Boscolo & Bertrando, 1992). These therapists have discovered an understanding of the reflexive character of time in St Augustine, among others. There are three forms of time, all of which have their point of departure in the present. The past does not exist for the individual as such; rather, it exists as the presence of things from the past, "the presence of past things"—this is the recollection. The present is direct perception, the presence of things here and now. The future is the expectation, a present that is about things in the future. The past exists by being constantly recreated in the present, which also implies that we do not have an absolute certainty about the past. This is why the issue of truth is so difficult. The past is not only recreated in the present, but it is also a collective creation, a social interaction where meaning is created. The past decides the meaning of present events, but the past is again defined through the present. The future also gathers its meaning from the past and the present. Past, present, and future are united by a reflexive loop in which one of them constantly gathers its meaning from the other two (Boscolo & Bertrando, 1992, p. 121). The same reflexive description of time is, moreover, described by T. S. Eliot in "Burnt Norton" (1963, p. 189), in which he says that time present and time past are perhaps present in time future, and future contained in the past, and that all possibilities point to one end: the present.

Systemic therapy is founded on an assumption that past and future can be brought into the present. There are no psychological problems that do not have a time dimension. Nor is there any form of psychotherapy that does not work in time and with time. Therapy consists of bringing problems and their possible solutions into the present. The present can change the past and create new alternative narratives that again will have significance for the future.

In Karl's narrative, we are first invited to a linear understanding of his anxiety. It is due to a difficult childhood. By introducing a new possibility—the narrative of a traumatic adolescence—more possibilities are opened up. The understanding of the anxiety is not locked up in a childhood that cannot be changed, but in a narrative of adolescence that one may dream of confronting. This does not mean that the narrative of a traumatic visit to the United States is replaced by the narrative of a traumatic childhood. The coinciding of the American experiences with the father's crisis—together with the childhood experiences—formed the plot that could give meaning to the anxiety. This opened up for another present and a possible future with possibilities for protest, action, and confrontation. This again gave an opening for seeing the past with different eyes, where the motive force was exploration and curiosity, and not guilt. Which experiences did the parents carry with them from their own childhood and adolescence to enable them to cope with anger and anxiety? What were the differences and what the similarities to Karl's experiences and reactions?

Karl's narrative also demonstrates how closely the experience of one's own identity is linked to one's own narrative. This also implies a conception of time.

Ingun's narrative makes the issue of truth more precarious and the ethical aspects more distinct. Ingun's desperate attempt to create narratives that will give meaning to her life also illustrates how self-narratives are closely connected to the experience of one's own identity. Identity is about being seen, both by oneself and by others. Language creates the ability, according to Stern, to narrate one's own life story, with all the implied potential for changing how one views oneself and how one has been viewed by others (Stern, 1995, p. 174). Stern goes so far as to maintain that "narrative-making" is a universal human phenomenon reflecting human consciousness. This is actually not so different from Bruner (1986), who also states that humans have an innate tendency to organize experiences in such a way that they create cohesion and meaning.

As regards Ingun, we can only speculate about the reasons that caused her to create for herself these marginal identities of an incest victim, a drug addict, and finally a maltreated child.

## *Conclusion*

Therapy can create new feasible explanations and—paraphrasing from Eliot's "Burnt Norton" again—can point to doors that were not opened and to roads that were not taken. Narrative therapy—whether within the psychoanalytic or the family therapeutic tradition—deals with topics connected to time, to experience, and also to identity. These topics raise more problems and possibilities than solutions and answers. What is our understanding of time? Is time a human construction or an objective feature of the external world? We humans move in time, but this time can be experienced, described, and understood in many different ways, as has also been demonstrated throughout the ages by philosophers, scientists, and poets. Our culture suggests an understanding of time as a linear causal event. Past, present, and future follow each other one by one, like a string of pearls. Time also leaves its mark through the events taking place, and the interpretation and meaning of these events is created or mutually created in a social interaction. The relation between time and experience is therefore not in the least uncomplicated. Should one emphasize the significance or belief in the individual's possibility to create a diversity of narratives, and believe that this multitude or multiverse is powerful enough to bring about liberation and change, as seemingly claimed by the social constructionists? The possibility of many alternative narratives seems to be more important to them than the extent to which these narratives are based on the experiences. Is this not rather relativistic? The discussion within psychoanalysis about the difference between construction and reconstruction, between narrative truth and historical truth, or the attempt to distinguish between a narrative and a historical point of origin for a problem, represents important and interesting challenges, but no clear solutions. Considering our current knowledge of memory and forgetfulness, the unreliable character of memory, and the different theories about how representations are formed, I still do not believe that there are clear and simple answers to these questions. The dilemmas and questions about the relation between experience and narration, about our views on time as linear and/or reflexive or circular, have consequences for our conception of our identity and contain a number of ethical dilemmas that must be kept open.

Even though this book argues in favour of the importance of psychological theory for family therapy, I would like to conclude this chapter by raising the issue of whether it is philosophy that can be of further help to us as regards our dilemmas. In the final chapter, the significance of ethics for therapy will be discussed, with a particular emphasis on the philosophical perspective.

CHAPTER SIX

# Self-experience, key metaphors, and family premises: the relation between common and individual stories

*Astri Johnsen*

Systemic family therapy is based on the assumption that the whole is more than the sum of its parts. Family therapists have been wondering what it is that characterizes this wholeness. Many different metaphors have been used to describe the common ideas, constructions, or representations that families have about themselves as families. Bateson (1972b) introduced the map metaphor that later became the point of departure in the Milan group's concept of family premises (Boscolo et al., 1987). The concept of family myth (Ferreira, 1963) was used to describe the set of conceptual beliefs the family has about itself. Family myths also give directions for actions, which are usually called family rules. Other concepts are family theme (Papp & Imber-Black, 1996) and family paradigm (Reiss, 1981), which refer to a central organization of shared expectations, experiences, and fantasies about the world.

Less direct attention has been paid to the individual's experience of this wholeness. However, family therapists have to deal with the wholeness as well as the parts—in other words, both with the family as a system and with each individual.

John Byng-Hall is a family therapist who has attempted to link the thinking on individual and family. He has studied the borderline between the intrapsychic, interactional, and intergenerational aspects in triads. As a family therapist, he makes use of script theory, but he is also interested in employing developmental theory, especially attachment theory (Byng-Hall, 1990, 1995b). Family script is defined as the family's shared expectations with regard to how the family roles are to be performed in different contexts. One differentiates between shared expectations and individual performance.

Like Byng-Hall, I have been greatly interested in connecting the thinking on individual and family, as is demonstrated in this book. In chapter 8, I refer to Judy Dunn's studies showing how siblings growing up in the same family are more different than one would expect. But do they grow up in the same family? We, as family therapists, constantly come across the fact that siblings experience their family very differently. In a discussion about autobiography and what characterizes the different concepts of self, Jerome Bruner takes his point of departure in interviews of members of the same family. After having collected their individual autobiographies, he invites them to a discussion where the topic is, "What it's like growing up as a Goodhertz" (Bruner, 1994, p. 123). Here he discusses how a shared premise about the significance of the distinction between private and public life leaves different traces in each individual. The family self, as Bruner calls it, is meted out over each individual; this viewpoint can remind one of Byng-Hall's use of the concept of family script.

Systemic family therapy as evolved by the Milan group also emphasizes the importance of differences. *Circular questioning* has been developed based on the idea that information is difference (Selvini-Palazzoli, Boscolo, Cecchin, & Prata, 1980). Without being explicitly formulated, this method of questioning serves precisely to elicit each individual's perspective and experience of the family and the relationships within the family. This method is thus suitable for promoting individuation, and it takes place in talks where the others are present.

The same reflections can be used with regard to the Milan group's concept of *neutrality* (Cecchin, 1987; Selvini-Palazzoli et al.,

1980). Respect for differences is central in the concept of neutrality and for the various versions of shared experiences. An individualization of the experiences is facilitated by an investigative attitude conveying respect for differences.

In this chapter, I take up some concepts in Daniel Stern's model and discuss their relevance to the issue of the relationship between the individual and the system, and between the individual and shared experiences and narratives. I shall do so by demonstrating how his theory has been an inspiration to me in my work with families, while at the same time being firmly rooted in systemic family therapy. I shall make special use of Stern's description of the five domains of the *senses of self* (see chapter 1) and his concept of *key therapeutic metaphor*, and I examine this in relation to the significance of the concept of *family premises* within systemic family therapy. The issue concerns both how an individual narrative can become a shared and common experience and how common experiences leave their traces in different ways in the individuals in a family. The two families I am discussing can shed light on these two different problems. In one family, one can see how a lonely and isolated narrative is given meaning when it is shared. The other family struggles with finding individual versions for a shared narrative. I shall begin by describing my conception of the concepts of *key therapeutic metaphor* and *family premises*.

## *The key therapeutic metaphor*

Daniel Stern has himself raised the question of how the developmental views he presents might affect clinical practice (Stern, 1985, p. 256). I would now like to bring up two aspects of Stern's theory that have clinical implications. Clinical topics such as dependency, autonomy, trust, and control do not originate in special developmental phases. They are not linked to sensitive periods and are therefore not the object of fixations. They are issues of life that are continuously dramatized across the whole range of modes of relating to others. The experience of being alone, for example, depends on which domain of the sense of self this experience belongs to. If it is connected to the domain of the sense of a core self, the pain of the experience can be soothed by being held or touched. If the experience of being alone is linked to the domain of the sense of a subjective self, then an empathic emotional response will be of help. As an example, Stern mentions how problems of control and autonomy have different significance, depending on which domain of the sense of self or of relatedness these problems are connected to. Are they connected to a relational experience where the control of physical acts has been most important? Or is the experience of being controlled linked to the type of feelings that can be expressed? Or is what is being said censured and controlled?

Another point in Stern's theory which has clinical consequences is the fact that the domains of the sense of self replace the traditional clinical developmental topics as points of departure for sensitive periods, but they are less vulnerable to irreversible early impressions. The domains of the sense of self are active and in progress throughout life. They are not relics of the past, nor are they terminated developmental phases.

These features in Stern's theory give the therapist greater freedom to listen to the patient's story and to reconstruct a narrative that can give meaning to the problems or to the symptoms. Stern's point of departure for therapy is a *narrative* approach (Stern, 1985, pp. 256–263; 1995, p. 37). In his understanding of symptoms or problems, Stern distinguishes between what he calls an assumed actual point of origin ("the historical point of origin") and the narrative that is told about the origin of the problem ("historical narrated point of origin"), or the narrative point of origin. This distinction is inspired by Donald Spence (1982) and his discussion about the relation between historical and narrative truth. According to Stern, the domains of the self are active and in progress throughout life and are therefore also vulnerable in times of crisis. Clinical topics such as autonomy, dependence, control, and trust are topics for life; they are not connected to specific phases but are vulnerable at any point in time throughout life (see chapter 1).

The clinical task is to find the narrative point of origin for a problem.

Stern emphasizes the importance of finding a *key therapeutic metaphor* containing a narrative that is sufficiently powerful to promote understanding and change. A key therapeutic metaphor is, according to Stern, a description using historical fragments as a representation (or metaphor) for experiences. The therapeutic effect of a key metaphor (or key narrative) lies in the *emotional* recognition that it really was like this, that this is correct.

In the search for a key metaphor, the therapist uses her/his clinical discernment. The therapist uses discernment to feel her/his way to the domain of the sense of self or the domain of relatedness that is most active or most noticeable. A clue to this, Stern says, may be the person's present life and transference reactions. In a family therapeutic context, I would search for clues first and foremost in the family members' relationship to each other (but also in the therapeutic relationship). The therapist looks for the affect-laden experience, which—when discovered—can function as a narrative point of origin. The *affective component* of the key experience usually takes place chiefly in one domain of relatedness (or in one sense of self) and often in one of its features.

The clinical question will be: which sense of self carries the affect? All the domains of the self will be active in relation to the symptom, but only one is usually experienced as the most painful one at a given moment.

The interesting part of Stern's model is that he coordinates a narrative approach to therapy with a study of which domain of the sense of self is active and is the carrier of the affect. The example later in this chapter of "The girl with the dog" shows how a story in the girl's development could serve as a key therapeutic metaphor. In the other example, "The price of loyalty", the key narratives are not rendered as a clearly delimited narrative but are central experiences, linked to a sense of self. The two stories thus illustrate two important aspects in Stern's use of the key therapeutic metaphor: reconstructing a narrative that is powerful enough to create understanding and meaning, an identification of the domains of senses of self that are activated, and the significance of the affective element.

Since an understanding of family premises is also a central issue in systemic family therapy, I shall comment briefly on this concept (see chapter 9; see also Johnsen, 1995).

## *What is meant by family premise?*

By *family premise*, we mean deeply ingrained or fundamental ideas that a family has about itself and the opinions they have of each other. These ideas (which others have termed "ideas themes" or "belief systems"), in turn, structure the interaction between the members of the family. The ideas decide the way in which a person or a family conceives, interprets, or reacts to decisive life experiences. Other terms are family ideology, family myths, or family motif. Family premises regulate the internal process in the family, decide on its traditions, rules, and values, and establish the quality of the interpersonal relationships. My use of the concept of family premise includes both *family myths* and *family rules* (Johnsen, 1995). The myths refer to a conceptual universe and to the implicit or underlying ideas influencing the conception of reality. They supply guidelines for action. These guidelines are also called family rules. As mentioned earlier, the concept of family script is also being used for describing these rules or guidelines (Byng-Hall, 1995b).

On the basis of an understanding of family premises, the symptom is not regarded as the result of a deficiency or error in the structure or organization of the family, nor is it regarded as serving a function in the family. Symptoms are looked upon as manifestations of a predominant theme, a message that the old ideas or premises are no longer useful in terms of a future development. The symptom can be a signal that the family's fundamental premises are in crisis and need to be re-evaluated. By understanding symptoms in relation to a central premise or predominant theme, the family is given an opportunity of broadening its conception of the symptom. Attachment and separation, autonomy and control, or the importance of gender can exemplify these predominant themes or premises.

## *Therapeutic consequences—two clinical stories*

### *The girl and the dog: a story about loneliness*

The father comes asking for help for his daughter Caroline. She is 17 years old. The parents are worried about her drug abuse, her money spending, and her truancy. It is also a problem that she herself does not feel that she needs help, and the father is uncertain about whether she will come to therapy. Which she does not, and it is the parents who come to the first therapy session.

They start off with a complaint and an accusation against their daughter, with whom they have lost all contact. Based on my first impression of the parents—who feel that, with a mean and impossible child, they have failed as parents—with the help of *circular questioning* I start exploring their experience of themselves as parents and their experience of their daughter. The first narrative they tell of her conveys the picture of a young girl who, since the age of 12 years, has withdrawn into herself, rejected her parents, and stopped taking part in the activities they approved of, such as athletics. She plays truant and frequents the drug scene. She is often stoned when she comes home. Their conclusion is that they do not understand her and consider her inconsiderate—rather wicked, actually.

When I ask the parents what kind of picture they think Caroline has of them, they become thoughtful, as they also do when asked how they think Caroline experiences them as parents. They themselves believe that they have no influence and therefore are of no importance to her as parents. When asked whether they think that Caroline experiences them like that, they become uncertain.

The question of how they believe Caroline looks upon herself also makes them wonder.

In the course of a number of circular questions, they begin to tell a slightly different story about Caroline, a story about a girl in search of herself. It happens, for example, that she asks her father what she was like as a child, she looks through the photo album, and she has a picture of herself and a dog on her wall, a picture that stands out from all the pop posters there. It turns out that this picture contains a story that took place when Caroline was exactly 12 years old. She loved the neighbour's dog, which she took care of and walked every day. She was given responsibility for the dog because everybody else was afraid of it. One day, when she came to take care of it, the dog had been put to sleep—without her being notified beforehand. She experienced this as a terrible *betrayal,* in addition to the *grief* she felt over her loss.

The parents begin to wonder in this session whether they may have underestimated this story.

The therapist concludes the session also wondering whether they may have underestimated their own importance as parents, and that possibly Caroline on her part may have underestimated the importance she has (had) for them.

Caroline comes alone to the next session, a sad girl with a tough façade. In this session, too, the therapist focuses on the experience of oneself in relation to others. How does Caroline think her parents regard her, and how does she think her parents believe she regards them as parents? These circular questions make her rather thoughtful, as they did her parents. She believes that her parents look upon her as bad and egoistical. She herself loves her parents, but she cannot imagine that they love her. She is curious about what they have said about her, thinks that they have only said negative things, and is positively surprised about their story about the dog. She confirms the experience of betrayal as described by her parents, and the grief she felt. The story had made her feel that she was of no importance in this world. She had no idea that her feeling and experience of worthlessness was something that could be shared. As Caroline tells the story of the dog, she becomes involved, her face comes to life, and she has tears in her eyes.

The therapist's intervention corresponded to the intervention given to the parents: a girl who underestimated her importance as a daughter, and parents who underestimated their value as parents—so they had something in common. The therapist also emphasizes the fact that they all attached special importance to the story about the dog.

All three come to the third session. Caroline still feels that therapy is not a good idea. The parents are still worried, but there have been some positive changes. Caroline has been at home more. They have talked more to each other, as well as about Caroline's childhood. Mother and Caroline have been to town together. Mother has experienced Caroline's asking for money for clothes not merely as an exploitation, as she had previously, but also as expressing that Caroline needs them as parents. The parents are still uncertain whether Caroline uses drugs. They have looked together at photos of Caroline and the dog and have thought and talked a lot about the story with the dog. They have also talked about what the therapist said to them: that they all underestimate how important they are to each other. We agreed that the parents would phone if they continued worrying.

This brief case history sheds light on how Caroline's narrative about herself, and the parents' narrative about her, did not contain her experience of loneliness, worthlessness, of one who loved her parents but was not worth their love—just as the parents' experience of themselves as unsuccessful parents did not contain the experience of the love and concern they felt for their daughter.

We may wonder whether in this family there was a premise about the relationship between parents and children that ruled out the possibility of sharing experiences of betrayal, grief, and uncertainty.

This case history can also illustrate Stern's recommendation to find a key therapeutic metaphor. As mentioned before, a key therapeutic metaphor contains a story that is sufficiently potent to create understanding and change. The story about Caroline and the dog served as such a narrative. It gave the parents a different experience and understanding of Caroline, and, above all, it gave Caroline an experience that they had nevertheless seen and understood her. This does not necessarily mean that this narrative was the only point of departure or the original one for Caroline's problems. But it served as an image—we can call it a metaphor—for the experience of betrayal and grief and of how important it is that these experiences are seen and understood.

### *The price of loyalty: a story about togetherness and separation*

The father in the family—we can call him Knut—makes inquiries about family therapy. The whole family has found it difficult to adjust after the death of the mother three years ago. Knut is worried about them all, but perhaps most about the youngest daughter, Ragnhild, who is 14 years old. She has not shown any emotional reaction after the death of her mother, although she had been very attached to her. The son Tom, who is 19 years old, is quiet and uncommunicative, sad, rather depressed. The daughter Else, who is 23, suffers from emotional instability, and Knut is worried that she may be too strongly attached to him. He himself has been depressed, has found it difficult to concentrate at work, and has felt apathetic and listless.

They all want family therapy because they are unable to talk properly to each other about what has happened. They believe that this is also why other things are not functioning.

At the first meeting, the family present a common problem, a common narrative, which is about the mother's death three years ago—a loss they all feel keenly, though in different ways: too much emotion, lack of emotion, sadness, incapacity to act.

Stern, as well as family therapists such as White and Epston (1990), are of the opinion that symptoms arise when the narrated reality does not tally with the experienced reality. Does that mean that the family's narrative, the approved version, does not tally with the experiences of each individual? Perhaps it is not a question of a common problem linked to the mother's death, but of four totally different experiences of this situation.

How are we, as family therapists, to understand the separate experience and development of each of these individuals and, at the same time, understand this in the light of the family system? Can Stern's theory help us to become aware of the unique stories?

In my talks with the family, I therefore wanted to be receptive for both the individual and the possibly common versions of their narrative. The Milan group's recommendation for *neutrality* can be useful here. A neutral attitude showing respect and interest for differences can, as mentioned earlier, be used to make room for the various versions of a common narrative or experience.

As a systemic family therapist, I also want to utilize circular questioning in order to grasp the relational interaction—the way in which the different persons and relationships are viewed by the others and, again, how each can contribute to supplying information about the others and about the relationship between them. Based on the information obtained by these methods, I shall draw attention to what may be the family's central or predominant *premise*. This can perhaps help us to understand why they still cannot talk to each other about the importance of the mother's death.

In the light of the referral and the opening line "We are quite unable to talk to each other about Mummy", we might perhaps be tempted to draw the (premature) conclusion that this is a family in which the domain of the self and the relational domain—termed the verbal self by Stern—is activated in everyone. They are unable to link meaning and coherence to what has happened: the loss of the mother. Ragnhild says: "It's as though she weren't dead, she's only still in hospital." They have not tidied up after her, her clothes are still hanging in the cupboard, the desk is still covered with all her papers.

When working to reconstruct a key therapeutic metaphor, Stern encourages us to look for the *affect-laden experience.* The affective component will take place first and foremost in one domain of relatedness—that is to say, in one of the domains of the sense of self.

So let us not jump to superficial conclusions but give ourselves time to get to know the family's narrative and each member's experience of himself/herself and the others.

We need to understand the ideas and the underlying rules that made it impossible for them to talk to each other about this central topic that concerns them all.

### *The family's premise*

They all agree that they are unable to speak to each other and share their experiences in connection with the mother's illness and death. The consequences this may have for the development of each of them may still vary.

We know from our own lives, as well as from clinical experience and studies, that siblings are different (see chapter 8). Family members have different conceptions about the relationships within a family. Each person has a unique position within the family system, and siblings will be aware of similarities as well as of differences in their relationship to their parents.

This is a family who feel that they are closely tied to each other. The siblings, for instance, say that they feel closer to each other than most other siblings.

The mother—we shall call her Inger—is described as the family's pivotal figure. Tom was the one closest to her. She was given a cancer diagnosis five years before her death. What was most painful, says the father, was that she would not talk about it. She did not want to show any weakness—she wanted always to be strong. But therefore Knut did not have an opportunity to talk about the illness, neither to her, nor to their friends, nor to the children. She wanted to spare the children, especially the two youngest ones.

There were five years full of crises, sudden hospitalizations, operations, and intravenous treatments. Else was let into the secret but was forbidden to say anything to the others. Knut himself thought that the children should be informed about the gravity of their mother's illness. He strongly disagreed with his wife. Also, Else disagreed with the imposed silence but remained loyal to her mother, except during the last months of her life.

Knut felt that he had to be loyal. He thought that he had no right to go against her will, that he had to respect her wish. It was her illness and her death.

When the mother became dependent on intravenous treatment, they decided to nurse her at home. Knut and Tom looked after her and learnt to give injections. A boy of 15 sacrifices his youth out of a sense of love and loyalty by nursing his mother. He can no longer ask friends to his house; he becomes friendless. No one must know how sick she is. "I felt that I was not alive", he says.

Else is given the task by her mother to see to it that the family sticks together—even death shall not part them. In fact, even after her death, the mother continues to be the family's central figure.

To speak about conflicts may cause division. Death is dangerous and does not exist in the world of language. It should not be talked about. Knut says that Inger would not accept that she would die, would not recognize it, would not talk about it. It was her way of keeping death at arm's length, literally speaking.

When Knut is asked what the most difficult thing for him to speak about is, he says that it is the feelings that are aroused. The most difficult part about talking is the fear that Inger will be blamed, that they will say nasty things about her.

So far I have made use of my general knowledge and experience as a family therapist. By listening to the words they use and to the family's narrative, I have outlined a family premise that is about loyalty and solidarity. This premise structures their conception of reality and who they are as a family, and it also controls the interaction between them.

In a crisis, when there is serious illness and death in a family, this premise is stretched to the very limit. Loyalty must be preserved at all costs. Disagreement, conflicts, and one's own needs can cause discord and must therefore go underground, be suppressed. We hear a narrative in which the premise of loyalty and solidarity has paradoxically turned into a scourge, leading to splitting, alliances, and secrets.

By challenging their premise with *hypothetical questions*, they gradually become able to talk to each other, including about their anger and disappointment and about their sadness at having been excluded from the secret or, conversely, at having to bear the burden of being let into it.

### *Key therapeutic metaphors*

I have raised the issue of whether psychological developmental theory can contribute to an understanding of the individual which can be useful in a family context.

Let us return to the problems of the different individuals we heard of at the beginning, and see if Stern's theory can shed new light on the understanding and treatment of these.

1. *Ragnhild and the key metaphor.* As we have heard, it is Knut who has been most worried about Ragnhild. She has not shown any emotional reactions and has not cried. What alarmed him most was to hear Ragnhild say on a certain occasion that she cannot remember anything about her childhood. Ragnhild's lack of emotional reaction is also totally incomprehensible to the other two siblings. In the sessions, Ragnhild gradually begins to formulate her problem clearly. What troubles her most is that she does not remember anything. "I don't remember the main features in my life. ... I remember nothing from my childhood. ... I clearly remember everything after Mummy's death, but not before it. One doesn't remember so much from the time before starting school, *but what I should have remembered, I don't remember.*" What she mostly wants from family therapy is "help to a bit of mapping out". When the family's homework is to reconstruct the course of events, the development of the illness, who remembers what, who got to know what, other events, good and painful memories, she becomes very eager and is the one who has the strongest wish to reconstruct the narrative. "Now I'm beginning to remember memories and

things like that. . . . What the others don't understand, is that one can't feel anything when one doesn't have the words—that's what the others don't understand."

Seen against the background of Ragnhild's lack of recollection—her lack of words and memories that could help her to have a narrative about herself—and her eagerness and involvement in the reconstruction of the past, I would presume that the domain of the sense of self most activated is *the sense of a narrative self,* and not the sense of a verbal self, as was indicated at first. She almost cries out for a narrative with a past, a present, and a future that can give her a clearer experience of herself and her relationship to the others, and also of the others' understanding of her. She would, for example, have wanted her mother to talk to her about what kind of a future she would have, what kind of advice she would have given her about school, and so forth.

We can say that the premise of loyalty has excluded topics that might threaten the premise. Death has been such a topic in this family.

The commencement of a reconstruction of the narrative has a special effect on Ragnhild. She begins to have a language and a narrative and, thus, also a possibility to feel.

In Ragnhild's developmental history, as told by her, her childhood is a blank, like a black hole. The narrative about an empty childhood serves as a key narrative—it is here that the affect lies.

2. *Tom and the key metaphor.* For Tom it is different. He is five years older than Ragnhild, and he painfully remembers the course of his mother's illness, the change in her, being isolated from his friends, and his loneliness.

How are we to understand his depression? Has it something to do with our assumption at the beginning about the sense of a verbal self—that he suffers because they are not able to talk to each other? He states this clearly, but is it here we find the strongest expression of the affect?

Tom is a quiet, thoughtful boy but is infinitely sad about having lost his mother, to whom he was strongly attached and whom he nursed faithfully at the end. He feels guilt because he was relieved when she died. Towards the end, he had also withdrawn emotionally from her. "I felt that I wasn't alive, I had to get out."

Tom reacts with deep despair as the course of the illness is gradually reconstructed and memories come forth. He feels guilty about having withdrawn, and he is jealous of his siblings, who had a closer relationship to their mother than he did during the last weeks. He is disappointed and in despair, yes, even uncomprehending that his mother, to whom he was so close, could not share her fear of dying with him. "That she was alone with her fear of dying was the worst part, and that she didn't want to share it," he says, crying.

On the basis of Tom's disconsolate reaction to being excluded, I would assume that it is primarily the relational domain connected to *the sense of a subjective self* which is impacted. He expresses grief and unhappiness because he and his mother were unable to share an internal emotional world. He would so much have liked to share her fear and certainly also share with her his own grief and anxiety about losing her. And he blames himself for not taking the initiative. Again we see here how the family premise about loyalty has ruled out the possibility of sharing some very important feelings.

It was a painful experience for Tom to express his despair and his realization of having been let down. But it made him feel freer to admit his right to take care of himself. The others in the family were relieved to see this kind and sad brother gradually becoming able to give such strong expression to his feelings of grief, longing, and growing anger.

When Tom tells his story, it is the situation with his mother, and his experience of loneliness and of not being able to share each other's sorrow, that becomes the central key narrative.

3. *Else and the key metaphor.* I have been more uncertain about which of the five domains of relatedness or domains of the sense of self it is that Else grapples with most. On the one hand, she is the one who most emphatically expresses her need to talk, to share meaning and coherence through language. At home, it is also mostly she who has taken the initiative to start talks. On the other hand, she is the one who is emotionally most unstable and least able to verbalize her feelings.

Can this possibly confirm our initial hypothesis about the sense of a verbal self? It is precisely the splitting that occurs through language that is described by Stern. But again—is it here that we find the strongest affect? When constructing a key metaphor, Stern urges us to look for clues in the person's life or in the transference relationship. We should also be able to find a basis for the affective experiences in the relationships to each other within the family.

In the sessions, Else's ability or lack of ability to control her feelings gradually becomes a challenge. She is overwhelmed by emotion. She is the one who is most verbal and yet also most emotional. I am beginning to wonder if her special position in the family as the chosen and trusted one has been a strain on her. An adolescent is drawn up to the level of adults. It overwhelms her, perhaps overstimulates her. She fights with her mother for her right to tell the truth to her siblings. She gives desperate expression to her sense of being overburdened, of not having established boundaries around her. "I am so insecure, there was no one who took care of me."

As mentioned before, this has made me wonder whether this young girl was actually overstimulated by this so strongly affect-laden information and not protected by it. This may have had consequences for her ability for affect regulation, which is a focal point in the domain of the self that Stern calls *the emergent self.*

It is a therapeutic challenge for me to find out how her outburst of feeling can be regulated. In her accusations of not having been taken care of, I can hear a plea to be taken care of, to be protected, and to get help to regulate herself. Or does she express a longing for a self-regulating other who is central for the regulation of feelings in Stern's description of *the sense of a core self*?

Else's narrative is about insufficient help to regulate feelings.

4. *Knut and the key metaphor*. Where Knut is concerned, it is easy for me to choose which one of the domains of the sense of self or the domains of relatedness is the most central one. He says that he is totally paralyzed. He desperately wants to be able to create a future for himself. He has a feeling not only of having been muzzled, but of having been tied up hand and foot. Inger forbade him to speak. He respected this wish out of loyalty and in spite of his own strong disagreement. Nor did she want to speak to him about their relationship, what it meant that she was ill and about to die. She was

unable to cope with the thought that he would have a future in which she was not included—that was too painful. She wanted to be the one who informed and was in control—"she begrudged me a future which she could not share with me", he says and cries. Again we see how a family premise excludes certain topics and thereby a possibility of common experiences, of sharing, of having an influence over one's own life, and oneself having an influence over one's own actions.

For me it is evident that this man is restricted in his possibilities to be the agent in his own life, which is so important in the development of the *core self*.

* * *

Based on Stern's theory, we have constructed four key metaphors:

- For Ragnhild, the key metaphor is a matter of being a person without a narrative and thus without an identity and ability to remember and to feel.
- For Tom, the key metaphor is linked to the painful experience of being excluded, of not being part of the mother's internal world and thus without a possibility of sharing some crucial feelings dealing with loneliness, grief, and anxiety.
- In the case of Else, we have been uncertain whether the key metaphor is about secrets, alliances, and an adult's role that has overstimulated her and destroyed her possibility of regulating her feelings. It is about needing help to regulate feelings.
- For Knut, the ability to be the agent in his own life stands at the centre—his experience of being a man equipped with both a muzzle, handcuffs, and ankle irons.

Common to these key narratives is a premise of solidarity and loyalty, which has excluded some central themes dealing with death (Ragnhild), anxiety and loneliness (Tom), insecurity (Else), and disagreement (Knut).

We can perhaps formulate like this: on the family level, the key metaphor concerns premises of loyalty and solidarity; on the individual level, the key metaphor has, for each family member, been given a special individual formulation and narrative.

## *Concluding remarks*

The topic in this chapter has been the relation between the individual and the system, between individual narratives and shared narratives. It has been a question of the type of concepts and methods that can be useful to family therapists for understanding the individual's experience in the family, while at the same time not losing sight of the system within which this individual happens to be. The concept of family premise indicates the shared ideas constructing the framework and supplying the rules for shared formulations. We can say that family premises function as filters both for the experiences that can be accepted and shared and for those that have to be suppressed and put away.

The topic about individual and shared narratives also invites questions and reflections about what it is that characterizes narratives, and what it is that causes the construction of certain narratives to lead to change and not others. We have discussed this issue in greater detail in chapter 4, where we have especially stressed the importance of emotional relatedness for giving meaning to a narrative.

Narratives are a matter not only of form, but also of content. The social constructionists, such as Kenneth Gergen, have emphasized that there is a diversity of narratives about reality and that no narrative has priority (Gergen, 1994). The discussion about narrative truth and historical truth, and about the criteria that can make one narrative more valid than the other, is the main theme in chapter 5.

Stern's theory has given me ideas for some topics (content) in the sessions with the two families I have described in this chapter. In my opinion, these topics focused very much on identity—who I am in relation to myself and in relation to the others. As we have already heard, this topic was formulated in different ways for each individual.

One of the stories ("The girl and the dog") was about sharing individual and lonely experiences. The other story ("The price of loyalty") was about how a shared narrative is given individual formulations and significances.

Stern's self-developmental model describes how the child creates meaning in its experiences and how the narrative one fashions about oneself is evolved in intimate interaction with other close partners. Stern shows how the narratives—the stories people make up about their lives—are intimately tied to the experience one has of oneself, of one's own affect state, one's ability to be an acting self, to share inner experiences and feelings with others, to be understood, but also to have the ability to understand others and to express oneself through language. This link between narratives and the sense of self can, in my opinion, represent a crucial contribution to family therapy and can give direction to some central topics during the sessions. This means that it is not just any narrative that gives meaning, as Gergen asserts, but only the narrative that is linked to a personal identity or sense of self, and in which it is the affectively laden experience that will hint at what is important in the narrative.

Systemic family therapy is well suited to enable one to grasp the predominant rules or notions controlling the interaction within a family. In its attitude to the individual, this method is, however, not as bad as it is made out to be. The circular method of questioning and the neutral attitude are useful methods for promoting the individuals' perspectives within a system.

CHAPTER SEVEN

# Senses of self and interplay as a metaphor for therapy with adolescents

*Rolf Sundet*

Working as a therapist means being regularly confronted with a wish that reality would follow the book a little more closely. Whether I work with drug problems, adult psychiatry, or child and adolescent psychiatry, there are always clients or patients turning up who are tangential in relation to what I have been trained to deal with. The common feature in these experiences is that the methods, approaches, or ways of understanding we are trained in do not seem to offer adequate help to the persons who have been referred to us or who have come to see us.

Kvale (1994) points to a state of tension between therapeutic practice and research on therapy. He compares it to being between Scylla and Charybdis: on the one hand, captured by exciting case histories "with the therapist in the role of the hero" (p. 31); on the other, being caught in a positivistic straightjacket "where the experience of personal interaction in the therapy situation vanishes into statistical significances ... rarely produces suitable knowledge about the inter-human situation in the therapy" (p. 32). In my daily clinical practice I am only too familiar with these dilemmas. Not letting oneself become aware of them is more a question of pushing them aside or repressing them in order to be left in peace than of the clinical situation itself letting one have peace. Yet the return of the repressed (Wilden, 1977) seems unavoidable. Clinical anecdotes about successful practice often stand out like lighthouses constantly tempting us to believe that all is well (Dawes, 1994), whereas the sphere of practice hurls in experiences that force us to recognize that getting an approximate outline of the factors producing change depends on more than merely clinical experience and well-told stories. As an example, I can mention a story about a successful treatment based on cognitive techniques where, during the evaluation phase, I was informed that the observed change coincided exactly with when Prozac could be assumed to have started having an effect—I had no idea that the general practitioner had prescribed it. What was it that had an effect: my treatment or the chemicals? Research seems to suggest that it is the interplay between them both that is important (Dawes, 1994). What will be important for me is that I depend on traditional research, but at the same time I am aware of the fact that, in my clinical everyday life, it is unrealistic to believe that I will succeed in taking a strictly scientific approach to acquiring knowledge. I depend on anecdotes and good clinical stories as a basis for clinical reflection and as a starting point for submitting problems for further discussion in traditional research.

Spence (1987) gives a description of the basic metaphors in psychoanalysis and argues that it is important not to forget that the forms of understanding suggested by psychoanalysis are actually metaphors. In Norway, Kirkebøen (1993) has drawn a parallel in relation to the field of family therapy. He argues that one should discover sources of metaphors other than those traditionally linked to family therapy—that is to say, systems theory, cybernetics, and so forth.

## *Some typical problems when working with adolescents*

The project for this chapter can be described as follows: based on clinical anecdotes about encounters with a therapeutically marginal group, I would like to suggest some metaphors for the therapeutic work with this group. Since they are clinical anecdotes, it is important to be aware of the implications. This is not a description of therapeutic practice based on a consensus between (non-participating) observers. It is more a matter of therapist-fiction created by the participating therapist. Moreover, it was recorded after the fact (Geertz, 1995). Finally, it must be added that this is an example of an attempt at a local form of understanding (Chaiklin, 1992; Kvale, 1992; Reichelt, 1995). It is connected to a group of adolescents in a special context.[1] It is not meant as an alternative to, or to be in competition with, other forms of understanding of this group or therapy in general.

The patient group I am presenting here is a group of adolescents who are often regarded, or presented, as "unmotivated" and "inaccessible" to therapeutic dialogue. The majority are boys, but there are also some girls. This group made me realize that my methods and my ways of presenting therapeutic work were most severely being put to the test. I found very little help in most of the therapy literature I have studied in recent years, within both psychodynamic thinking and a family therapy orientation.[2] This group can be described by the following clinical anecdotes:

> There was the boy who had been referred because he beat his mother. His smile was friendly, he was polite, and he voiced the famous words "I don't know" when asked about his problem and what he thought about having been referred to the outpatient clinic and to me.
>
> There was the girl who arrived dressed all in black, including black mirror-reflex glasses, and who with an "impudent look" asked me what the hell I wanted from her. She was about to be thrown out of her foster home on account of drugs and so-called manipulation.
>
> There was the boy whom I met together with a colleague at a school. He had thrown a teacher to the ground, threatening to cut him up with a knife. After a while he quietened down and came with me for a walk. I asked if he would be prepared to have some sessions with me. He said the typical words: "It's all the same to me." I said: "Let's do it then."
>
> There was the boy who was referred because he had knocked down a pal. He agreed to sessions. In the following session he

said that he had a pal who needed a psychologist just as much or even more than he did, and could he take him along. I said yes.

It is typical for this group that they do show up. They do not actually reject the offer, but they are passive or apparently uncomprehending about what they are supposed to do here with me. This was what the adolescents offered me as a starting point for going ahead with psychotherapy. The challenge was both obvious and frightening.

I felt certain that it was possible to work with these adolescents, but I had problems imagining what this work would consist of. It did not resemble what I was accustomed to think of as psychotherapy. In addition, I saw that these adolescents changed, but it was difficult to give a good description of what the changes consisted in and why they came about. This involved a need for models or metaphors that might help me to understand what was going on with these adolescents and might perhaps give me some clues for further work with them. Furthermore, one might possibly be helped by alternative formulations to discover unseen or unregistered aspects in a different theory.

In this chapter, I use parts of Daniel Stern's (1985, 1990) developmental theory as metaphors for therapy, as discussed in chapter 1. It is the five senses of the self and the relational forms attached to them that I wish to use as a metaphor for being together therapeutically and for dialogues with adolescents. I am searching for a figurative expression of being-together. This means that I accept his description without problematizing it as developmental theory. Developmental psychology, which can be seen as naturally including Stern, is undoubtedly not unproblematic (Burman, 1994; Cushman, 1991). Chapter 1 gives a brief summary of some of this criticism.

## *The emergent self as a metaphor for work with adolescents*

Stern emphasizes that the experience connected to the emergent self bears a certain resemblance to a *déjà-vu* experience, or an experience of correspondence or familiarity. Adolescence is often described as a period of reorganization (Wrangsjø, 1993). This implies a period marked by changes as regards physiology, biology, and psychological and social circumstances. Adolescence can therefore be looked upon as a period in life mainly characterized by the emergence of something new. Themes and dilemmas that are connected to the known and to the unknown, the old and the new, can therefore be regarded as crucial issues during this period. Stern states that the experience of the emergent self is also created through amodal perception and vitality affects. According to him, this implies experiences that are more comprehensive than those expressed through the verbal and narrative self. Since this period involves a reorganization, one has to expect that it is the experience of something new emerging that is more total than what is verbalized. A feeling of unease is characteristic of this period. As in the infant, affective activation needs to be regulated. If the level of uneasiness becomes too high, one may feel "driven" to do something. It can be experienced as something negative rather than a positive restlessness. In infancy, the responsibility for regulation rests with the carepersons. A change in adolescence means that the responsibility for one's own life becomes clear and that the environment expects one to cope with the regulation of one's own affective states. One can no longer expect others to take care of the regulation. Moreover, helping to regulate one's affective states during this period is often mistaken for interference with adolescent autonomy. "You must do this and that" is readily conceived as taking control, interfering, and impeding autonomy. The task of the parents in this period is therefore to find out how to help adolescents to be able to regulate their own affective states without interfering with their autonomy.

In child therapies, after a certain age one can simply say that symbolic play is the chief material given to therapists to work with. Dialogue is the medium in adult therapy. The time of adolescence is a "halfway-between" period. What kind of material do we actually get from adolescents? Taking the experience of the emergent self as a starting point, one may hypothesize about the following part-characterization of the adolescent material for therapy: experiences filled with uneasiness, connected to an area of tension regarding the known and the unknown, the old and the new. This has to do with topics such as autonomy, dependence, closeness, distance, revolt, and adaptation. Taking the emergent self as an image, these topics will unfold and present themselves nonverbally. The physically awkward, anxious, restless, and verbally "contact-weak" signifies that it is an adolescent who has entered the office and not a specific pathological formulation.

What are the implications for therapeutic work (together) with adolescents? Characteristic for this group is that they are "unmotivated" and not very "accessible". Based on my therapeutic experiences with this group, I would here like to hypothesize that concepts such as "unmotivated" and "inaccessible" reflect therapeutic practice and thinking about therapy rather than qualities in these adolescents. Therapeutic practice must, of course, be adapted to the person one works with. If the sensing of an emergent self implies an experience of wholeness and affective experience, then this must be the starting point for the therapist's experience of both the adolescent and his or her own self. The therapist must focus on becoming aware of and keeping an eye on the affective content perceived in the other and in his/herself and on the affective climate that becomes characteristic of the relationship. This will be made clearer when we examine the subjective self and the concept of affect attunement. It is a matter of relying on the affective content and becoming familiar with it. The relational theme is *regulation*. It becomes important to regulate the affective state of the client, of the therapist, and of the relationship. What we see in the interplay between the infant and its careperson is a regulation that aims at keeping the affective content at an optimal level. Needless to say, it is not optimal to stimulate the child to play and be active when it is supposed to go to sleep.

What would the optimal affective state be for an initial meeting with "unmotivated" adolescents? Their state must be presumed to involve feelings of rejection, anxiety, humiliation, and so on. If it is to be at all possible to establish an interaction and a being-together, one will have to try as a therapist to facilitate the emergence of other affects and experiences. Time and time again I have experienced that talking about problems makes adolescents feel uncomfortable. The natural thing would then be to take this feeling seriously and not talk about problems. I call this being *sensitively insensitive*. Most of the adolescents I have worked with showed signs of discomfort, shyness, and withdrawal when asked about their problems, their families, and what they were feeling. My reaction was then to look away and to speak of something else. I encouraged problem-free topics that were of interest to them, such as what they were doing and so forth. This sensitive insensitivity had a regulating effect. They became more relaxed and more focused on interests. At first there would be a lot of talk about motorbikes, rock 'n' roll, the opposite sex, teasing, "so what were you doing yesterday", film and video, and other small talk. This was especially the case with the boys. The girls were more accessible to problem-talk, but here it was also important to try to regulate the intensity of feelings that became too troublesome, be it fear, shyness, or other feelings. One way of doing this was that I "talked my head off", another was that I let silence and tranquillity prevail. Whatever has a regulating effect is relative.

Generally I can say that I am willing to do all I can within ethically justifiable limits to attain regulation—that is to say, that the adolescents show signs of relaxing and not feeling pressured, anxious, challenged, or having other experiences of a negative nature. Without regulation being shown, attained, and experienced in the session, one gets nowhere, with the result that the adolescents do not return. It is by permitting and experiencing regulation of inner states that these adolescents can begin to "become themselves in the session", whatever that may mean for each one of them. Of course, I know that there is a great deal I could ask and explore, but I also know that doing it would heighten their level of anxiety and discomfort. It is necessary to contribute to a regulation of the affective state when dealing with adolescents, even if it may seem to lead one far away from one's ideas about therapeutic dialogues. If I get the feeling that talking about mother and father will lead to a body posture in the adolescent expressing "I don't want to talk about it", well, then I don't talk about it. But if the word motorbike makes a face light up, then the topic for the session is clear. However, if it is uncomfortable for me to talk about a topic because I have a problem with it myself, well, then I must be permitted to avoid it, even if the adolescents want to talk about it. Regulation in the relationship as a mutual phenomenon causes me to let myself be regulated too. By being considerate of myself and letting the adolescents be considerate of me, I help the adolescents to become considerate of themselves. I shall return to this later.

Metaphorically speaking, the key concern in the therapeutic relationship is the regulation towards an optimal state of being-together and having a dialogue. In the therapy literature, this has been expressed in terms of concepts such as security and respect (Hougaard, 1995). Another formulation is to speak of something that is not too different (Andersen, 1987b). Let us now pass on to the experience of a core self and what type of metaphor can be generated about the therapeutic process.

## *The core self as a metaphor for therapeutic work with adolescents*

In the following, I use two main components in Stern's description as metaphors for therapeutic work: the four self-invariants and their establishment through the theme-with-variations format and the setting up of an evoked companion. By carrying out a number of everyday routines in the sessions, one can create a repetition and a variation of the type of theme-with-variation that can be experienced as though self-invariants are emphasized, developed, or created in the direct contact.

Stern states that *self-agency* contains two elements: *volition* and *mastery*. We are all familiar with the rows about what adolescents want and do not want, at what time they must be back, housework, school, and so on. Mastery shows itself in all types of activities: sport, skateboarding, dance, parties, school, work, and social situations generally. In the therapeutic work, this is expressed by giving them permission to want, letting them decide as far as possible if they want a session, when they want the session, what they should talk about, and what we shall use the session for. I would like to emphasize the aspect of determination by referring to two rules. First, I only talk to people who want to talk to me. Second, I want people to phone me if they cannot show up at the session, or if they wish to drop me. My experience tells me clearly that if adolescents are permitted to want, then they want—including therapy. This does not only apply at the start of the relationship. Wanting becomes a central factor in everything during the sessions.

Stern underlines the fact that mastery implies an experience of proprioceptive feedback and predictability. For me, this necessitates the use of one or other form of activity in the sessions. One may say that adolescents are midway between play and reflection. This midway point can be created through action or activities that suit the adolescents. By carrying out activities, they can experience concrete mastery, they can be aware of the feedback from their bodies, and they can have an experience of being able to predict the action and the result. This implies having one or several activities that can be repeated time and time again. The type of activities I have used are throwing darts, building with bricks, chairs, tables, and the like, targeting the dustbin, making paper aeroplanes, demonstrating martial arts, drawing, games, walkie-talkie, playing music, and listening to music. In the course of these activities, I had a clear feeling that what we did was functioning "therapeutically". The adolescents became involved, and they displayed themselves actively, affectively, and verbally in regard to what we were doing. This was particularly reflected in their sense of humour. The same happened to me because they permitted me to be this type of therapist. My sense of mastery rose. The most exciting thing was that I felt the participation of both parties to be the most important part—far more than our tendencies to reflect.

*Self-coherence* deals with the experience of being physically coherent and experiencing coherence in form and intensity. An example of this are three boys who formed part of a therapeutic group. All three of them tried to enter my office simultaneously, with great physical intensity, and then they seated themselves in a physically clumsy way while their fingers and hands wandered restlessly about and seemed in many ways to live their own lives. This was again connected to activity and action. Another example is a boy who was referred for aggressive behaviour. For a long period, we used the session for having contests in throwing darts. He was physically clumsy and had difficulties concentrating. On account of this, he often missed the bull's eye, thus losing the contest. This often annoyed him. We changed the situation from being a contest to being a training situation, where one aspect was to begin by standing close to the board and then increasing the distance. Now he managed to hit the bull's eye more often. He became less irritated and more involved and concentrated more when taking aim. After a while we were again able to have contests, and gradually he became able to win and to lose. Of course, there are several aspects to this anecdote. But what I would like to emphasize here is that a necessary aspect for progressing was a training situation that heightened the experience of body control. Training to improve a coordinated movement—aiming, changing the position of the body in order to have better control, then throwing and seeing the result—can be looked upon as heightening the feeling of being physically coherent.

The focal point of *self-affectivity* is to let the adolescents express their affects in their own way, whether it be through activity or verbalization. The crucial point is not the content, but expressing oneself or showing affects. This may, of course, be done in many ways, from cursing and swearing when the dart gets stuck in the wall over and over again instead of in the bull's eye, to physically accompanying wild school stories with "arms and legs", with shrieks from cracked voices, laughter, and so on, to positive teasing of me—"Has your car broken down again now?"—to use of dialogue about video and film—"What do you think of the *Evil Dead*?" By letting affect become visible in the mode of adolescents, it also becomes possible to express negative affect: "Damn it, I'm fed up with school!" At times even I could come out with some of my negative affects, with my more or less wild everyday stories: "There was this idiot today whose car nearly crashed into mine." What is important with these verbal stories is not their content, but the affect they express.

The experience of continuity in time is the key point in *self-history*. During the course of a series of sessions, a joint interactional history is established. One can think back and remember happenings and see how one reacts differently to them now. One can experience oneself as similar and different and also experience the therapist as similar and different. Suddenly, the therapist speaks in a different way than he/she has done before. Something has happened. Perhaps he/she has learned something new, has had new thoughts, or been inspired by an everyday occurrence. Adolescents take note of this and make comments. The self and the other become clear through the variation of being similar and different over time. "Earlier I was angry, unhappy, but now I am feeling a bit ok." There were many times when I experienced that the adolescents got involved in my stories, that they returned to them over and over again, and I had to report my changes and experiences to them. As I have mentioned, I talked with a group of boys. At that particular time I had bought myself an electrical guitar as a belated realization of my boyhood dream. The boys became intensely interested and wanted to be told again and again how this had come about, what had made me want to buy one, and so forth. I also experienced that being allowed to ask again and again created a continuity, not only in our relationship: it also legitimized them as something continuous. There was one boy in this group who returned again and again to his relationship to a teacher in primary school who had pointed him out as being stupid. This memory became his opening for looking at himself as one who had a previous history, as one who existed over time, who took with him things from his previous history, and who perhaps could now create for himself a new and different history.

This type of activity can be described as fortifying and developing self-invariants. This is a sense of self, expressed as being able to want and to master, to cohere as a physical unit with the ability to feel, and existing over time. It is through a variation of the theme that it is strengthened and developed. The three boys who continued to enter my office simultaneously were expressing mastery, volition, and that they were physical units. They also expressed an intense affectivity through these actions and their expressions, and they established time as a dimension by repeating their actions, almost like a ritual that says: "Here we are again, and we are."

If we make use of Stern's description of the core self as a metaphor for therapeutic work, we get an image of concretely being-together as a place where self-invariants can be permitted to show themselves through variation in the activity and through expression of feeling and forms of being-together over time. The exciting aspect here is that it can be used to demonstrate aspects of therapy other than the ones that are verbal and insight-oriented or reflection-oriented. To the extent that one uses words of praise as a support and confirmation to demonstrate a "good" therapeutic relationship, this can be visualized by concrete forms of being-together.

According to Stern (1985), the experiences of interplay with another person can be internalized as an *evoked companion*. Examples of states that are often intense and, via regulation by the other, create an experience of being-together are affectivity, security, attachment, attention, curiosity, and cognitive involvement. This means that creating evoked companions is an important aspect in the therapeutic work with this group—that is to say, positive episodes of interplay that can be evoked if one aspect of the episode is present. Furthermore, it implies that repair work or some kind of solution, marked by security, is connected to interplay episodes that are difficult for adolescents. Let us look at some examples.

A boy was referred to me who had knocked down a pal. This type of episode contains a number of possibilities for getting attention, for affect and reactions. It was quite obvious that to talk to the boy about hurting someone would have created an affective intensity that would have overwhelmed or frightened him. It was all right to talk to him at first about what the other one had done to provoke this action. After that, it became possible to approach violence as an expression of affect. This exemplifies the point about dealing with negative feelings and experiences in such a way that it creates an episode that is marked by security.

According to Stern, an evoked companion implies a subjective experience of being-together with a historical self-regulating other. In other words, the regulation that has taken place in the session can be evoked in another situation. If one has spoken about "the forbidden" while anxiety has been regulated to a bearable level, then Stern's account suggests that the client will be better able to face "the forbidden" outside the session. In my experience, a great deal of the therapeutic effect when working with adolescents has to do with establishing the interplay between client and therapist as an evoked companion. This is dependent on a concrete history of interactions where the therapist has functioned as a self-regulating other.

The examples mentioned here were connected to verbal topics. I would like to mention an example where action is also in focus. It is about a boy who had great difficulties verbalizing. He had reported an assault and was terrified that the assailant would come and punish him for talking about it. He was anxious and watchful and did not quite know what he wanted, but he was fascinated by the large building cubes. He had turned 14 and was embarrassed about wanting to play "children's games". The compromise was to build towers. We decided to build a tower right up to the ceiling and fasten it there. He struggled hard but did not manage it properly. I spoke about stress and about trembling hands and also about the good effects of breathing slowly down into the abdomen. I breathed, and he breathed, shoulders down, steady now, "we are building"—and of course he managed in the end. He had a great ability to cope when he was relieved from his anxiety.

Once more, I like to imagine that the metaphor of an evoked companion can be used to describe this type of episode. Gradually he began to appear more secure during the sessions, and he reported that he felt more secure in his school situation. The odd thing is that since then, a number of the clients I used to work with have contacted me about further sessions. When returning to me now, they are more direct about their wishes, and they verbalize far more than before. This is probably due to their having greatly matured, but I like to think that the reason for contacting me was that we had interactional episodes functioning as evoked companions. When a new problem arises or they are in difficulties, then the therapist is partly present in these episodes, and they phone me. The key issue is participation in concrete action episodes. The work of experiencing a core self and of being related to others in the sense of having experiences that form an evoked companion is connected to being directly together in an actual relationship.

## *The significance of the subjective self-domain in the work with adolescents*

In infancy, the focus is on sharing attention, sharing intentions, and sharing affective states. In connection with the latter, I would like to deal with affect attunement more specifically as a metaphor for processes in the therapeutic work.

One element in the *sharing of attention* is, for example, to follow hand movements but also glances in order to see or experience what the other sees or experiences. The infant also checks via glances for confirmation that the common focus has been attained. The encounter with adolescents in the sessions is often chaotic, unstructured, or hampered by scant "material". It is possible to come into contact with something or other that will catch the interest of the adolescents by observing what they fix their eyes on, what their hands are doing, and which words they are using. If an adolescent looks at the picture of John Cleese hanging on the wall of the office, well, then the topic can be *Monty Python* or *Fawlty Towers*. One can focus on experiences related to these TV shows. If the adolescent plays with his pencil, Lego cubes, or his cigarette lighter, then this can become a starting point for sharing experiences. A 17-year-old boy I talked to was interested in Zippo lighters. I had been given one for Christmas. He borrowed it to light his cigarette and continued fingering it. It turned out that he knew a number of tricks inspired by having seen the film about the rock 'n' roll detective Ford Fairlane and his tricks with a Zippo lighter. Again, this resulted in a number of experiences we were able to share, both verbally and nonverbally.

The *sharing of intentions* can be exemplified by an anecdote about the 14-year-old mentioned earlier and his work with the cubes. He drew my attention over and over again to the box with big wooden cubes, but at first I did not attach much importance to this. He continued coming back to these cubes. He put them on top of each other and asked me what they could be used for. The sessions with him had been rather sad for me; he was halfway between childhood and adolescence, and I was wondering how to make our encounter meaningful. At one point, I did then give him an answer about his strong interest in the cubes. His questions about the cubes had not only been prompted by curiosity, but were also an invitation for me to share his interest in the cubes. I realized that his intention was that we should do something together, and so we started on our tower-building project.

Stern (1985) refers to an experiment with the "visual cliff". Here, the infant's "investigation" of the affective state in the care person seems to me to be a good metaphor for what happens when adolescents attempt to find topics for dialogue or activities during the session. The topic is the *sharing of affect*. They look at me and check my reactions. There was a couch in my office, and a 15-year-old boy with an extremely tough background had a tendency to lie down sideways on the couch when he began to calm down. I noticed his glance and understood that he was checking if that was all right, and so I asked him if he wanted to lie down. He then lay down, stretching himself and smiling: "Well-being feels good." Other examples of this kind of "checking behaviour" are connected to putting feet on the table, smoking, "dirty talk", and so forth. Stern calls attention to the implicit message here: it is my inner state that is checked, my attitude and feelings connected to the other's behaviour. The adolescents thus use my expressions in a purely bodily and behavioural sense to check how I feel about what is going on, exactly as I am doing. This inter-affectivity, as Stern calls it, also permeates the entire session. This kind of nonverbal communication seems to clarify a great deal of what one can permit oneself to do or not to do in the sessions. I have also experienced that adolescents have been so chaotic and anxious that they are unable to check me out. I have to do something to help them check me out. This implies affect regulation. Moreover, it is not only a matter of affect regulation, but also to feel that one's inner state becomes known to the other, that it can be shared, and that one can receive feedback on whether it is all right or not.

*Affect attunement* can be used in the session to help one establish the existence of a subjective inner experience and that it can be shared nonverbally. What types of actions and processes signal to others that one feels something similar to what they are feeling? How can one "get inside" other people's subjective experience and then let them know that one has arrived there without using words? Three processes must be present to facilitate an intersubjective exchange of affect between client and therapist: (1) The therapist must be able to read the client's affective state by his/her visible behaviour. (2) The therapist must behave in a way that is not strictly imitative and yet corresponds in one way or another to the client's visible behaviour. (3) The client must be able to read this corresponding behaviour by the therapist as being connected to the client's own original emotional experience, and not as a mere imitation. What does this imply?

When I was on emergency duty, a teacher brought in a pupil, a boy of 16. He was totally disintegrated and, at the same time, angry about having been taken to the clinic by the teacher. The teacher had informed us by telephone that the boy had broken down in class. Sobbing loudly, the boy had told him that he had been summoned to the local psychiatric hospital, where one of his close relatives had been admitted. He had been asked a number of incomprehensible questions about this family member, formulated in words he did not understand. Expressions like "psychotic" had been used that he did not understand the meaning of. Being questioned like that made him somehow feel that he was to blame for this person's illness. In the session, he retreated to a corner and sat hugging himself, sniffling and crying and being angry with me, with the teacher, and with the psychiatrist, one after the other. One could single out several emotional states here, but the one I felt important in this situation was that he felt humiliated and wished me or himself to be gone. My response was to withdraw to my chair and to make a movement with my hand which cursorily imitated being grabbed by the throat, conveying to him that when people are taken and humiliated like he was, I have to avoid doing the same, and that is why I wondered if he wanted to leave. There are several elements here, both verbal and nonverbal ones. In my opinion, it was important to indicate my understanding or to share his feeling of wanting to withdraw by withdrawing myself a little. And it was important, furthermore, to symbolize his humiliation by my hand movement signifying "to be grabbed"—because I felt that he had been psychically "grabbed" in his encounter with adult psychiatry. Even though words intensify the meaning, I experience time and time again that it is the body language that conveys the affect, perhaps because body is affect. If we consider this in regard to Stern's criteria on affect attunement, the following can be stated:

1. The acts I carry out (withdrawing physically and the "grabbing" hand movement) are a kind of imitation of his emotional expression. This emotional expression—his sensitiveness and distancing himself through aggressivity—emerges most explicitly in his tone of voice or his way of vocalizing, while at the same time it is also conveyed physically by hugging himself, a sign of both withdrawal and protection.
2. My manner of expressing myself nonverbally can be seen as a cross-modality to his vocalization.

3. Matching our behaviours is not the point here, but, rather, my way of expressing withdrawal and humiliation. It is not his behaviour that inspires or controls my own choice of behaviour; it is his affective state that I take in and wish to express in my way. One might say that this was my way of symbolizing his state.

Needless to say, this description is only a very small part of what actually happens during a session, and—as we shall see from the next sense of self, the verbal self—nonverbality is not the only factor in an encounter like this one. The point here is to give a description of the nonverbal aspects in the session and to emphasize them as a crucial part of what happens in a therapy and, as we have seen here, when being in contact with individuals in crisis. The end of the matter was that we agreed not to meet again. He conveyed very strongly that having to talk to a new person would mean another humiliation for him. He said that he had people who were better to talk to. I felt deeply in my "soul" that this was right for him, and I tried to convey this to him as well as I could, both verbally and nonverbally. His response—which I took to be a confirmation that he realized my genuine sincerity—was a smile and a thank you when he was leaving. I never saw him again and do not know what became of him.

The above was written after the fact (Geertz, 1995), and therefore it contains clear elements of reflection and thinking. In the actual episode, however, there were no such clear elements of reflection—there was only interaction. In video recordings of current therapy sequences, one might be able to point out a number of these interactions that resemble affect attunement, and one would expect that these were non-conscious or unreflected at the moment of interaction for both the client and the therapist. In places where one sees that being-together develops into a meaningful and sound form of being-together, one may assume that this is in part due to affective interaction.

The concepts used for these interactions in the clinical literature are acknowledgement, recognition, support, gratification, and so forth. All these concepts have, in my mind, a tendency to point to a reflected form of being-together on the part of the therapist. This does happen, of course, but my point is that something far more than that happens, perhaps something even more fundamental—that is to say, an actual affective being-together that does not need to be called anything but, precisely, an affective being-together. That would be sufficient. This affective being-together implies a shared experience of what exists and, thus, an affective reality. We can therefore speak of a shared reality, and, regarded as such, the affective being-together deals with something as fundamental as sharing a reality and experiencing it as real. The alternative would be an experience of unreality, of being psychotic, and finally of being negated as a person. I once worked at a psychiatric hospital in England, and I met there a young man who said: "I am not." When I pointed out to him that I could see him, he laughed and said that I had a big problem. Since then I have been striving to understand how he could experience that he did not exist—especially because, if he was right, then I really did have a problem.

### *The possibilities and limitations of language when working with adolescents—putting into words*

One of the reasons why I was fascinated by the thought of using Stern's theory about the senses of self as a metaphor for therapeutic work is his distinction between senses of self linked to the nonverbal as direct and immediate experiences and those linked to the verbal as versions and representations of, among other things, these immediate experiences. Stern's descriptions of the preverbal self-domains offer material and a basis for formulating therapy as an immediate being-together. This is what in the clinical literature is often termed the establishing of a working alliance, or relational work. In my account, I have attached importance to the immediate, perhaps unconscious or in any case nonreflective, form of being-together, as a special and independent therapeutic aspect. If I am to comment on therapeutic work based on the experience of a verbal self, my point of departure will be that one must make use of *negotiations about meaning and the importance of words*. Descriptions of adolescents as being "little motivated" and perhaps "unsuited" for psychotherapy may signify that this type of negotiating work has not been carried out, or that it has been conducted in an inadequate manner. I have often, while doing therapy with adolescents, had the feeling that this negotiating work about meaning has been continuously in progress, so that in many ways the issue of suitability for therapy becomes meaningless. Stern views language as a new form of relatedness. If we use this as a metaphor for what goes on in the therapeutic work, this will greatly resemble what has been called support. When we have established that we will talk to each other or be together once a week, and we have begun our being-together in the way I have described, then the word will become both a comment on what is happening and a mode of expressing topics of special interest to adolescents. This becomes "support" because it is mostly about being there where the young ones are. We talk, for example, about "Satanism" while the adolescent is drawing the symbols that he dreams will be seen on the cover of his first CD. I can talk about my scepticism about the satanic scene and, at the same time, take part in his interest in the uncanny. He lets me share some of his interests, and I can share my experiences with him. It is particularly important that I share mine, not as something normative, right, and correct, but as my true experience. I am actually frightened when people write about sacrificing other people, but at the same time these verbal accounts in magazines and so on give rise to experiences that are important to the person I am talking with. The first step is to put a name on the experience, so that it can be shared. Turning words like anxiety, worry, anger, irritation, humiliation, honour, pride, jealousy, and so forth into words that indicate experience is necessary for seeing connections between experiences, actions, and events in the outside world. These concepts must become meaningful both to the adolescent and to me.

A girl I spoke with complained that she had difficulties breathing. Her throat tightened, and her heart began to pound. She was afraid that something was wrong somatically. She had seen a doctor several times, but he did not find anything. I said that I was not a doctor, so that if she felt like it, we would have to check with the doctor whether there was anything physically wrong with her. I asked her at the same time how she felt when she had these attacks. Well, she was scared. I asked her what it felt like in her body when she was scared. Well, she had shivers and shudderings in her stomach. I asked her if she had ever felt greater fear. Yes, she remembered once when the car she was in nearly crashed—she had stopped breathing then, and her heart had pounded like a drum machine. I asked her if it resembled a bit what she was feeling when she had difficulties breathing. Yes, a little, but not quite. I said that sometimes one can have difficulties breathing and palpitations without knowing the reason for it, and that some people call it anxiety. It is anxiety precisely because one does not know the reason for it. Had one known it, one might perhaps have called it worry or fear. She said that this distinction was relevant to her. With this, we had succeeded in negotiating that something could be called anxiety. I did not know whether it was anxiety she had, but if it was, then it was important to look at what happened before the fit, what happened afterwards, and what she was thinking and feeling before, during, and after the fit. The crux of the matter here is that I do not know, and it is she who has to find out. But through her descriptions I can share with her what I have experienced in myself and others, and there may perhaps be something common to us here. This can be a further basis for dialogue that is best described under *the narrative self* (see further on). Her experiences can be shared through words, and we can create reciprocal meaning. This dialogue can also become a topic. How does it feel to talk about it? Can it be of any help? If it can, then we are about to create a being-together or a reality where we can create, for example, possibilities of change. She can be created as a person who starts coping with her own life. By using and exploring words, a being-together or a type of reality is generated or created. What we are doing in this type of sequence is, of course, producing a linguistic version of the immediate experience. We are grappling with the existential paradox in which she and I are living. Language can distance us from what is experienced. On the one hand, we try with words to bind together this split. On the other hand, we attempt—in line with the subjective self—to attune ourselves to each other's experience.

Since Stern indicates that language is generative, it also becomes an immediate activity. Language is not only reflection and creating versions of experiences. It is also actions that we carry out in relation to each other. For example, in my work with suicidal young people I use direct questions in order to find out if there is a danger of suicide. If I have a feeling that there is a danger, even though the youth denies it, then I have to make a choice. Should I hospitalize the youth or not? I have said many times: "If you behave like this, well, then I shall have to hospitalize you." In this way I insinuate a world—a world of force—for the youth. The same applies to getting stoned. "I shall call the Child Welfare" implies a special future for the youth—a world in which one no longer has one's parents as daily care persons. This may make the youth furious and sad, but he may also feel relieved. All this is often expressed in words. These words have an effect on my life. The fury of youths about being coerced naturally makes my life different from how it would have been if they had felt relief. Even though these words express the experience of youth, they also have a "rhetorical" or pragmatic effect on my life as a therapist and on our relationship.

Two processes in the therapeutic work have so far been focused on. The first one concerns the immediate being-together between the adolescents and the therapist. The second deals with the ability to find words, to make it possible to share one's own world through words, and to create a common meaning in our being-together. These two processes are intertwined, and over time they constitute our common interactional history. Elements in it can be named by the youths and the therapist, and one can begin to create a narrative about our being-together. A part of this narrative can deal with the youth's and sometimes the therapist's own life history outside and before our being-together was established. With this, we have reached Stern's last self-domain: the experience of the narrative self.

## *The possibilities and limitations of language—telling one's history*

At the start of the chapter, I mentioned a boy who hit his mother. He had great problems with aggression, and he found it very difficult to talk about this aggression. Mother was stupid—this was the nearest he came to an explanation. His father had died when he was a year old. Since then he and his mother had been living with his maternal grandparents. The area where I found that it was possible to contribute to a regulation of what he felt was when we talked about and did things with vehicles of all kinds, though which he could express his volition and carry on with coping and also through which we could share experiences. Keeping to the topic—by studying brochures, drawing bicycles, motorbikes, and cars, describing how to drive them—increased his feeling of security, his focusing, and his vitality.

Gradually a story developed about the "stubborn mountain-bike". Bit by bit his activity with this bicycle began to take a special course. He is busy with it. Something is broken or does not function, so he tries to fix it, his attempts are unsuccessful, and he becomes angry; he kicks and hits the bicycle, which results in even more damage to it. There are two actors in this story: he and the bicycle. His motive or aim in the story is to "get a good relationship to the bicycle" or to "get a good bicycle". The bicycle becomes the stubborn one. Its "motive" is "not to want to" or "to be stubborn".

The context in which this is happening is always his home. This directs my attention to the fact that the story takes place in the most central sphere of his life. This underlines the importance of the story and opens it up for dialogue about it and similar episodes with, for example, the mother or the grandparents. The dramatic line or the story's climax is at the point where he attacks the bicycle. This story is used by the people around him to indicate the boy's problem. The story is interpreted by Child Welfare and his family as an example that the boy is in a bad way. In the session, it leads to talking about experiencing problems, trying to solve problems but not succeeding, and about aggression as an expression of helplessness. "I can't manage to cope with the stubborn bicycle." The part of the lived story that this boy cannot tell is that he is helpless and that this is terrible. The told story concerns itself with the boy's pathology, his aggression, and the despair felt by the people around him. This means that the boy becomes part of a "misery-story".

The therapeutic work here was at first to clarify the story. Moreover, it implied starting the construction of a new story. This had to be something other than a misery-story. The story that was created was about coping—his ability to cope with the bicycle and to cope with his own aggression. Both the bicycle and his stubbornness should be transformed. In session after session, we went on talking about what could be wrong with the bicycle, and we talked about what he himself could do instead of hitting and kicking. He became a person who was about to cope. In this story, he became a hero—a hero because he tried, did not manage, became upset. Instead of becoming angry, he began to talk about being upset. The other topic was control of aggression. What could he do instead of getting even with the bicycle—for example, kick the wall? It could tolerate more than the bicycle. He could swear. We talked about swearing. I told him about my father and his rich vocabulary and so on, and so on. The amusing part was that the bicycle always got the problems. I have been periodically in contact with him for the last five years. He has a car, and the last time I spoke with him the car was stubborn, but he was coping in the sense that he did something other than smash it. The last aspect here was that after a period with the story about the bicycle, one could begin to approach the story about him and his family—the stubborn and defining others who made him powerless, just as the bicycle did, and his own reactions, which created problems for him. Again, the focus was on coping and thus on the development of a story of a hero.

This boy, and several others of those I have mentioned here in anecdotal form, I have met again after I stopped working at the outpatient clinic. These meetings are brought about by phone calls from them saying: "I have a problem now", or "there is something I am wondering about", or "can I speak to you about something, Rolf?" They get a session, and their point of departure is something we did or talked about in our previous meetings, which they connect to their problem and ask if we can talk about it. Previous interactional episodes and stories can be viewed as calling up an "evoked companion" for adolescents. The being-together we have shared facilitates an approach to our own present situation because we share a story that can be verbalized. There was the boy who knocked down a pal—he phoned one day saying that it is starting to happen again. I said: "What is?" "Well, what made me come to you, the fact that I was angry." This boy had a long story of coping within an institutional framework. By talking about this story, about what he had done, and what he had succeeded with, we were able to approach the present situation.

The above are examples of how one can spend time creating narratives. This can be explained and formulated from many different viewpoints (e.g. Freeman, 1993; Schafer, 1992; White, 1993). My own point is that this type of verbalization and narrative writing is facilitated by having an affective, direct, and real relationship to each other—that is to say, sharing an interactional narrative that can be verbalized and can form the basis for creating and viewing narratives that reach beyond the therapy-room. So "adolescents have at last become accessible to therapy". In many ways, the important job has already been carried out through a real and affective relationship implying a direct change-promoting being-together.

## *Concluding remarks*

The intention in this chapter has been to provide some metaphors for therapeutic work with a treatment-marginal group of adolescents. The material has been Daniel Stern's presentation of the five senses of self and the relational forms that are connected to these. I have attempted to make this abstraction easily accessible by way of clinical anecdotes. The material is not presented in competition with other presentations, but as a supplement. At the same time, it also has its roots in some of the issues connected to modern presentations of therapy, especially those with a family-therapeutic orientation (e.g. Friedman, 1993; Gergen, 1992; Gilligan & Price, 1993; McNamee & Gergen, 1992). These issues are linked to a biased linguistic focus. Here one of the cues is narrative. Creating new, rewritten narratives characterized by solutions, exceptions, and unique results (de Shazer, 1994; White, 1993) is the dominant factor on the scene presented to therapy. All is language, and only what is depicted in language is or exists. Language becomes like a black hole devouring everything. Since we cannot evade the issue of linguistic presentation and communication, all that is presented as non-linguistic will become language-determined, because it cannot be presented without language. As far as verbal language is concerned, it results in a word- or verbal-centrism that can prevent us from exploring other modes of understanding and experiencing. Every form of centrism or privileged standpoint creates marginal positions. Therapy formulated within a philosophical tradition that focuses on (verbal) dialogue will create its marginal groups. I have here given prominence to one special group. It is a group of adolescents who do not seem to have verbal language as their strong point. They are more action-oriented and more oriented towards a being-together where language primarily generates experience, and where there is little orientation towards reflection or insight. It is a group that is quickly labelled as "unmotivated" and is little accessible to therapy. This chapter has attempted to indicate metaphors that are not based mainly on language, even though language obviously is a part of the interaction.

## NOTES

1. This article is chiefly based on work at the Child and Adolescent Psychiatric Outpatient Clinic in Drammen and on the work of the Psychiatric Adolescent Team in Drammen.

2. Family-therapeutic orientation here stands not only for work with families and family therapy, but for the entire tradition of thought and understanding associated with modern (system-oriented) family therapy.

CHAPTER EIGHT

# Differences and similarities: the relationship between siblings

*Astri Johnsen*

As one of seven siblings and as a twin, a mother of one child, a psychologist, and a family therapist, I could not help being particularly intrigued by an article I read in *Family Process* about siblings and sibling differences (Dunn & Plomin, 1991). And when one of the authors—Judy Dunn, mother of three children, two of them twins—also presented herself as a developmental psychologist who combines the knowledge gained from reading fiction with scientific studies, my interest was truly aroused and I eagerly delved into her work.

The article—"Why Are Siblings so Different?"—was published in 1991, at a time when the issue of the relationship between the individual and the system had begun to appear on the agenda, while family therapists were still pursuing their theoretical interests in cybernetics, linguistics, and philosophy rather than in psychology. Like Daniel Stern (see chapter 1), Dunn poses questions that are phenomenon-related and recognizable and are immediately experienced as meaningful. How do small children develop their social understanding of others and their surroundings (Dunn, 1988, 1993)? What is the significance of sibling relationships for the social understanding of children? What can studies of siblings teach us about what it is like to grow up as an only child? Why are some sibling relationships characterized by love and harmony, whereas others are characterized by conflict and hate (Dunn, 1988; Dunn & Plomin, 1990)? These are issues that have relevance to scholars, therapists, and parents. I myself had become engrossed in the study of *family premises,* the shared myths and rules characterizing a family, which are usually passed down from generation to generation. But what on one level—the family level—is common to all can yet be experienced very differently on the individual's level (see also chapter 6). Life within the same family often turns out very differently for the different participants. Jerome Bruner (1990a) gives a very apt illustration of this in a study where parents and their four children are asked to characterize their family from their own personal point of view. In therapy, we try to put emphasis on the different experiences that family members have within their family. Nevertheless, our understanding is influenced by our thinking that siblings growing up in the same family are exposed to the same influences. I would like to state here that we have made little use of children's different positions as useful information in therapy. We have also taken it for granted that the personality of the parents, their background, and their education has the same effect on all the children in a family. The study of the significance of the social environment has been permeated by an idea that environmental influences vary between families and not within them. For this reason, most of the goals of the family milieu as regards the child are *general* and not *specific*. One has, for example, compared families in terms of the parents' caring ability and its significance, but not how this caring ability can be practiced differently with different children within one family. Neither has one focused on how this ability is experienced by the child(ren) within the family—in other words, the child's *subjective* experience. The importance of the children's own experiences and their conception of events is just as decisive for their development as "factual" events. Dunn shares her interest in the child's subjective experience with Stern (1985), which is precisely what gives her studies this vibrant and recognizable quality.

The interesting feature in Dunn's studies is that, apart from her references to fiction and her studies of children in their natural milieus, she has collaborated with scholars within a field that has been given the name of *behavioural genetics*. Besides studying the importance of genetic factors for development, genetic research can also shed light on the environment's impact on personality and on psychopathology (Dunn & Plomin, 1991). This is of interest particularly in relation to the tendency to biologize behavioural sciences, with a focus on genetic and biological explanatory and therapeutic models.

The combination of behavioural genetic research and developmental psychology sheds new light on the influence of the environment on individuals. Studies of what has been termed *non-shared environment* show that processes within the family lead to sibling differences. In this chapter, I examine how the study of sibling relationships and sibling differences can shed light on individual differences, the individual's development within the family, and the family's influence on the individual. I also discuss possible theoretical and practical implications for family therapists. The study of siblings is also useful for throwing light on the development of the social understanding of children. The manner in which Dunn's studies of children have changed our conception of children's social understanding and close relationships has been discussed elsewhere (Johnsen, 1997).

## *Families make siblings different, not only similar*

The following statement is repeated almost like a magical jingle or a hypnotic induction in Dunn's and Plomin's writings. "The environmental factors important to development are those that two children within a family experience differently" (Dunn & Plomin, 1991, p. 272, see also pp. 273, 280). "Family influence works to make siblings different, not similar, and the salient sources of the influence that affect development are specific to each child in a family, rather than shared" (Dunn, 1993, p. 52). I went around for several months contemplating these assertions, repeating them as if they were a kind of mantra that would finally reveal its secret to me. How was I to understand that families make children different rather than alike, that a shared childhood and adolescence with shared parents and with shared rules and values would create differences rather than similarities? I am used to looking upon my own family as special and different from most other families. None of my friends or classmates had six siblings and a father who travelled around collecting money to build a psychiatric clinic. However, having something in common as a group does not necessarily mean being alike as individuals. I also struggled to comprehend that it is the *non-shared* experiences that are significant for development, not those that children/siblings experience together. I return to this point later in the chapter.

Mythical revelations cannot supply answers to the question of how similarities and differences develop—only scientific studies can do so. It is here that behavioural genetics presents sophisticated analyses of similarities and differences and a theory of non-shared environment. Modern behavioural genetics makes a distinction between "shared" and "non-shared" environmental experiences and influences, to indicate *the conditions experienced respectively alike and differently by individuals in the same family.* By studying identical and non-identical twins, biological and adopted siblings, one was able to differentiate between genetic and environmental factors and their influence.

Behavioural genetic studies demonstrate that:

- in spite of genetic influences, the environmental factors play an important role in development;
- environmental factors do not necessarily cause siblings growing up in the same family to become similar;
- the salient environmental factors are those that make children in the same family different, not similar.

Even though siblings share half of their genes and grow up in what has traditionally been conceived of as a shared environment, siblings are extremely different with regard to personality and psychopathology. Studies show, for example, that siblings correlate only 0.15 for personality. In terms of psychopathology, sibling concordances are less than 10%. The resemblance one finds between siblings as regards personality is due to hereditary factors and not to the experience of growing up together. One refers here, for example, to studies of non-related children growing up together. They almost do not resemble each other. Another example is twin studies. Identical twins are 100% genetically alike. Yet they are only 50% alike in terms of personality, and this likeness is mainly genetically determined. Why, then, are they so different? Since twins are identical in genetic terms, there must be environmental influences causing twins to differ so much from each other. But how can they be so different when they grow up in the same environment, which we believe is even more similar than the environment for siblings? But is it the same environment? In order to find an answer to this, one has to study more than one child per family and to identify the non-shared experiences that are decisive for development. This implies a shift from one frame of reference that compares family with family to a perspective that focuses on the different individuals within the family. Theories that rely on more general and undifferentiated conceptions of the family need to be replaced by a more nuanced analysis of the micro-environments that each one of the siblings experiences individually in a family. This implies that it is the child's *subjective* experience of events in the family that is decisive for its development. Dunn emphasizes that she uses the concept of environment in a broad sense. It is the non-genetic influences, both within and outside the family, to which she refers. As an example, she mentions physical illness, accidents, random occurrences, peers, and so forth, in addition to psychosocial environmental factors.

Behavioural genetics research, however, says nothing about which of the specific processes in the family make siblings different. Dunn's longitudinal studies of siblings have proved to be an important contribution in this respect. It is precisely the combination of behavioural genetics research and developmental psychology that can shed a light on the environment's influence on the individual.

Dunn and Plomin (1990, 1991) discuss two potential sources of experiences that are different for siblings:

1. The *parent–child relationship*—children who grow up in the same family can have different relationships to their parents.
2. The *sibling relationship*—this, too, represents different experiences that are significant for development.

## *The attitude of family therapy to differences*

Practising family therapists have been aware of the fact that family members have different perceptions of the relationships in the family. *Circular questioning* has been evolved precisely in order to facilitate awareness of these differences. The "invention" of the circular method of questioning by the Milan group was inspired by studies carried out by Gregory Bateson. Bateson asserts that we perceive a world of differences. Our sensory apparatus is constructed in such a way that we register differences rather than similarities. Information is difference, and this was the Milan group's theoretical justification for the circular method of questioning (Selvini-Palazzoli et al., 1980). Through circular questioning one can receive information about the relationship between two persons, as it is perceived by a third person (triadic questioning). One can gather information about differences in explanatory models or maps ("mind reading"), or differences in relationships ("who is most worried about . . .?"). Dunn's and Plomin's research offers an empirical justification for the circular method of questioning, which—in my opinion—can benefit family therapists.

The fact that differences are important for development becomes more understandable viewed in the light of Bateson's emphasis on the significance of differences. Perhaps the reason why Eskimos have so many different words for snow is precisely in order to create differences in a reality that to us looks rather homogeneous. We only see snow, or perhaps three or four different forms of snow (wet snow, newly fallen snow, etc.), whereas the Eskimos see something like ninety different forms of snow.

Families where similarity is an important family premise can illustrate the importance of differences for individual development. Families like these are described by Salvador Minuchin in his book about psychosomatic families, which are characterized by conflict avoidance, rigidity, overprotection and fusion (Minuchin, Rosman, & Baker, 1978). Differences in these families are looked upon as rejection, betrayal, and disloyalty. In his research of families showing signs of centripetal or centrifugal forces (binding or expelling families), Helm Stierlin (1981) shows that self-delimitation and self-differentiation are essential for individuation.

### *The price of similarity*

In Ida's family the premise of similarity became an obstacle for further development both for herself and her brother, who was three years older. When she was 11 years old, Ida developed serious anorexia, which led to hospitalization in a somatic hospital. The 14-year-old brother was described by his parents as a kind and quiet boy; he was almost considered an adult after a brief and scarcely noticeable period of puberty. During Ida's hospitalization, he became even kinder and more well-adjusted. The family describes itself as a family without conflicts, where agreement is taken for granted and showing consideration for each other is an indisputable virtue. In this atmosphere of harmony, kindness, and relatedness, there is not much room for individuation or for development. This example shows how development can stagnate when there is no room for differences.

## *Differences in the parent–child relationship*

In order to investigate the importance of differences in the parent–child relationship, Dunn and Plomin (1990) refer to different types of studies: interviews in which children and adolescents were asked about their family relationships and about their parents' relationship to them and their siblings, and questionnaires (Sibling Inventory of Differential Experience [SIDE]) in which adolescents and young adults were asked to compare the treatment of themselves and their siblings. These studies show that children experience great differences in their parents' treatment of themselves and their siblings, whether it goes in favour of themselves or in favour of their siblings. Interviews with mothers also show that in spite of strong norms about equal treatment, these mothers report differences in their feelings, attention, control, and discipline as regards their children.

Other studies (e.g. Colorado Adoption Study) show how decisive the children's developmental phase is for their parents' behaviour towards them. Mothers are more consistent with children on the same age level than with the same child over time. The child's developmental phase is determinative for the mother's behaviour towards it. Siblings in a family are at any given time on different age levels and in different developmental phases. Witnessing differential behaviour towards oneself and one's siblings may possibly be of greater significance than the uniform experiences of direct interaction with the parents (Dunn & Plomin, 1990).

Children's sensitivity to differences in their parents' behaviour is also expressed by their own behaviour. Dunn refers here to her longitudinal studies of two-children families from the time each second child is 1 to 3 years old (Dunn, 1988), with a follow-up when the child is 6 years old. These studies show that children at an early age observe and react directly to their parents' interaction with their siblings. Children are also sensitive and react to the relationship between their parents. From the age of 18 months, children comment and ask questions about the actions and feelings of others. For instance, they compare their own relationship to their mother with the relationships of their siblings. Social comparisons and self-evaluations appear early in childhood. Children are particularly aware of interactions and react to them where *emotions* are expressed.

In developmental psychology, it is the direct interaction between parents and children that has been the object of attention and exploration. In this respect, Dunn stands out in two ways: she goes beyond the dyadic relationship and direct interaction to study how the relationship between two persons is experienced by a third person. This turns it also into a study of triadic relationships. The relationship between two is always influenced by a third factor—a wisdom we already find in the Oedipus myth. In conformity with Stern (1985), Dunn (1993) emphasizes the fact that children are active interactional partners and active participants in their own construction of reality. This means that there is a reciprocal influence in the relationship between parents and children.

The differences in the parent–child relationship described by Dunn and Plomin give rise to two questions: (1) Are the differences the consequence of individual differences and not their cause? (2) And which consequences will these differences have for the child's subsequent adjustment?

The first question is difficult to answer. Differences in temperament between siblings will instinctively set off different reactions in the parents. But in terms of the child's adjustment, experience of competence, and self-esteem, the studies show that this is a result of—and not a cause of—differential treatment (Dunn & Plomin, 1990; 1991, pp. 296–297).

### *Differences in sibling relationships*

Clinical experience, but also our own lives, will have taught us the painful fact that the experiences of relationships are not necessarily alike. This is obvious in terms of the parent–child relationship, where the description of the relationship from the point of view of parents and children will necessarily contain some differences that we know tend to create misunderstandings. From couples therapy, we also recognize the phenomenon of the parties giving different descriptions of their relationship. In friendly relationships we can feel surprise, hurt, or anger about the difference that may lie in the importance and evaluation of the relationship and about the fact that our feelings of love, admiration, and respect are not reciprocated. This also applies to siblings: there can be quite a difference in the importance and evaluation of the relationship. It is not a good experience to feel that love and devotion are repaid with rejection and jealousy. When the discrepancy in the experience of the relationship is too great—whether it be loving or hostile feelings—then this may be connected to problems on the part of one of the parties. For example, the greater the difference between the love shown by an older sibling for the younger one and the love returned by the younger one, the more likely it is that the older one is depressed or asocial. Self-esteem and competence are also linked to differences in the relationship between two siblings. Dunn and Plomin (1991) point to many different forms of studies verifying these differences.

For me personally, this has been an exciting topic to explore in therapy. Through circular questioning you can obtain information about how siblings experience each other. Questions to two siblings such as "How do you think your brother/sister would describe the relationship between the two of you?" can often give surprising information to both parties, as would the question "How do you think your brother/sister experiences you?" These can be effective ways for oneself and others of working with the relationship, and they can be useful in talks with one person, with siblings, or with the whole family.

In addition to the importance of differences in sibling relationships, Dunn and Plomin point to a more indirect form of influence—the importance of growing up and observing a child that is different from yourself. Children become aware, surprisingly early in their development, of the difference between themselves and their siblings and will compare themselves to them.

### *Appreciating each other*

Hanne is a woman of 30 who has struggled with eating problems for the last twelve years. Her older sister, five years her senior, is experienced as successful in every way—professionally, in her appearance, and in her private life. Hanne experiences herself as unsuccessful and worthless in relation to this sister whom she loves very dearly. In the last session before a holiday, she cries out: "I do look forward to being together with Hilde, but I also know that I shall be comparing myself to her all the time and feeling unsuccessful." In a subsequent joint session with both of them, I ask Hanne what she thinks her sister appreciates about her. Hanne says it can't be much since she has always felt herself to be fat and stupid in relation to her sister. When asked, the sister says that what she appreciates in Hanne is her ability to listen, that she is a good person to talk to and loyal. Hanne had clearly underestimated her own importance to her sister, but also the sister's importance to her. Family therapy can help to clear up and change these deadlocked conceptions and to negotiate new ways of comprehending each other.

## *Consequences for family therapy*

Even though therapists, as already mentioned, have been aware of the fact that different family members may have different conceptions of what goes on in the family, this knowledge has not been based on theory or empirical data. I have already mentioned how the theory and research done on non-shared environments can offer an empirical justification for the circular method of questioning. Children's early social understanding and observation of relationships can also justify the circular method of questioning and its importance for promoting the ability to understand the perspective of others (Johnsen, 1997). Children are, already at an early age, observers of the relationships of others, and they are sensitive to the quality of these relationships. They show an interest in the feelings, intentions, and worries of their parents and siblings. This heightened social understanding makes them capable of fighting for their own interests and positions. The criticism levelled against systemic family therapy—that children cannot answer questions about relationships—can be invalidated also on the grounds of this knowledge about children.

The study of micro-processes in families, showing how small differences in children's differential experiences can have a self-reinforcing effect on children's development, can also empirically justify the importance of feedback processes. The question of why one child in a family develops symptoms while the others do not can become more easily understandable when examining the non-shared environmental factors in the family. Perhaps these studies will inspire new research into the issue about choice of symptom.

The significance of children's subjective experience and the specific environmental factors are therefore relevant to the development of all children, including those who are only children. Even though only children do not witness differential behaviour between themselves and a sibling, they will still register and react to the relationship between their parents and other significant persons. This can apply to the mother's or the father's relationship to his or her own siblings, parents, or other children (male and female cousins or the children's friends).

The study of siblings has also shown that not only do children register the way parents relate to the child, but they are sensitive to the relationship between the parents and others, and not only siblings.

The perspective has changed from studying children in relation to one parent to seeing the child as a member in a family.

An understanding of the non-shared environmental influences will also be significant for the therapeutic process. I at least have experienced that attaching importance to the micro-processes—in accordance with both Dunn and Stern—has made me more accurate, precise, and detailed in my talks with families.

The importance of siblings in family therapy has also been underestimated in terms of both being informants with nuanced experiences and being possible assistants in the therapy. The focus on the parent–child relationship has deflected one's attention from the fact that siblings can also be of importance, for better or for worse. The sibling relationship has great potential, and this can be made use of therapeutically.

The following vignette may serve as an illustration.

### *Common fate, different experience*

The twins, Mette and Mari, aged 13, were referred to the Nic Waal Institute, an outpatient clinic for children and adolescents, together with their sister, Kristina, who was three years older. Child welfare was worried: as small children, all three had been sexually abused by their father, just after the parents had separated. The abuse had taken place for more than one year, and the sisters had been partly abused together and partly individually. Kristina had finally alerted her mother, who reported the matter to Child Welfare and the police. The police did not take the case any further.

Child welfare workers who have been in regular contact with the mother and the daughters are now very concerned. The girls have reached puberty, and all three display sexualized behaviour and signs of promiscuity; there is a suspicion of drug abuse, and they are doing badly at school. They think that the girls need to talk about their traumatic experiences in childhood. Could it be that they feel badly about the way the case had been handled earlier?

The mother and the three girls have different concerns. They worry about their quarrels and fights and that they always have troubles and problems. They would like to get help to reduce their quarrelling.

In the therapy we started off with the mother, the girls, and Child Welfare, and later we had sessions just with all three girls together. We also had various couple combinations and individual sessions. The thread running through the entire therapy, also for the therapists, was joint talk and sibling talk. The individual therapists were also team members in the family therapy. The structure of the sessions—joint, individual, or couple—also reflected the content: what was shared and similar in their narratives, and what was unique and distinctive? This example can also serve as an illustration of the book's views on family therapy: the main issue is not who comes to the session at any given time, but the type of predominant thinking governing the therapeutic process.

I shall present a few examples of sibling sessions to illustrate the significance of differences and similarities.

Their shared experience—sexual abuse by their father—had in one sense made them alike: all three competed with each other, mostly about boys and getting the attention of boys. This caused conflicts, quarrels, and jealousy, since they fought for the same boys. The twins also competed for their mother's new live-in partner, and one of them emerged victorious. This victory was dearly bought—she was abused. But they could also be generous and loyal to each other, and they take over each other's boyfriends.

Their common fate also created loyalty and a notion that they should all be in the same boat. There they might assume slightly different roles, but the framework was erected, the pattern could not be broken, and the boat could not be abandoned. As they gradually dared to start talking about their abuse, this also became the object of competition. Whom had the father most abused—this also meant having been the most preferred one. What had taken place when the other two had not been present? Was one allowed to experience the shared situations differently? As the shared narrative was gradually mapped out, room was also left for nuances and for individual narratives. We can say that a process of individuation had begun. However, each time one of them expressed a difference—for example, in her evaluation of boys—it turned into two against one. It was just like a betrayal.

The twins began to dress differently, to wear their hair differently, and to chose different friends or gangs. As the differences slowly progressed from being about external things (clothes, boys) to being about opinions, choice of different milieus, and so forth, there came a period of increased conflicts. The main task in the therapy now was to negotiate about which of one's own experiences, opinions, or feelings was legitimate and could be shared even if it was different. Precisely by legitimizing and problematizing similarities as well as differences, a process of individuation took place that enabled them to have a more active attitude towards their shared—but also particular and individual—destinies. Their case was reopened, they obtained redress and ex-gratia payment, and they all embarked on their various educations. And they were always ready to help each other if one of them needed help.

## *Discussion and some problematic issues*

As mentioned initially, Dunn and Plomin's article (1991) came at a time of growing focus on the individual's place in the system. Even the leading article in the issue of *Family Process* in which their article was printed had the heading "Finding a Place for the Individual". This is precisely what Dunn's and Plomin's studies are aiming at. Through precise argumentation, they demonstrate how differently life turns out for members within the same family. It is precisely the non-shared environmental factors—the specific experiences lived through and interpreted by the individual—that are crucial for development and can explain how and why children in the same family are so different. Their strong point lies precisely in their exploration and emphasis on the special and distinctive quality of the environment's impact on the individual. Seen from this perspective, their focusing on the individual and individual differences can contribute to an understanding of the individual and his/her place within the system. However, their research leaves us with both new and old questions. For example, it does not solve the question I raised to begin with—about the importance of family premises, shared ideas, belief systems, traditions, and values, all of which characterize a family. There is also the question about the importance of family premises for understanding the similarities and differences between members of a family. One important premise in my own family was that one should mean something to others. Six out of seven siblings are doing one or another form of therapeutic work within the health system—a striking similarity in terms of choice of career and choice of values.

My own family and circle of friends also show that the educational level in siblings is fairly similar, and likewise their life style, values, and attitudes. In some of my client families, I can see how the same symptoms sometimes appear in several members of the family. I have several clients with eating disorders where it emerges that the sister too has or has had an eating disorder. Or there are families who all have somatic symptoms such as, for example, high blood pressure. This may be due to the genetic similarity between siblings, and yet the incidence of symptoms they share is higher than one would expect in terms of heredity estimates. Can it be that some types of family culture or premises make siblings more alike than other types of culture or premises? For example, will a premise of loyalty create a higher degree of identification with each other and the community than a premise of "being the master of one's own fate"? Do families who have strong traditions and a sense of solidarity have a different impact on the development of differences and similarities from families in which there are signs of dissolution? Dunn's studies and clinical experience demonstrate at the same time that differences are important for development. Too much stress on solidarity, similarity, and loyalty can also be an impediment to development, as shown for example by both Minuchin (Minuchin, Rosman, & Baker, 1978) and Stierlin (1974; Wirsching & Stierlin, 1982). Self-delimitation and self-differentiation is required if individuation is to take place. Families characterized by centripetal forces—called binding families by Stierlin—may inhibit development, while families with too strong centrifugal forces—the expelling families—may promote chaos and dissolution.

It is tempting to speculate about the phenomenon of *affect attunement* in relation to the importance of similarities and differences. For affect attunement—the experience that feelings are understood and shared—to take place, the shared experience and feelings must be communicated in a way that also creates a difference (see chapter 4).

Dunn and Plomin (1990) underline that their material comes from studying normal families. They raise the question of whether the experiences of siblings are more alike in families living under extreme conditions, such as grave pathology, violence, or other traumas. There are, however, indications that such extreme conditions may have different consequences for the different children. This touches upon the issue I raised earlier regarding the choice of symptom and why one child develops serious symptoms and the others not. Dunn and Plomin recommend a systematic examination of more than one child in these "families at risk", as this will contribute to a better understanding of the factors of protection and vulnerability.

I cannot see that Dunn and Plomin have raised the issue of the size of the sibling group and in what way this may be significant for the development of similarities and differences, nor have they discussed marginal groups. A large family of children often develops a special culture, with its own rules and norms—for example, that it is cowardly to tell on someone, that one must not cry, that sticking up for each other is important. Special alliances, roles, and identifications are also developed. Marginal groups—groups that are endangered in various ways—are also more concerned with solidarity and a sense of community than with being different from each other. In some cultures, identity is connected to the group and not to the individual.

Even though Dunn and Plomin maintain that their material is compounded as regards culture, class, and so forth, many of the studies they refer to are of middle-class and working-class families in England and the United States with two children. One exception is their material from the biographies of famous writers, where families with, for example, five children are also referred to. Even though these siblings show similarities—for example, all the Brontë sisters had literary talents—they believe that their personalities were extremely different.

The question I ask myself is whether siblings really are as different as Dunn and Plomin will have it. The answer is probably that it depends on which parameters one uses. Dunn and Plomin have examined sibling differences in terms of personality and psychopathology. Other parameters would perhaps have led to somewhat different answers—for example, that siblings are more alike with regard to cognitive development and scholastic achievements, physical aggressiveness, and certain forms of criminal behaviour (Dunn & Plomin, 1990).

However, Dunn and Plomin have made an important contribution to the understanding of the development of the individual within the family, and they have directed our attention to the significance of specific rather than general environmental factors. In conformity with Stern, they indicate that the child is an active participant in the interaction and in its conception of reality. The emphasis laid on the child's subjective experience underlines the fact that the child is not a passive passenger in its own life, a victim of circumstances or of biological programming, but is, on the contrary, an active participant.

Systemic theory has contributed to an understanding that the whole is more than the sum of its individual parts. This has revolutionized the understanding of the family as a system. The interest in the whole and the relation between its parts, and the innovations this created for therapeutic practice, caused the individual and its specific place and importance to be overlooked or forgotten. The issue of the relationship between the whole and its parts—between the family as a system and the individuals—has not been solved by Dunn's and Plomin's contributions. At a conference in Heidelberg in 1981, attempts were made to address this issue in two ways: (1) the viewpoint that the family level and the individual level represent two logically incompatible levels; (2) the viewpoint that argues in favour of individual and system thinking being compatible (Stierlin, Wynne, & Wirsching, 1983, pp. 245–251). Both Dunn and Stern have contributed to a thinking on the subject of individuals, relationships, and families that is useful for family therapists and many other clinicians. But this does not mean that the problem concerning the relation between these levels has been solved.

CHAPTER NINE

# Together or alone: a both/and approach in work with eating disorders

*Astri Johnsen*

The phrase "together or alone" in the title points both to a dilemma that confronts the young girl/woman with eating disorders and to the choices and dilemmas confronting the therapist in terms of understanding and choice of method.

The young girl's/woman's longing for togetherness, belonging, or relatedness is intense. But she is at the same time caught up in a notion about control and autonomy: one can only exist alone, only rely on oneself. Relatedness implies a sense of community, but it also implies a threat of losing oneself: being together is always on other people's conditions. She expresses both her hunger for love and her need to control.

Traditionally, therapists have had a choice that represents an either/or. Either one should come to therapy together as a family, or one should come alone as an individual. Either one should attempt an understanding of the young girl and her symptoms from a systemic perspective, or one should attempt it from an individual, psychodynamic perspective.

---

This chapter is an adaptation of a lecture given at the Second Nordic Congress on Eating Disorders, Bergen, 1998.

Seen in this light, the eating disorder and the therapy tradition reflect ancient cultural premises: either Jew or Greek, either heathen or Christian, either hell or heaven, either ill or healthy, either dependent or independent.

In this chapter, I wish to move beyond the cultural premise and try to regard eating disorders in the light of both systemic thinking and (modern) developmental psychological theory. The consequence will be a therapeutic approach with an interplay between the thematic and the contextual. The topic determines the context—that is, whether they should come together or alone: if they come together, then with whom (mother, father, siblings, etc.)? The context will then, up to a certain point, determine the topics that are taken up.

The experiences I build on are based on my work with eating disorders within a child and adolescent psychiatric context, the Nic Waal Institute, Oslo, and my private practice at the Institute of Family Therapy, Oslo, where the clients are mainly women between the ages of 18 to 35. I have little experience with boys/men with eating problems. Nor do I have any experience with children (under 11 years) with eating disorders. I shall therefore start with the family-therapeutic approach and indicate in what way and why modern developmental psychology can contribute to an understanding and treatment of eating disorders. I shall illustrate some of my points with clinical vignettes.

## *The family therapeutic approach*

Families with eating disorders have been described according to certain characteristics. Most widely known is Salvador Minuchin's description of what he calls the "anorectic family", characterized by a merging of boundaries, over-involvement (especially on the part of the mother), rigidity, and conflict avoidance; he also describes triangulation, which means that the child is drawn into the parental conflict (Minuchin, Rosman, & Baker, 1978). The psychoanalyst and family therapist Helm Stierlin and his research group in Heidelberg have also attempted to systematize the characteristics of families with eating disorders (Stierlin & Weber, 1989), the similarities and differences between families with anorexia and bulimia, and what distinguishes families with these symptoms from families with schizoaffective psychoses and manic-depressive illness. Both Minuchin and Stierlin caution against linear causal thinking and emphasize the mutuality in the interaction and complexity of the contexts in which these symptoms must be seen. However, many families have also felt incriminated by these descriptions of family dynamics, believing that they themselves were to blame. The focus in family therapy has also gradually shifted to the possible impact of a dramatic symptom on the interaction.

Eating disorders have, moreover, dramatically increased since Minuchin's description of the "anorectic family" in the 1970s. Hilde Bruch (1985) has described how anorexia—as a form of expression—has lost some of its psychodynamic specificity; the background for developing eating disorders is now more varied than the picture of symptoms. The same will also be true of the picture of families: it will make it less relevant to search for specific characteristics in families with eating disorders.

In spite of problems (concerning cause and effect, guilt, etc.) arising when one tries to understand symptoms in a family context, I would like to assert that this can nevertheless be both useful and necessary.

Inspired by the family therapists Luigi Boscolo and Gianfranco Cecchin from Milan, the Stierlin group in Heidelberg, and the Swedish child psychiatrist Kjerstin Laurén, I found it useful to understand eating disorders in the light of what I have termed central family premises (Johnsen, 1995). The Milan group looks upon symptoms as attempts at solutions—they must be understood as indications of antagonisms and dilemmas in the family that find their expression through symptoms (Boscolo et al., 1987). Families have their own inner logic—a set of premises or basic conceptions about themselves as a family and about each other (e.g. "in our family we have no secrets", "you must mean something to others", "separation represents betrayal").

Family premises are not a pathological phenomenon. Every family has to cope with some basic issues requiring solutions. One of these issues is attachment and separation. Another topic is the importance of gender—what it means to grow up as a girl as distinct from being a boy. In my experience, these topics are crucial in the work with eating disorders. Other important topics can be similarities and differences, justice and power.

Symptoms or problems may arise:

1. *When the premises come into conflict with developmental needs.* In a family that has experienced traumatic losses, solidarity can become identical with survival and separation can be connected to betrayal and dissolution. The premise of solidarity can come into conflict with an adolescent's necessary need for separation as an important part of development. The balance between attachment and separation requires different solutions, depending on the developmental phase in which the family happens to be. If this balance becomes rigid, then there is a loss of flexibility or elasticity and problems may arise.
2. *When different premises exist simultaneously and come into conflict.* This occurs when the premises have become rigid and are not open to negotiation. There can, for example, be a command that one should help others and, simultaneously, a demand about not burdening others. If one gets problems oneself, then one can be faced with a dilemma, with difficulties, and the solution may then be to hide one's difficulties.

Symptoms can be understood as transmitting a message that the old ideas or premises are no longer useful for further development. Premises are passed on through the generations and may have been useful for coping with earlier conflicts and difficulties. They may have slowly become rigid and will no longer be useful in terms of new challenges.

Regarding symptoms as attempted solutions and linking symptoms to family premises is one way of giving meaning to something that seems meaningless to oneself and others or that is perceived as an illness having struck a person. This perspective can be useful in relation to the narrative wave within family therapy in particular, but it can also be useful within psychoanalytic therapy, where creating meaningful narratives is of crucial importance.

### *Issues for discussion*

A family therapeutic understanding and approach to eating disorders will nevertheless comprise a number of dilemmas and problems, as I have indicated in my introduction. Are there, for example, some topics that are more difficult to become aware of in a family therapeutic context, or is it more a question of timing? An example here is Kari, who contacted me two years after ending family therapy and said: "Family therapy helped my parents, and that was good for me. I need no longer watch out and feel responsible for how they are. We also talk better with each other. But it did not help me with my feelings of being worthless." How are we to explain that a change at the family level does not always lead to a corresponding or adequate change at the individual level? Is it that the verbal dialogue does not pick up certain relational experiences that are communicated through nonverbal channels? Or did she have to relinquish her task as her parents' helper before she was able feel who she was herself? What is the significance of the experience of emotional sharing and exchange for our ability to create our own narratives? This is a central issue in a narrative tradition, but it is also a central issue in terms of eating disorders, which many regard precisely as expressing a lack of feeling-language.

Systemic family therapy has examined how symptoms can be understood in relation to others. It can often be sufficient to deal with this aspect of the symptom. Something happens to the interaction. The premises are changed, the symptom is resolved, and the girl gets started on her further development.

But the symptom can also be understood as an expression of a relationship to oneself, a window into oneself, becoming acquainted with aspects that have gone underground. The person has fallen silent but may again begin to find a voice of his/her own after a family therapy or a few hours of individual therapy. But how are we to understand this person? What are the therapist's ideas about the individual and the family, about separation and attachment, about dependence, independence, control, and autonomy—issues that I believe to be crucial for the understanding of eating disorders. Modern developmental psychology represents a fruitful viewpoint on these issues. This is also demonstrated in Vigdis Wie Torsteinsson's (1995) chapter on relationship and sense of a self as central concepts in work with eating disorders. However, before presenting some crucial points in modern developmental theory, I would like to return to some of Kari's experiences.

## *Control has its price*

Kari, who is now 20 years old, has gained control over her eating problems which started as anorexia when she was 12 years old. By the time she turned 14, they had developed into compulsive eating, and then bulimia became a sort of solution. She was 16 years old when I met her and her family, who came together to family sessions over a period of two years, all in all twenty times.

When she contacts me at the age of 20, although her eating problem is no longer the dominant factor in her life, she now has feelings of worthlessness and loneliness and thinks that she is someone whom no one can understand. As it is for many other girls with eating problems who have gained control over their symptomatic behaviour, her worries about food and body continue to occupy her thoughts and feelings. The eating disorders have moved up into her head.

One day she sits in my office, sad and empty. She complains that no one—not even I—is able to understand her. How can anyone understand how she feels when she no longer has visible symptoms, visible signs of her illness? (These girls mistake attention for understanding.) It is worst during the weekend. She is alone then, and her head is filled with food, and her body feels far too big. When I question her further about the weekends, it emerges that she receives many invitations to spend time with friends, acquaintances, and family, but she declines them all.

I say provocatively (I have known her for a long time and have learned that I can be quite direct with her): "No wonder you still have eating problems. You reject everyone who wants to come in contact with you, you do not trust anyone, not even me. Relationships are the nourishment which you do not dare or want to have. The eating problems merely express that the relational nourishment does not function. The price you have to pay for the control that you regard as so important is loneliness."

The example of Kari demonstrates several points. She is caught up in the idea of an autonomous and independent self, which is essential for gaining control, a caricature of the self-concept in Western society. Love and the feeling of belonging represent a threat of losing oneself: either she loses herself, or she loses the others. Dependence and independence are an incompatible pair, similar to attachment and autonomy. She also expresses what we all want—to be understood. In my experience, this is a recurring theme in those suffering from eating disorders. Symptoms are a signal—they represent a wish to be seen and understood. "I almost yearn for the time when my eating problems were visible, to the attention I then received," says one of these girls. However, attention is not the same as being seen and understood, and neither is it a simple matter to translate the symptom into the dilemmas and problems it conceals. Modern developmental psychology has been useful to me in my further exploration of these difficult issues. Kari's dilemmas call into question the types of notions we humans have—whether as therapists or as clients—about the sense of self and interaction, attachment and detachment, and above all what we actually mean by understanding each other. As Signe, one of my other clients, said: "I haven't the faintest idea what you could say or do to make me understand that you had understood."

## *Modern developmental psychology*

The infant researcher and psychoanalyst Daniel Stern has formulated a developmental theory in which the sense of self constitutes the organizing principle for development (Stern, 1985) (see also chapter 1). I shall take up some points that I believe may be relevant to the work with eating disorders.

1. From the very start, there is a social communication in which the infant is an active partner in the interaction. The infant is an active participant in constructing its own world. We should remember this point whenever there is a tendency to blame

mothers/parents. Both infant and caregiver are active interactional partners. In terms of Kari's lonely weekends and my challenging comments, I wanted to convey to her that she too can be an active participant in her own life.

It is easy—in any case, it is for me—to find oneself trapped in a position where one feels sympathy instead of challenging and exploring the possibilities of not being a passive victim.

2. Self-development is not characterized by phase-specific issues. Clinical issues, such as dependence and control, trust and autonomy, are not linked to age-specific phases. They do not define specific developmental stages. They are central issues right from the very start and are worked through and repeated at each developmental phase and are shaped and developed on the basis of developmental competence. They are life issues. Here Stern differs from other (psychoanalytic) developmental theory. Development is defined not from the point of view of phases, but from the point of view of developmental lines. Development does not take place from symbiosis towards individuation or from dependence to independence. Dependence and autonomy, attachment and separation, are not opposites. They are pairs following us throughout life. As shown earlier, these themes are central in the work with eating disorders.
3. The constitution of the sense of a self will always be based on the interaction with others. The sense of self is formed from within, but it is based on the subjective experience of being together with an other. The development of the self and the development of relationships are two sides of the same coin. A competent, autonomous self, detached from all relationships, is at best an illusion and at worst a tragedy.

Stern conceptualizes five different senses of self, each with its parallel forms of relatedness and special forms of communication linked to these. I shall not enlarge on the different self-domains here, but merely emphasize those forms of communication that are linked to them. For the first three of these senses, this is a preverbal form of communication; and for the last two, it is a verbal or narrative form. The Norwegian psychologist Bjørg Røed Hansen has termed them affective and narrative dialogue, respectively (Hansen, 1996a, 1996b).

In work with eating disorders, it is precisely the affective form of communication that has been silenced, gone underground, or not found its form of expression. I have therefore been interested in this form of communication and in what way it may help us in the sessions to get a better grasp on the affective exchange and the sharing, both between the family members and in relation to the therapist. Can it also help us to understand the question that Signe is struggling with—what can the therapist (or the parents) do to make her feel understood?

## *Affects and the affective dialogue*

Family therapists have given a great deal of thought to the communicative aspect of feelings, primarily the impact that an expressed affect has on the others, but they have also become interested in the meaning that is communicated through feelings. Only a small amount of attention has been given to the experiential aspect: the strength, tone, and intensity of the feelings. I believe that this is because we have been thinking in terms of the categorical affects—anger, joy, grief, disgust, and so forth. Stern makes a distinction between what he calls vitality affects and categorical affects (see chapter 4). Vitality affects accompany every experience and come together with or without a categorical affect. The vitality affect describes the frequency, intensity, form, the very rhythm in the experience.

### *Attuned or out of tune?*

Line, who is 14 years old, is hospitalized for serious anorexia nervosa. She comes to the session together with her mother and her sister Anne, who is 18 years old. Like many girls with similar problems, Line states that she does not feel understood. In the session she seems cross and uninterested, averting her eyes, looking away, and giving only reluctant answers to my questions. Anne, on the other hand, is lively and contact-seeking, smiling and involved; above all, she and her mother are in contact. After the session, I am left with an unpleasant feeling of having made a fool of myself by putting eager questions to a person who most certainly wished me to go to blazes.

A close study of the video of the session gives a surprisingly different picture. To start with, the mother and Line do in fact look at each other, but never simultaneously; it is as if they are completely out of step. Line is not uninvolved—on the contrary. True enough, the content of what she says is often critical, but she is involved. By studying the frequency, intensity, and form of her statements (the vitality affects), we get a different picture, a different story—that of a desperate girl trying to express herself, to be heard and understood, but without succeeding. She cannot achieve a meeting, not even with her eyes. With the mother and Anne it is different—they look at each other, their eyes meet, smiles appear when they recognize a common experience.

This video taught me two things. Feelings are about something more than a special affect, it is the pattern (frequency, intensity) I should see and listen to. I also witnessed two different mother–daughter relationships. One relationship demonstrated mutual exchange and attunement. The other showed signs of the opposite; it was out of step or out of tune. Therefore, it is not a question of a mother who has no ability for empathy, but that this ability was connected to the relationship. She expresses empathy in one relationship but not in the other. She herself says: "I would so much like to understand Line, but I don't know what I can do to understand her."

Stern, however, makes a distinction between empathy and what he calls affect attunement, a distinction that I believe to be useful to us when we need to grasp the simple—and yet so complicated—question of what it means to understand each other. How can I know that I have understood the other? Can she see it on me? Can she feel it deeply inside her (Johnsen & Torsteinsson, 1997)?

Affect attunement resembles empathy in that it presupposes an emotional resonance. In addition to the emotional response, empathy also implies a cognitive communication. Through affect attunement, the original emotional resonance is automatically recreated in another expression, and it is this recreation that establishes affect attunement as a phenomenon of its own. Affect attunement is a nonverbal communication of having understood the child's inner experiences. The adult uses a different modality for expression from that used by the child, but the experiential pattern is the same. Affect attunement is a concept that Stern uses to describe the early interaction between parents and infant, where the focus is especially on communicating and understanding inner experiences. The early interaction is precisely about regulation, modulation, sharing, and integrating feelings.

Affect attunement does not only characterize the early interaction; it is a phenomenon that characterizes all human interplay and is particularly important in close relationships. When, for example, Line's sister Anne talks about a special experience, she looks across at her mother, the tone of her voice rises, her eyebrows lift, and her eyes sparkle. A smile lights up the mother's face, and she says, "Oh, how lovely," in a tone that reflects the same intensity and movement as in Anne's expression. They look at each other, share something, and understand each other, at least at that moment. The emotional interaction is also crucial to the therapeutic relationship.

The importance of an emotional involvement on the part of the therapist has been emphasized by several authors (Bruch, 1988; Burbatti & Castoldi, 1994; Torsteinsson, 1995). In this connection I would like to mention the Canadian psychologist Peggy Claude-Pierre (1997), who demonstrates the importance and power of emotional involvement in her treatments of eating disorders. In her work at the Montreux Clinic in Victoria, Canada, she shows how decisive an active emotional attitude can be for coming into contact with a rigid and almost dead internal world. To me, her therapeutic work represents a demonstration of the use of developmental psychological principles, even though on her part this has not been explicitly formulated. The regulation of physical and affective states is a central principle. Her work can also illustrate the importance of love as a guiding principle in the treatment of eating disorders—a treatment based on love and unconditional support and on a confirmation of the uniqueness of the patients' lives.

Inspired by Peggy Claude-Pierre's work, the Swedish paediatrician Olof Ulwan has worked out a plan for patients with serious eating disorders at the children's unit at Ullevål Hospital in Oslo. The framework of the treatment plan is acceptance, care, and support. Seen with the "eyes of Stern", the main concern in the treatment is regulation, as opposed to control (which in the past had been one of the main features in the somatic treatment of eating disorders).

### *The narrative dialogue*

As mentioned earlier, Stern distinguishes between the preverbal and the verbal domains of the sense of self.

The onset of the verbal stage in the life of the child (15–18 months) creates new possibilities of communication, of self-reflection, and of creating its own narrative. Stern, however, points to the duplicity of language: it offers new opportunities for communication while at the same time causing a split from an immediate experience and from preverbal or nonverbal experiences.

Young girls and women with eating disorders are often apparently good at expressing themselves verbally. They may sometimes seem older and more reflective than other people of the same age. But when it comes to communicating their feelings, they are often at a loss. When constructing a narrative together with a girl and perhaps also with her family, a narrative that will be meaningful to them and give them a sense of cohesion, we must meet the challenge of connecting it to something with an affective content. It is precisely at this point that metaphors can be useful. The family therapist David Epston from New Zealand uses a flowery metaphorical language in his work with eating disorders (e.g. anorexia is called the executioner, taking one to a concentration camp, leading one to the gallows, etc.). In her book *Nattmennesker* [Night People] (1996), Anne Røer, a Norwegian psychologist, gives several examples of how metaphors can be useful in the treatment of bulimia. The very title of the book is a metaphor for a person whose vital aspects have been blacked out.

Personally I have used metaphors such as that bulimia is like a thick fog making a person invisible. It can also be compared to a parasite who knows how to exploit its host, a tyrant, but also a friend in need. I have also used theatre as a metaphor, where one is caught in a role, where the script has stagnated and forced one to repeat the same lines. Therapy can also become like a stagnated play, where the therapist is caught in the role of helper and the client in the role of passive victim.

The work with family premises can be useful when one needs to link cohesion and meaning to the symptom. Stern and other developmental psychologists—for example, Jerome Bruner (1990a)—maintain that the need to organize experiences in meaningful and cohesive narratives has been handed down to us humans as a genetic disposition. Symptoms can be seen as signifying the breakdown of such an experience of cohesion and meaning, and therapy can be seen as a way of rectifying or creating a new narrative with meaning and cohesion.

In family therapy, it will be a question of which narrative should be given priority. A family's shared narrative may give meaning on one particular level, but perhaps not on another level. Take the differences between Line and Anne, for example: their narrative about the mother–daughter relationship, and what it was like to grow up in the same family, must necessarily also contain essential differences.

This is also the point made by the developmental psychologist Judy Dunn, who has carried out research into children's close relationships and social understanding (Dunn, 1993; Dunn & Plomin, 1990). She finds that siblings growing up in the same family have greater dissimilarities than one would have expected considering their common heredity and common social environment (see chapter 8). But do siblings grow up in the same social environment? A great number of experiences are extremely different for siblings, and it is precisely these differences that are important for their development. According to Judy Dunn, the environmental factors important to development are those that two children in the same family experience as different. A therapist must therefore attach importance to these differences and make room for both the shared and the individual narratives.

This is most important in the work with eating disorders. According to Minuchin's descriptions, there is very little room for differences in many of these families. Similarity is equivalent to solidarity, and differences to rejection. If we are to take Dunn's experiences seriously, then emphasizing and legitimizing the differences will be of importance for further development.

## *Therapeutic implications*

In the same way as premises can stagnate or reach a deadlock in a family, so too can our therapeutic premises reach a point of stagnation. I am, for instance, doubtful about the expediency of continuing to think in terms of categories such as family therapy or individual therapy. Personally I feel more comfortable in a family therapy setting where—together with the family—one is free to decide who is to come to the sessions at any particular time; likewise in individual therapy, where I want to have the possibility of drawing in the whole family— parents, siblings, or girlfriends— whenever it can be useful for the process.

I have stated earlier that it was natural to start with family therapy in cases where the girl lives at home, as we generally find is the case in a child and adolescent psychiatric context (Johnsen, 1995). I still believe this to be helpful and necessary when we are dealing with an unwilling anorexic girl and with parents/family who are distressed. It is often a disheartening experience to offer individual sessions to many of these girls. They themselves have no problems other than people telling them they are too thin. Working with family premises and creating meaningful narratives will here be useful. Modern developmental psychology at any rate can put us on the track of topics that are important in these narratives. It can also remind us of the importance and necessity of grasping the emotional interaction, or its absence, as was shown in the example with Line. I have also begun to think more in terms of phases—for example, one particular phase where family therapy can be useful, another phase perhaps where sessions with parents are appropriate, and perhaps later some individual sessions where the focus can be on the sense of self and the experience of others.

With the unwilling bulimic girl, it is a different story. She hides her symptoms from her parents, and it is often her girlfriend who is the first to discover them. The health visitor is involved, and the health visitor and the girlfriend are the worried (and motivated) parties. The girl herself usually thinks that she has found the perfect solution for regulating her weight. At this point, motivational work is most important, and this may not yet be the right moment for therapy. In cases where the girl herself is worried but does not want to involve her parents, it is necessary to consider flexible solutions. The health visitor and the girlfriend can be useful helpers, but usually, at some point, the parents find out about it and can then be involved in the treatment. The bulimic symptom often requires a different approach from that with the anorexic symptom. A cognitive, behaviour therapeutic approach with symptom registration can often initiate work where the symptoms are gradually invested with meaning. It may, for example, emerge that overeating and vomiting are linked to special, concrete situations. Later in the therapy, these can again be linked to thoughts and feelings that are connected to significant other persons.

One is faced with great challenges when the anorexic symptoms are combined with severe obsessional problems. In many cases, hospitalization will become necessary (somatic or psychiatric ward). In a context of child and adolescent psychiatry, the family work will be important, and individual therapy will often also be required. Some people are convinced that the effective method here would be cognitive behaviour therapy using exposure techniques, while others claim that the combination of eating problems and obsessional symptoms requires a more diverse approach.

In the case of the worried, adult bulimic woman who is engulfed by her bulimic everyday life, it is useful to start off by mapping out the symptom, as I have described above. As the symptoms gradually recede into the background and life themes such as dependence/autonomy and trust/control present themselves, it may be most interesting to involve the family in different ways. Having the courage to accept help from a sister, a mother, or a father can often create dramatic turning points in a therapy.

In the case of the anorexic woman who is "on the wagon" and no longer has visible symptoms, a combination of individual and family therapy will be an interesting and exciting challenge. It can be especially fruitful to work with the mother–daughter relationship. The Swedish psychologist Mia Andersson (1995, 1997) is an enthusiastic exponent of this form of therapy, connecting it to the problems relating to dependence and independence and to a sense of belonging and autonomy.

It can be added here that follow-up talks we have had regarding family therapy for eating disorders also demonstrate the impact that the mother–daughter relationship can have on the process of recovery (Johnsen, 1995).

## *Conclusion*

In this chapter I have presented and discussed a perspective in which eating disorders can be understood and worked with, based on an affective and cognitive viewpoint, but within a relational context involving the young girl/woman and the therapist and also in which the family (one or more members) is in the background or steps forward onto the scene, depending on where one is at any given point in the therapeutic landscape. Metaphorical language will form the bridge between the bodily, preverbal experiences and the verbal world of experience. The family therapist's use of the circular method of questioning will link the individual and the relational reality.

The work with family premises offers opportunities for putting the symptom into a context of cohesion and meaning. Similarities, as well as differences, will be crucial ingredients in the narrative.

Another significant contrast in this work is the relation between passive and active. The client often presents herself as a passive victim, struck down by illness, with difficult family relationships or other troubles. I have experienced that therapy can reinforce this type of victim role. In her or his desire to understand, the therapist may accidentally underline this role. Modern developmental theory has reminded us that the child is an active interactional partner from the very beginning. A therapeutic goal must be to turn all parties in a therapy into active collaborators who can have an influence over their own lives.

Eating disorders have been conceived as expressing a lacking ability to find words for feelings. Developmental psychological thinking makes it possible both to understand and to act differently in relation to emotional problems (see chapter 4). This will have consequences for our understanding of the interaction in the family, as well as for our therapeutic attitude in relation to eating disorders.

*PART III*

# WHAT NOW? THEORETICAL PERSPECTIVES AND REFLECTIONS

CHAPTER TEN

# Involved thinking and concept formation as an aid in therapy

*Rolf Sundet*

An exciting experience when I was a patient was that at one point my therapist changed his questions to me. Having previously often asked what I was *feeling* now, he began for some reason to ask me what I was *thinking of* now. He had originally presented himself as a body-oriented therapist, in the Reichian tradition. Becoming aware of one's tensions and feelings that emerge during the work with one's body and muscles had been one of the approaches. At a certain point, the work with the body diminished, and instead I became aware of his interest in my thoughts, and I noticed that my thoughts were coming. I had an experience of doing what one might call mental work: producing words, experiences, sentences, images, sensations, and stories.

One experience I have had as a patient, a therapist, and a supervisor is to get stuck and not to know what to do. In the position of a patient, I experienced that directing my attention towards thinking offered more possibilities in situations like these. What I learned in this position of thinking and producing thoughts has been of invaluable importance to me as a therapist and supervisor. Chapter 7, which deals with the use of Stern's descriptions of the senses of self and relational domains as metaphors for therapeutic interaction with adolescents, evolved precisely from a deadlocked situation. I was working in a child and adolescent outpatient clinic, in which I was looked upon as a family therapist. My own conception was that I was an apprentice in the field of family therapy. In this encounter between expectation and reality, I withdrew to my office wondering how I could be useful at this outpatient clinic. I had one advantage: I was a male, and it was thought that boys between the ages of 12 to 18, who often acted out, needed a man to talk to. It was when meeting these youths that I was first confronted with the experience of not quite knowing where to go. Responses such as "I don't know", "It's all the same to me", or "What do you think?" when invited to participate in a therapy that was based primarily on language and verbal activity proved to be a somewhat unfamiliar starting point for a therapist who had heard a great deal about motivation and accessibility on his road to learning.

Chapter 7 describes the use of Stern's concepts as a means of providing an outline of the practice that evolved with these adolescents. The present chapter is about thinking and conceptualization. When working with this group of adolescents, it became necessary to develop thoughts that could legitimize a practice that often went beyond what I used to consider as psychotherapy. At that point, I was not accustomed to and had no theoretical evidence for considering my participation in affect regulation as necessary therapeutic work, nor when it was a question of action and activity—for example, karate training or folding paper aeroplanes. This practice evolved as a result of a necessity of the moment rather than as a result of planned and carefully considered rationality. A gradual reflection as a comment on this practice grew in strength and intensity in the encounter with Stern's descriptions of the interaction between the infant and the caregiver. The experience of this encounter was precisely characterized by being right in the middle of mental labour that gradually yielded products that could further contribute to the process. Chapter 7 is an attempt at formulating a product that tries to grasp a certain part of this practice through Stern's concept of the senses of the self and the interactional domains. Summarized, the attempt has been to grasp this practice through affect regulation and action orientation, with an emphasis on mastery and volition, sharing of experiences, expressing oneself in words, and putting these words to work through thinking, narratives, and stories. It is my concern here to develop a sequence of thought. Its topic is to find out whether it is possible to develop thinking about thinking as an aid, or as an activity that may help the therapist in his subsequent work.

## *Thinking*

> Philosophical thinking for Gilles Deleuze and Félix Guattari is not primarily "about something"; thinking is something in itself: a mental event with its own dynamics and intensity, which precedes both a metaphysical transcendence and a reference to something actually existing. [Madsen & Tygstrup, 1996, p. 8]

Michel Foucault (1977) has characterized Deleuze's philosophy as theatre. The reality of the theatre has connections to a world outside, but it is not this reality. What happens on the stage exists in its own right. It can be used to say something about or point to something out there in the world, but it follows its own rules of the game. They can be similar to those in the outside world, but they can also be different. "Philosophy as theatre . . . is the invention of conceptual rules of logic and relationships dramatizing thought" (Madsen & Tygstrup, 1996). Philosophy for Deleuze and Guattari is about creating new concepts or giving old ones a new content. It is a matter of putting these into play and seeing what kind of relational forms and social arrangements they will facilitate (Deleuze & Guattari, 1996). I like the idea of looking at thinking and the producing of thought as any other kind of production that produces an object, a product. One can interact with them and avail oneself of them in everyday life for whatever use one finds can be made of them. One can use them for decoration or for pleasure, if that is convenient, or else they can be discarded as useless. These thoughts are not only *about* something, they *are* something. In our context, the issue is the ability of the concepts to be the point of departure for new relational forms. It is the creation of new forms of being together and conversing that is our concern.

Clinical everyday life is full of events and happenings. They appear as both known and unknown. They can cause certainty in the therapist about what to do, and they can cause uncertainty. My concern here is with situations and events that are experienced as unknown and where there is uncertainty about what action to take or how to deal with them. These situations can be characterized by ambivalence, uncertainty, and doubt. The professional approach implies availing oneself of theory and research.

When recalling my introduction to clinical work, I am struck by one difference in today's attitude to practical and theoretical knowledge. In the light of retrospection, the 1970s and the beginning of the 1980s seem dogmatic, with a situation where one could easily let oneself be identified with theoretical positions—for example psychoanalysis, operant analysis, or systems theory. Today, one speaks more of diversity in terms of approaches and theories. Attention is not so much directed at predominant theories as at isolated formulations and findings. It is not the loyalty to theoretical positions that prevails today, but formulations and conceptualizations that are reported to be useful from the point of view of the users, therapists, and scientists. In this situation, one is oriented towards theory as a variety of possibilities, where one can permit oneself to use elements from different theoretical orientations.

In my view, it is important to pass this development on. This chapter argues in favour of the fact that clinical everyday life always presents one with new, unknown, and unfamiliar situations in which established theoretical and research-based knowledge is not adequate as a directive for action. One must, in addition, try to establish ways of working that will facilitate access to knowledge in the actual situation one finds oneself in. In a potentially uncertain work situation, it is important to have conceptual resources that will help one to maintain theoretical and clinical flexibility and offer opportunities for developing concepts, thoughts, and perspectives that can aid clinicians in the situations that may at any time arise.

## *The supplement*

When theories and clinical approaches are seen as alternatives, one can easily end up in contrasts where adopting one perspective will exclude others. The fact that something is an alternative can often make one believe that something else is excluded. What is excluded no longer has any place or use and is pushed out to the extreme edge or margin of the professional field or the theory. I have found it useful to include other perspectives and concepts, which does not mean that what is exchanged will disappear. The word that represents the aid here is "supplement". Considering something as a supplement implies taking with one something of the old (what is supplemented) while at the same time bringing in something new. Supplements (Derrida, 1976) are both *in addition to* and *a substitute for* or something *instead of*. Supplements can be looked upon as passing on something from what is supplemented, while at the same time bringing in something new. Let us look at this in a clinical context.

### *"The patient"*

She came to the session clearly in the throes of an inner storm. There was something she wanted to say, had to say, but which was difficult, threatening, and potentially destructive. She had to say it—"I'm in love. With you." I felt my whole body going into a state of alert: an alertness not to destroy, trample on, not to put a stop to her communication—an alertness to receive, listen, accept, and understand. This was the first task. For both of us to be present in what was—the falling in love, the feeling, the anxiety, the vulnerability.

She had a question: "What shall I do about it?" Our dialogue is more directed at understanding, grasping what kind of feeling this is, and what it means when it is directed towards her therapist. We get a distance to the feeling. In my body there is an uneasiness. It has been there since the falling in love was voiced. This uneasiness has to do with the question of what is triggered off when I become the focus of this feeling. Professional reflection takes over. The uneasiness is there. The thought becomes clearer that this is an important point. We can now approach her inner motivation for the feeling. Who do I become for her? Whom and what does the feeling in reality deal with? What is it that is being repeated now? The professional reflection brings up an early acquired aid: to think of the phenomenon as *transference*. She senses that I have an understanding. She asks me what I am thinking. I am thinking aloud about transference. She stops me, almost abruptly, which was very unusual for her. She says loudly and clearly: "I won't have it that this feeling is changed into something different than it is. I am in love with you. What our talks have made possible is that at last I am able to bring out my feelings, become acquainted with them and show them. They have been locked up, buried, changed, concealed. Now they can come out into the open. When I am feeling something now that I have never felt properly before, then it should not be turned into something else than it is."

Suddenly I can understand my uneasiness. It was fearful for me to be confronted with such a frank and intense expression of falling in love.

It could be subdued by distancing myself from the feeling. To regard it all as transference took the feeling away from me. Countertransference? Shall I look at what it brings up in me, my repetitions, my previous relationships? I am doing it again. I am running away from it. Running away from what? Running away from being a therapist for one who is in love with me. I am running away from being a therapist in this kind of situation.

The other part of the job was to agree that she is right. We shall not change the feeling into something else. We shall not spend time thinking about the origin of her falling in love and my uneasiness. We shall spend time thinking what it means to have this feeling in the room. My other uneasiness is about how to work with this. I needed words to interact with, which would give me other options than transference. The focus is not on what is transferred from a different period or a different relationship; it is on what is presented in this relationship at this point in time, here and now. It is about a *presentation*. What we find ourselves in is a real situation. The focus of attention is on us and our relationship. What kind of relationship is it? It is a therapeutic relationship. We are working with therapy where one is the patient and the other the therapist. What matters is the client's development and recovery. Falling in love enters into this relationship, and one has to deal with it. What should one do about it in this relationship? One might say that it does not belong to this relationship and should therefore be kept out of it. One might say that the chief concern in this therapy is to look at the etiology or the origin of the feeling: how it has become what it has become, what it is that makes it come alive, and why—all the while with a focus on a historical understanding, and on what has turned it into what it is today, a learning about why I have become what I have become. This is an aspect in the perspective of transference. There is no excluding factor between transference and what I have called presentation. These two concepts or perspectives supplement each other. In order to become better acquainted with the perspective of presentation, I will let the perspective of transference, as a contrast, remain in the background.

After several sessions she gives us an answer to what it means to work in this perspective. She says: "You are a mirror. I'm sending my feelings towards you, and I get no response to them. They are reflected back, and I can get to know them. It feels good and bad at the same time." Responding to love, becoming a couple, lovers, boy- or girlfriends, implies stepping out of the therapeutic domain and entering the domain of the couple, of romanticism, passion, and love. This relational domain has different tasks, different goals, responsibilities, and commitments from those in the therapeutic domain. Not to give an answer means receiving, listening, noticing, verbalizing, but it never means entering into a relationship where the demands or desires of the feeling are satisfied. It means being open to the feeling, confirming and accepting it and what it leads to—for the patient. Of course, falling in love and its disclosure leads to a number of events for her. A number of other feelings emerge in its wake. She is worried about how I will react to it when it is disclosed. She is ashamed of having fallen in love. She has feelings of guilt about throwing it at me. She becomes angry because she is rejected. She grieves because this is how things are. She is glad that she is rejected, because it gives her a possibility she says she has never had before—to become known to herself without others interfering.

Two concepts have been demonstrated here: transference and presentation. One way of seeing transference is as emotional reactions towards an other that originate not from the way the other actually is or behaves, but from the patient's earlier experience and interpersonal relationships. Killingmo (1971) defines transference as "all the feelings and behavioural patterns which the patient shows in relation to the therapist, and which are unconscious repetitions of relationships he has had to other persons in his earlier life history" (p. 124).

In the case outlined above, the first part of this was considered, inasmuch as the therapeutic relationship has the patient as its focus. The issue is not whether the therapist is one to fall in love with, or whether he has special qualities—everyone is potentially just that. In addition, the special point about the therapeutic relationship is that the therapist shows only a limited part of his personality. What can be emotionally difficult and potentially a strain for the therapist is that he is aware of the fact that the other—the one he is to help—is in love with him. The patient goes through a number of painful and difficult feelings precisely because the therapeutic situation and relationship is about not responding. The patient's suffering is no longer caused by the others outside the therapy-room; the therapist is himself one of the conditions that cause suffering. It was in this situation that I found it helpful to work with the concept of presentation. The other part of the concept of transference—that the other's reactions stem from earlier experiences and interpersonal relationships—opens the door for creating another concept for oneself: presentation. The phenomena we see should be worked with as they are presented or as they appear. Attention is not directed at the history of interaction and experience, which is concealed. It is the surface and not the depth that is our concern here. Let us form an image. We can speak of breadth and depth as aspects of our experience. Depth as an experience in time (e.g. as history) and in space (e.g. as inwards in a landscape or downwards in a psyche) are all well-established metaphors in the psychoanalytic metaphor apparatus. Spence (1987) refers to Dreyfus and Wakefield (1987) regarding the use of breadth as a metaphor. One can speak of a breadth-psychology on a level with a depth-psychology. The latter often has archaeology as its image. For breadth-psychology, the image of a clearing in a forest is used. In line with this, I find that depth-psychology brings associations about a focus kept steadily at one point, where one uncovers layer after layer while maintaining the same focal point. This point is pictured as the individual, and we get classical depth-psychology.

In breadth-psychology, many objects and phenomena present themselves in the clearing. One sees a panorama of events and objects and their relationships to each other. Breadth-psychology has the relationship as its main concern—not how it has been deposited as a point covered by new deposits, but how it presents itself and takes shape here and now. We have to think of the individual in a connection, in a situation or context characterized by heterogeneity and complexity. In therapy, this situation includes the therapist and the relationship between the therapist and the client. In depth-psychology, the focus is held as the therapist limits his or her involvement. The therapist can register his or her reactions and make use of them, but strictly speaking it is important that he or she is kept out of it as much as possible. In breadth-psychology, the emphasis is different. The central issue is the current relationship and what is presented in it. In order that this may turn into a relationship that can be used to become acquainted with oneself, the patient must meet relational phenomena involving the therapist's reaction–action register in a personal way, but not beyond the domain of the therapeutic relationship. The clinical problem will be to explore and find out what this implies in terms of concrete being-together and interaction. The issue about boundaries and delimitation, and about letting oneself become involved in and by the other, becomes a concern for both the patient and the therapist. Let us look at an example.

### *"The therapist"*

She came and wondered where I would go when I was on leave. What I would do, and whom I would meet. She dwelt on the thought of whom I would meet. I changed focus and asked her how the week had been for her. She returned to her question about whom I would be with, and whom I might meet. My response was to say that this was not the topic here at this moment. We started working with her material.

In the next session she began by saying that it was good that I had become angry. She had understood that she had gone too far, and that it was important that I had put her in her place. This had made her realize that I, too, was a person. I was dumbfounded and amazed. I had not been angry, and I said so, but she strongly maintained that I had been angry, but that it was fine. I began to feel that this was all wrong. I had not been angry. She responded with a smile expressing that she knew I had been angry. It did not matter what I said. My uneasiness became strong and persistent. The previous session and its feelings returned to me. I thought I had brought back her topic, and not that I had been angry. Yet there was something there. Gradually it came to me that—yes—I had felt that there was something I had to keep to myself. She had experienced her falling in love with me as a preoccupation about whether I would see other women. Had this not become too intimate for me? Had I not wished to avoid this topic? Had I not felt something like a hint of anger? Suddenly it became clear to me that even if I found it difficult to call it anger, I still had to admit that she was right. I tell her this, and I continue by saying that it was precisely this that I did not manage to feel properly during the session. It would have been too difficult to admit anger towards one who was a patient, who was in love with me, and who was interested in whom I was meeting. It was also difficult to acknowledge my anger openly, because it would reveal something about myself. It felt too private both to admit feeling angry and not to have been able to own up to it. It felt anti-therapeutic to become angry and to reveal oneself.

She said it was not her business what I did with my feelings. She said this in a caring way. It felt good to her that she had known how I felt. My denial did not threaten her. She had not become confused as she had always done previously. That was a good experience. But, in addition, she felt that it had been good to experience me as a person through my anger and through my admission that I had wished the feeling to go away. It was good for her to experience that our relationship could also be a place of learning for me. This feeling was mutual. An exciting event had been experienced by both of us as filled with a forceful intensity. For both of us there were personal histories linked to this intensity, but the central issue was that this intensity was experienced, examined, and talked about as something to do with both of us and our relationship.

### *Closure and contamination*

In the first clinical vignette, one can say that the theme was delimitation. The therapeutic element in this situation is not to respond to her feeling. Responding to being in love means leaving the therapeutic field. There is a limit to the types of relational forms that can occur and where the relationship can still be called therapeutic. In the second clinical vignette, the topic is of a different nature. A kind of grey zone is created where the therapist's feelings become the topic, and where the therapist does not delimit his emotional life from what is happening in the therapy. One assumes that the therapeutic element here is that the therapist lets himself slide into precisely such a grey zone. Again, I feel the need for a concept that would enable me to enter here and examine these relational forms as therapeutic ones.

To enter into an area of grey zones, ambivalence, and vague limits makes one feel fearful. It feels like walking on shaky ground. One can lose one's footing. For a therapist to lose his footing can often entail that he no longer experiences himself as a therapist. The characteristic experience of these situations is that different phenomena overflow into each other. The one becomes a part of the other or is mixed up with the other. It results in contamination, contagion, or diffusion. If closure and delimitation is the topic in the first vignette, then one can say that contamination, pollution, and contagion are the topics in the second vignette. "I know that you are angry", while the therapist experiences contamination, through his private feelings overflowing into a space that he has been trained to keep out of.

I shall use the concept of *closure* about what happens in the first vignette and the concept of *contamination* about what happens in the second vignette. The rationale of the choice of these concepts is that they point both to something that one could call good or positive and to something one might call bad or negative. The positive part about closure is the setting of a limit that makes it possible to be delimited. One can set up a wall against being invaded. The negative part is that one can let oneself be isolated. One can shut oneself off from the outside world, one can try to step out of relationships, and one may end up excluding dependence.

The positive part about contamination is that one lets oneself blend with the other. One can let the other's feelings and experiences reside in one. One can attune oneself to other's affects, and one can let oneself be affectively attuned. Dependence is not a menace, it is security and safety. One lets oneself be enveloped and involved in the other. The negative part is that one can be invaded, polluted, and destroyed. To be or not to be as a person is at stake. Closure and contamination implies an existential field of tension in which we are all living and with which we must cope in all kinds of circumstances. In therapeutic relationships, this becomes especially important and difficult since this is not a symmetrical relationship: the therapeutic relationship is a relationship with an unequal distribution of power. One has to tread particularly cautiously because of the therapist's superior position of power and the patient's vulnerability on account of her or his position and suffering. In my experience, most therapy theories and clinical descriptions give clear instructions as to how to act in order to avoid invading and impinging on the autonomy of patients. Here, the way in which I have used the concept of closure makes it into a central aspect of autonomy. By definition, dependence and contamination represent a more opaque area. One therefore needs concepts and thinking about how to proceed within this area. This chapter and chapter 7 attempt to show that there are situations and modes of acting that cause the therapist to set out into these difficult waters, where action, personal and emotional involvement, and participation are crucial for the therapy.

## *Technical terminology as a problem*

In today's family therapy, the central focus is the client and the client's perspective (Anderson, 1997; Duncan, Solovey, & Rusk, 1992; Miller, Duncan, & Hubble, 1997). Traditionally, an important part in the development of technical and professional skills has been to develop a conceptual apparatus and technical terminology. To be initiated into a profession and a professional orientation is linked precisely to acquiring this terminology. One way the profession or the professional orientation delimits itself from others is, among other things, the way one speaks. The result has often been alienation and marginalization of "the others". Even though the concepts basically invite new relational forms, one sees that they can easily become signals pointing to a conservation and fixation of relational forms. They have become signals affirming a perspective or a theory. They become increasingly decontextualized; they are given significance not through the context in which they appear, but from earlier contexts or connections. They bring forward a repetition of an already fixed context, and they maintain and function as a conserving element. The good part is that they represent a fixed perspective from which the world can be viewed and experienced. This perspective implies order and a firm point of departure from which one's own clinical practice can be evaluated. The danger is that the concepts in themselves can be given a status of importance and that they begin to appear disconnected from a concrete interaction or meeting between the client and the therapist. We get a mystified technical terminology that does not exist in a local context in which it could promote life and possibilities. Instead, it creates compulsion and limitation. Technical terminology has become an instrument of power.

In my clinical practice and also in my work as a supervisor, I feel that I have often been confronted with the above. In my work in an adult outpatient clinic, for example, I was struck by the fact how easy it is to regard everything the client presents as transference. Transference has become a kind of template for interpretation on the basis of which everything is explained and understood. Psychotherapy has become synonymous with working with transference. In the context of family therapy, one finds the same phenomenon—namely, that new words begin to live their own lives and fill the clinical space. Concepts such as *solution* (de Shazer, 1994) and *narrative* (White, 1993) are on the verge of getting a hypnotic aura, where the word itself seems almost to guarantee change. One way of reading the history of family therapy is precisely to follow the development of concepts that have had clear meanings in certain contexts but gradually begin to show greater promise. They develop an aura of being final solutions.

Implicit in this discussion is the aim to develop a context-sensitive technical terminology—an involved conceptualization in the sense that the words that are used are linked to concrete interactions. This also refers to the fact that developing concepts that can supply alternative or supplementary perspectives in the work one is doing depend on functioning as a difference that makes a difference (Anderson, 1997; Bateson, 1972b; Keeney, 1983). Seeing and experiencing differently requires different conceptualizations. Bringing up unfamiliar and diverse concepts forces one to think again over one's situation and perspectives. When this is done, the next step will be to see if the options made possible by the concepts can be conveyed in a language that does not promote mystification and affiliation to the field, the theory, or the profession. This implies that it is not the aim of the concepts used here—for example, closure and contamination—to survive other than what is remembered as having once been useful. They should remind one of possible relational forms that have been useful. Developing as a therapist means, therefore, being someone who collects relational forms and forms of being-together. These, again, can be useful in concrete contexts, but otherwise they imply a kind of nostalgia. They are what one might call *memorabilia,* which invite themselves to be understood and discussed in everyday language. It is as a part of everyday language that they can avoid becoming alienating instruments of power. In everyday language, the relational forms and the social arrangements that are encouraged by the concepts are further developed inasmuch as this language is accessible to more people than those belonging to the limited profession or theoretical schools.

In this chapter I have attempted to argue in favour of the notion that conceptualization is an important part of the work of thinking and an aid in clinical work. This applies especially to contexts where the clinician finds him/herself in unknown territory or areas where he/she is uncertain about what to do. These are situations where local knowledge must be developed in the very interaction with the patient. I have maintained that the goal of such conceptualization is to facilitate and create new and supplementary relational forms and forms of being-together. What is it about relational forms and forms of being-together that can promote change and have a therapeutic effect? Let us look at this more closely.

### *Corrective and supplementary emotional experience*

This chapter deals, and does chapter 7, with a closer look at client groups and situations where the traditional approach to therapy does not seem to be sufficiently helpful. Both chapters have the here-and-now-relationship as a recurring issue. In chapter 7, the keywords are affect regulation, mastery, volition, and intersubjectivity and then putting into words and using these in a narrative form in attempts at specifying the content in the client–therapist relationship. This chapter has continued this task by presenting the concept of presentation as a way of pointing at and giving substance to the concrete relationship between client and therapist. The concepts of closure and contamination have been introduced in order to direct attention to the relational and existential dilemmas that confront both the client and the therapist. The concepts have also been chosen because they point towards possibilities as well as dangers in the landscape in which client and therapist move together. Both chapters have been inspired by family therapy thinking and psychoanalytic thinking. These theoretical approaches are to be seen as conceptual backgrounds from which I have either collected ideas or which have functioned as contrasts that have made it possible for new concepts to come to my mind.

Both family therapy and psychoanalytically oriented therapy have relationship as their key concern (Gullestad & Theophilakis, 1997; Reichelt & Haavind, 1996). The concern of family therapy with a relational understanding of the phenomena and the psychoanalytic focus on the therapeutic relationship, as well as the significant relationships that have contributed to our development, can all be seen as different facets shedding light on what one could call the *relational perspective.* Based on the thinking in this chapter, one can say that these theoretical perspectives supplement each other. Traditionally, the psychoanalytic perspective is historically and ethologically oriented in terms of emphasis on the transference here and now. Naturally, this does not mean that the main concern of psychoanalytic thinking is not the current relationship between client and therapist (Zachrisson, 1997), but that, in the last resort, the work with transference represents a cornerstone in the therapeutic work.

Alexander and French (1946) make a subtle distinction here through the concept of corrective emotional experience. This concept clarifies the relationship between transference and the current or real relationship between client and therapist. They point out that traditionally there has been a tendency to emphasize the repetition of an old conflict in the transference relationship; it is the similarity between the old situation and the transference situation that is stressed. The significance of the difference between the original conflict and the current situation in the therapy is, however, often overlooked. Alexander and French maintain that since the therapist's attitude is different from that of the significant others in the past, the patient is given the opportunity to approach difficult feelings under new conditions. In this way, the patient can cope with these feelings in a new way. The concrete experiences in the therapeutic relationship make this possible. Alexander and French emphasize the difference between the contribution of the original significant other in the interaction and the therapist's contribution to the interaction. The concept of presentation also points to the relationship between patient and therapist. On the other hand, the attention is not primarily directed at a correction of an earlier experience.

In my experience, adolescents seldom described their relationship to their parents as traumatic or pathological. They were sometimes angry or dejected, but in the last resort they would describe the relationship mostly as being good. In relationships where the parents had carried out severely traumatizing and offensive acts, these acts were indicated and talked about, but other aspects of the relationship continued to be regarded as good. The content of the stories told by these adolescents was that their relationship to their parents had been both difficult and good. Of course, one could choose to regard this as a defence against and a denial of difficult realities. One might regard their loyalty as a reaction to fear or as an understandable reaction of young persons who had no other choice but to support difficult parents.

However, I have found it important and useful to accept their reactions as factual descriptions of their relationship to their parents. As a consequence, in therapeutic work correction is not the primary necessity. Correction might easily bring the therapist into a competitive relationship with the parents, and this again might stigmatize the parents as generating pathology. This does not seem to conform with the adolescents' own experiences. Apart from that, the parents are naturally important elements in the external and internal lives of these adolescents. If the therapist presents the parents as generating pathology, he or she may add to the adolescents' burden: "I am a child of bad parents." Of course, what these adolescents are describing is that they sometimes experience their relationship to their parents as difficult. Issues concerning limits, performance at home and at school, and potentially risky behaviour with drugs, driving, and other youthful activities are for most young people central areas of conflict.

The assertion in this chapter is that emotional experience is a central aspect of therapeutic work. For a number of patients, I do not repudiate the importance given by Alexander and French to corrective emotional experience. However, my own experience points to an additional fact—namely, that a great deal of emotional experience in therapy is of a different nature. The emotional experience taking place in what I have called presentation is supplementary, in the sense of being both similar and different. Parents and therapists are different persons, and they have different roles. Together they offer a diversity of modes of reaction and action which supplement each other. For adolescents, they can represent a repertoire of possible actions from which they can choose. They also offer a diversity of emotional experiences. In my opinion, this makes it possible for them to experience options where neither the parents nor the therapist need to be disqualified.

In cases where abuse or traumatizing actions have been committed by the parents, it appears that it is still important to maintain a relationship to the parents without denying the abuse or the trauma. The idea of a combined corrective and supplementary emotional experience seems to facilitate this. Correction is given to the traumatic events. Important and significant parts of the parents' modes of acting are confirmed through similarity with the therapist's modes of acting, while at the same time new ways are offered via supplementation. The message is that each situation can be confronted in different ways. Some of these are traumatizing, others are not. Some of the parents' ways of acting are traumatizing or hurtful, others are not. The relationship to parents can be maintained without a denial of traumas and mortifications. One can get on with one's own life.

The concepts of corrective and supplementary emotional experience have been useful to me. They have made it possible to enter into dialogues and to be with both parents and adolescents. Similar to the other concepts and thoughts mentioned in this chapter, they have sprung up when working with patients and their families in situations where there was uncertainty and confusion about how to proceed. The actions or forms of being together that the concepts have given rise to, or which have arisen through these concepts, are acts and forms of being together that have made me feel involved in the patient and the family. What does this mean?

## *Sensations, involved thinking, and concept formation*

In this chapter, it has been my wish to let a chain of thought unfold itself. The point of departure is the clinician's experience in his practical everyday life. It is the clinician's subjective experience that is the point of departure. Special attention is also directed to situations where the clinician is uncertain of how to understand what is happening and how to act as a therapist. The encounter with the client—the therapeutic relationship—presents itself as a multitude of relational and actional opportunities that fill the therapist with uncertainty and ambivalence. Here, I raise the issue of the use of technical terminology in this type of context. New concepts and new meanings of old concepts included in the thinking around the clinical situation have been the tools that I have attempted to exemplify. "Involved" is the term I have given to this conceptualization and thinking. Here, the term "involved" implies that as a therapist one lets oneself be touched, that one experiences, senses, or feels one's encounter and one's relationship with the client. Daniel Stern has presented a hypothesis about the infant's experience, sensation, or perception in the encounter with itself and the outside world. In this book, we describe this from many different angles. I shall examine here two aspects of these senses of self. First of all, it is their emphasis on immediacy, on the here-and-now, on the temporal closeness when encountering others; second, their two-sidedness as both nonverbal and verbal.

Stern says that the five senses of self exist side by side in the adult. They appear directly in one's own and others' contribution in the interaction, and they are both verbal and nonverbal. Let us have a look at the encounter with the client in interactional episodes that are uncertain, as I have described above. It is my experience that word and non-word appear in the immediate encounter. Words can have something to do with both immediate and earlier experiences, while the nonverbal has to do with sensations in one's own body. Uncertainty and ambivalence manifest themselves in the insecurity of both the body and the words. Are the words relevant to the situation? Are they involved in the significance of having to deal with what is happening here and now, or has their significance been transferred from other situations? In the terminology of this chapter, transference and presentation are supplementary perspectives, but it is presentation that has been brought into focus. This means that one first and foremost wishes to emphasize what presents itself in the encounter, or to understand in the sense of creating concepts and thinking that emphasize the here-and-now. "Involved" implies, therefore, directing one's attention to bodily sensations and experiences, to see which words, concepts, and trains of thought these will bring forth. In constructivistic-oriented therapy (Anderson, 1997; McNamee & Gergen, 1992), one has traditionally been interested in the question of how language brings forth, creates, or constructs experiences and sensations. This chapter has argued in favour of the idea that bodily sensations, perceptions, or experiences of relationships and situations also bring forth, create, or construct concepts and thinking. I find it useful to think that language and non-language are circular phenomena.

Daniel Stern (1985) uses two particular concepts to refer to the nonverbal experience of coherence and organization: amodal perception points to an immediate perceptual unity or coherence across the sense modalities, and affect attunement gives an experience of coherence and unity across persons. Intersubjectivity and understanding appear as possible nonverbal phenomena. Both these concepts refer to bodily processes—the first to perception, the other to affect. The first points towards individual experience, the other towards a common or shared affective experience. Verbalization can be enforced by clinical judgement in the sense of a perception of oneself and others and by having contact with it through affectively registering and perceiving the other—that is to say, through affect attunement. It will be experienced or sensed as a bodily state that forces or elicits words—not any kind of words, but words that "cover" or point to something similar to what the bodily state comprehends. This occurs within a common language in which some conversations or discourses are preferred or else are dominant (White, 1993). This implies that common language and culture set limits and directions for how bodily sensations are to be expressed. For this reason, therapeutic work has to deal both with expressing the bodily sensations and experiences of the client in his relationships, and also with elucidating the discourses restricting the client's possibilities of action and experience in these relationships (White, 1993).

I shall let this passage put a temporary stop to this train of thought. It does not stop here, of course, but in order to evolve it will depend on continuing in a different medium from the written one. It must continue to be experienced in clinical practice. Through involvement in concrete relationships with a client or clients, new concepts and thoughts will be formulated. The practice or the interactions included in this text can already now be looked back on in order to see whether some of the words, concepts, or thoughts that have been used to present and comprehend this practice can still be used in a form presented here, or whether they have already turned into memorabilia. Have they become reminders about something that was helpful once upon a time but that is now about to be formulated in new contexts in new ways?

CHAPTER ELEVEN

# Opposite and dilemma: reflection on therapy as a meeting place between psychoanalysis and family therapy

*Rolf Sundet*

The attempt to create conceptual aids in one's own practice can sometimes lead to a short-lived experience of having come across something new—short-lived, because a search in the literature quickly places the "findings" in an established therapy tradition. Chapter 10 can be read as reporting on a work of conceptual development linked to a particular clinical situation. Especially at the outset of this work, I experienced a new mode of thinking and acting connected to the concept of presentation. One aspect in this work was using the concept of transference as an opposite in order to bring forth and clarify this mode of thinking and acting. This use of the concept of transference brought about a search in the psychoanalytic literature. Reading about modern psychoanalytic thinking soon taught me that my current thoughts were not particularly new. It seems that in modern psychoanalytic thinking, the problems I was confronted with by my client are dealt with in discussions about the concept of transference. In what follows, I would therefore like to pursue the development of this concept. This review will lead to a way of thinking about opposites and dilemmas. I wish to apply this thinking to parts of the history of family therapy and today's positions in the field. The aim is to point to challenges and developmental areas for therapy.

Family therapy refers to formulations and practices that have their origin in communications and systemic theory (Hoffman, 1981; Sundet, 1993). One perspective in this field is that one of the driving forces in its development was antagonism towards psychoanalysis (Hoffman, 1981; Schjødt & Egeland, 1991). The field developed as an opposite and alternative to psychoanalysis. They were competitors in the therapy and theory markets of the 1950s, 1960s, and 1970s, and this antagonism is still kept alive today in many clinical and theoretical contexts. My concern here is not to confront or resolve this antagonism. From my point of view, these are two independent theoretical and clinical approaches to psychotherapy. I see no reason why they should "be unified" in one single approach.

My concern in this chapter is to pay attention to theoretical formulations connected to what goes on in therapy. This means that my primary sources here are not actual experiences in therapy, but experiences connected to reading theory—that is to say, to the encounter with and experience of the text. Needless to say, this is something other than experience with clients, even though the texts are dealing with such experiences. I find it natural to emphasize this divide by making use in this chapter of direct quotations from original texts.

One of the concepts that is about to be included in the everyday language of therapists is *discourse*. The concept is often associated with Michel Foucault, but it can be linked to a number of sciences and approaches (Mills, 1997). Foucault (1972) speaks of "practices that systematically form the object of which they speak" (p. 49). He emphasizes at the same time that the concept cannot be reduced to one meaning. Sometimes he treats the concept as "the general domain of all statements, sometimes as an individualized group of statements, and sometimes as a regulated practice that accounts for a certain number of statements . . ." (p. 80). Psychoanalysis and family therapy have, as mentioned earlier, been traditionally opposed to each other. However, I wish to argue in favour of their both being part of a discourse, in Foucault's sense, dealing with all statements on the whole, but also with special statements and practices connected both to our culture in general and to the specific cultural practice called psychotherapy. My concern in this chapter is therefore to see how these opposites might shed light on some of the dilemmas that every psychotherapist in our culture group will have to face.

## *Psychoanalysis*

My role in relation to psychoanalysis will be that of the visitor. I have no training as a psychoanalyst, but am fascinated by the literature and the thinking this field has produced and is still producing. My relation is also influenced by my critical attitude, but always in such a way that every time I try to delve deeper into the material in order to clarify my criticism, I tend to become interested and caught up in it. My critical point of departure is soon forgotten, and I am fascinated. As soon as I gain a certain distance to the field, especially through my clinical practice, the critical part in me is revived. This implies that I am both "familiar with" and "unfamiliar with" psychoanalysis. I am quick to assume a negative and critical attitude, but I am also easily fascinated. This makes one take "big" words into one's mouth, but one always ends up being reality-oriented. If I become critical and point to deficiencies in psychoanalysis, I soon discover that I have been unaware of the debates that may have existed already from the very beginnings of psychoanalysis. If I become enthusiastic and get carried away, I most often face a clinical reality or experience that brings me back from the sphere of psychoanalytic mysticism.

Psychotherapies based on psychoanalytic theory can be said to be characterized by the fact that they "aim at a thorough working through of unconscious conflicts and character attitudes. The central therapy concepts are free association, resistance and transference/countertransference" (Zachrisson, 1997, p. 25). It is the relationship between the client and the therapist, the analysand and the analyst, that is the central focus in the therapy. Transference is emphasized as one of the most important aspects. In its most general form, transference is "displacement of emotional attitudes from one psychic situation or representation to another" (Killingmo, 1971, p. 122). In this form, the concept of transference is not linked to the therapy situation. It is a normal reaction in the sense that in all psychological reactions there are degrees of transferred material from other situations and representations. When asked why I am doing what I am doing, or experiencing what I am experiencing, I might answer that it is because I am the person I am; furthermore, that I am the person I am because I have lived the life I have lived, because I live in the context I am living in, and because I have the genes that I have. Psychoanalytic thinking stresses here the importance of life experiences as a focal point, and it indicates that all experiences continue to remain with us in life. Killingmo (1971) speaks of "fundamental patterns of affect ... a model for how the person will later react to and become attached to other people ..." (p. 123). These fundamental patterns of affect can be changed under conscious control. The greater the unconscious part, the less flexible will the person become. Where fundamental patterns of affect have been repressed due to conflicts, they will "be repeated undiscriminately later in life" (p. 123). In therapy, transference will be increasingly marked by regression as the therapy progresses.

In addition to displacement, the central elements in the transference are repetition and projection of inner representations. The concept of transference connected to the psychoanalytic therapy situation can therefore be defined in the following manner: "all the feelings and behavioural patterns which the patient displays in relation to the analyst and which are unconscious repetitions of relations he or she has had to other persons in his or her earlier life history" (Killingmo, 1971, p. 124). Laplanche and Pontalis (1980) indicate that the concept of transference is difficult to define because a great number of authors have given it a very broad meaning, inclusive of all the phenomena that constitute the patient's relationship to his or her therapist. Bateman and Holmes (1995) emphasize that the concepts of psychoanalysis are characterized by "elasticity". Psychoanalysis and psychoanalytic thinking is a heterogeneous domain with diversity and controversy attached to all its aspects. Psychoanalysis is not a static domain. As all other theories, it exists in a social, scientific, and cultural context. Psychoanalysis has been evolved and is still evolving within this framework or horizon of understanding. Binder, Holgersen, and

Høstmark Nielsen (1998) underline the relational perspectives as the most prominent ones in today's psychoanalytic psychology; the focal point in this development is that "psychoanalysis must be firmly rooted as a theory of people's relational life" (p. 1151). The interesting part in our context of their examination of the psychoanalytic field is an increasing emphasis on the emotional here-and-now.

Chapter 10 made a distinction between transference and presentation. The aim was to make possible a here-and-now that would not let itself be disturbed by the there-and-then in the therapist's reflections. Attention was transferred from depth to breadth, and from archaeology to clearing: the surface is the area one wishes to examine. The metaphor of depth and archaeology invites one to search beneath and behind. It underlines the immediately given as the façade, and this always invites one to search behind this façade. It also seems to invite an inquiring attitude marked by suspiciousness, a kind of friendly paranoia. What presents itself is never what it pretends to be. The metaphor of breadth with the clearing—that something is shed light on—invites an exploration of any perspective that is brought forth, without there being an assumption that it is anything other than what is presented. The predominant attitude is reflective naiveté rather than friendly suspiciousness.

I would like concepts to facilitate relational forms and forms of being-together (Deleuze & Guattari, 1996). Implicit in this—in our context—lies an assumption that these forms of being-together and relational forms are central elements in psychotherapy. The emotional here-and-now is one way of speaking about this. One also speaks about the relationship as being real or factual (Binder, Holgersen, & Høstmark Nielsen, 1998). What one sees is that the distinction between transference and presentation seems to be approximated within psychoanalysis, and that this happens within different understandings of the concept of transference. I would therefore like to continue exploring this concept. The point of departure is to use a distinction between *classical* and *modern* practice and thinking as regards the concept of transference (Bateman & Holmes, 1995).

The classical meaning, as presented by Bateman and Holmes (1995), is synonymous with the already mentioned definitions. The patient transfers onto the analyst earlier experiences and strong feelings that he or she has experienced earlier in his or her relationship to mother, father, or siblings. The patient is not conscious of this and experiences the feelings as being connected not to the past, but to the actual here-and-now situation. The therapy is about interpreting the transference in such a way that the past can be revealed and reconstructed. Insight helps one to get over earlier traumas. The analyst must be seen as a neutral screen or background onto which the patient projects his or her infantile wishes. This perspective emphasizes the reconstruction of the past.

The modern meaning of the concept of transference is displaced from being seen as an expression of unconscious mental forces to what Bateman and Holmes (1995) call "the emergence of latent meanings" (p. 97), which is awakened by the intensity of the therapeutic relationship. Bateman and Holmes portray transference as a far broader concept involving the interaction between the patient and the therapist, where it represents both mental conflicts and the interaction between internal representations. It is the "medium" in which the patient's internal drama is played out together with the therapist. It deals with "a new experience influenced by the past, rather than a repetition of an earlier one" (p. 98). The image emerging here is that "the classical" and "the modern" interact and together form today's psychoanalytic understanding of transference. This appears as a kind of heterogeneous matrix that covers and evolves a number of aspects of the therapeutic relationship. I prefer to understand this in the perspective of a supplement. It concerns supplementary ways of describing and creating the therapeutic relationship. Bateman and Holmes's discussion of this issue is based on three questions. The first is whether one should regard transference as a distortion of reality or as a tenable representation of a present unconscious situation, coloured by experiences from the past. The second is whether transference is a general or a specific analytic phenomenon. The last question is whether transference is the whole analytic situation or just parts of it. I would like to have a closer look at the first of these three questions.

The development of different understandings of the concept of transference can be described as a movement away from focusing on the distortion of an objective reality, towards regarding reality as (inter)subjective. The analyst moves from being a neutral or empty screen towards being regarded as one who contributes through the interaction. In addition, there is a movement away from the historical perspective with its focus on what happened there and then, towards a focus on what is happening in the relationship here-and-now. Bateman and Holmes (1995) emphasize that what is happening here and now is often only vaguely influenced by events and internal constellations from the past. The modern psychoanalytic concept of transference appears to have been radicalized in different ways. It is no longer a specifically delimited concept but, rather, an underscoring of the fact that what a person brings into a situation has many sources, but the decisive factor will be the here-and-now relationship. The psychoanalytic focus is maintained since the concern is unconscious fantasies and conflicts in the here-and-now situation. In the modern perspective, the way in which the patient reacts to the therapist must be seen as representing what one might call a current fantasy or expectation that is inaccessible to consciousness and therefore requires a transference interpretation in order to bring it out into the open (Bateman & Holmes, 1995). We can see here that the depth metaphor is still valid inasmuch as the focus is on making conscious what is unconscious, and what is made conscious is only indirectly linked to earlier experiences.

On this basis, in terms of the concept of transference, psychoanalysis can be seen as existing in a field of tension. This tension area exists between a there-and-then orientation and a here-and-now orientation. Fields of tension like these can often be characterized as dichotomies or conceptual opposites. When working with the concept of presentation, I experienced how easy it was to place it in contrast or opposition to the concept of transference. There would also be a sneaking tendency to rank or emphasize the one as positive and the other as negative. One might almost say that one concept was labelled as "all-good" and the other as "all-bad". I think it is important and useful to me as a therapist to reflect on my own tendencies to produce such opposites. It is also my opinion that it is necessary and useful to see these dichotomies and opposites as expressions of the culture we are living in (Griffiths &

Whitford, 1988). These issues are under discussion in most specialist fields. Luce Irigaray (1985a, 1985b) and Jessica Benjamin (1988, 1998) are two examples in the field of psychoanalysis.

### *Dichotomies*

The French philosopher Jacques Derrida (1981; Norris, 1987) asserts that the structure of the Western way of thinking is based on these dichotomies or polarities: good versus bad, being versus nothingness, presence versus absence, truth versus error, identity versus difference, soul versus body, man versus woman, life versus death, nature versus culture, and so on (Johnson, 1981). According to Johnson, these are not independent and equal. The second term in the pair is seen as "the negative, corrupt, undesirable version of the first . . ." (Johnson, 1981, p. viii). These concepts must be seen as standing in a hierarchical relation to each other, which gives priority to the first term. Whitford (1988) presents Irigaray's criticism of the Western concept of rationality. Like Derrida, Irigaray understands Western rationality in a similar exclusionary perspective. In Irigaray's opinion, the man–woman symbolism is used to present human nature as characterized by these relationships of dominance and subordination. She attacks these presentations and, according to Whitford, presents thoughts conveying that "psychic health may be conceived of . . . as a state in which both parents, i.e. both the male and the female elements, are felt to be in creative intercourse within the psyche" (Whitford, 1988, p. 111)..

Jessica Benjamin is interested in the same type of dominance perspective on the relationship between the sexes. The crucial point for her is that the woman, as in Irigaray's presentation, functions as the man's primary other. In this landscape, one suspects that there may be a series of opposites that also cause problems. Let us first take our point of departure in a psychoanalytic understanding that has often been formulated as: "where id was, there ego shall be" (Freud, 1973, p. 112, quoted in Frosh, 1997). This sentence carries the seed to problems. One can say that this sentence expresses "the advocacy of meaning over chaos, thought over suffering, integration over splitting, symbolization over symptom, consciousness over unconsciousness . . ." (Benjamin, 1998, p. 115).

In many ways, this is a description of the ideals of the Age of Enlightenment: "the autonomous, coherent, rational subject" (p. 115). The criticism of the ideal of enlightenment points precisely to the problem in the sense that it implies preferring one element in an opposite or binary opposition. A metaphor used here is that it or the other is marginalized. It is pushed out of the field of vision or is concealed behind or under the dominant element in the conceptual pair. We then have the situation that "repressed parts" stand central in this perspective. The criticism of this perspective also implies that "the repressed" always can or will return. The return of the repressed is a key element in all psychoanalysis (Wilden, 1972). As a defender of traditional rationality, psychoanalysis is therefore in danger of "losing itself".

In the 1990s, both within family therapy in particular, but also in our culture in general, the concepts of postmodernity, postmodernism, and postmodern thinking (Kvale, 1992) have increasingly become key concepts. One can speak of the postmodern moment (Marshall, 1992), where postmodernity can be regarded as the era we are living in, postmodernism as the cultural expression of this era, and postmodern thinking as this era's scientific and critical thinking (Kvale, 1992). The postmodern criticism can be seen as representing "a crisis of authority for the western knowing subject posed by the refusal to stay silenced on the part of those whom this subject has cast as Other; natives, colonials, woman and all who are placed in a client relationship to expert, professional authority" (Yeatman, 1994, p. 187). One problem here is that one might easily place postmodern thinking in opposition to modernity. In my estimate, the central element in postmodern thinking is precisely to approach dichotomies and opposites in a different way from turning them into opposites that always seek to exclude one of the parts. In this perspective, postmodern thinking does not become something that is in contrast to modernity. It is more a question of this thinking being seen as a part of modernity's critical reflection on itself. For psychoanalysis this implies, for example, that the rational and the irrational do not exist as exclusionary opposites, but that it is more a question of the elements existing in an existential area of tension. They represent dilemmas. The *Concise Oxford Dictionary* defines a dilemma as a "situation in which a choice has to be made between two equally undesirable alternatives". Etymologically, dilemma is derived from "*dilémma*, a double (*di*) *lémma* or assumption" (Partridge, 1979, p. 156), a double assumption implying an experience of discomfort, of being put in a predicament. I shall therefore, in the following, use the concept of dilemma about these fields of tension between concepts that are often regarded as opposites or binary oppositions and are experienced as uncomfortable.

### *Deconstruction*

Let us have a closer look at this via the concept of deconstruction. Deconstruction is one of the concepts that have attached themselves to the name of the French philosopher Jacques Derrida. I do not wish to start a debate on this concept here but will, instead, present an interpretation of it. Norris (1987) writes that to deconstruct a piece of writing is to undertake a kind of strategic reversion that reaches out for details that one has not paid attention to in the text. These can be metaphors, footnotes, and other details that are always and necessarily skipped by orthodox interpreters: "For it is here, in the margins, that is, as defined by a normative consensus—that deconstruction discovers . . . unsettling forces at work" (p. 19). Culler (1989) maintains that what has been relegated to the outer edges or set aside by previous interpreters can become important precisely because of the reasons that led to its having been relegated. To interpret means to discover what is central in a text or a group of texts, similar to the practice in scientific tradition. On the one hand, the marginal works within this understanding against a reversal of a hierarchy, against showing that what had been thought of as marginal previously is actually important. On the other hand, this reversal bestows importance on the marginal in such a way that it not only leads to the establishment of a new centre, but to an undermining of the very divide between what is essential and what is non-essential.

I have chosen to give an interpretation of deconstruction here that lays emphasis on not letting anything take precedence, or on the fact that two concepts in such a relation shall combine into a higher unity. It is a matter of bringing out aspects or elements that have been concealed from or been outside the field of vision of those reading the texts. It also implies that both of these elements must be permitted to exist in the text, albeit in a reversed form.

Deconstruction presents and clarifies conceptual pairs that in our culture tend to become opposites. Deconstruction does not remove them or turn them into something else, but clarifies them as aspects or elements that cannot exclude each other. Their degree of importance can be reversed, but one cannot escape from them or get out of them. My interpretation here will therefore be that deconstruction can be seen as a kind of descriptive activity bringing forth and clarifying double assumptions, to which one can link experiences of discomfort because one is put in an awkward situation. I will use deconstruction here as a metaphor for bringing forward and clarifying dilemmas in our lives. This mode of defining deconstruction does not make the dilemmas disappear. This way of viewing dilemmas also attempts to demonstrate that they are not necessarily something that can be solved in the sense that the conceptual pair is dissolved or turned into something else, but that, instead, the dilemmas may just have to be lived. To confront and work with dilemmas is to find ways of living with tensions that can be portrayed in conceptual pairs or "dichotomies". In my thinking, the dichotomies mentioned above represent existential fields of tension that can be lived in many different ways and in which some ways are more suitable, function better, or are easier to cope with for the person faced with the dilemma.

Benjamin (1998) points to an opposite that arises in connection with the psychoanalytic therapeutic relationship. She asserts that attaining autonomy is a product of a "discourse that situates the subject in the oppositional complementarities—subject and object, mind and body, active and passive, autonomously rational and irrational . . ." (p. 116). This follows the above-mentioned perspective where one aspect is split off and devalued. Benjamin's point is that the feminine is linked to the devalued aspect. The feminine is thus connected to being an object: bodily, passive, and irrational. Feminist theory and philosophy (Lennon & Whitford, 1994) support this and show how women are placed in a marginal position, not only economically and socially, but more fundamentally within the mainstream of both philosophy and psychology/psychiatry (Griffiths & Whitford, 1988; Seller, 1994). Women or "the feminine" are often placed within these fields, on the border between the rational and the irrational. Frosh (1995) maintains that this is at that particular point or border that defines the symbolic from what is outside it—for example, the normal and sensible from the abnormal and psychotic. This brings a duality into the feminine. On the one hand, a woman is always close to madness; on the other hand, she can protect herself against it. She offers "a boundary of containment, something protective allowing what is inside to survive" (Frosh, 1995, p. 293). This duality often results in women belonging neither "inside" nor "outside". Moi (1985) writes: "It is this position that has enabled male culture sometimes to vilify women as signifying darkness and chaos, to view them as Lilith or the whore of Babylon, and sometimes to elevate them as representatives of a higher and purer nature, to venerate them as Virgins and Mothers of God" (p. 167).

Benjamin (1998) exemplifies this by showing that Freud's client Anna O—in real life Olga Pappenheim, who later achieved recognition as a well-known feminist—can be used as a metaphor for this tension between the helpless, passive, and non-speaking hysteric on the one hand, and the articulate and active feminist on the other. This tension does not only exist in the analysand, but also in the analyst. Benjamin points out that in psychoanalysis one can see the problems connected to constructing the encounter between the analyst and the analysand as one between "the Analyst-Subject who already speaks and the Patient-Other who does not yet speak" (p. 116). The one who suffers needs recognition from the other, from the therapist. According to Benjamin, this recognition is only effective if it incorporates one moment of identification. One must feel what the other feels as his or her own. In Stern's (1985) terminology, one can speak of an attunement. The delimited subject must admit the other's state, and one is no longer delimited. (Using the terminology from chapter 10, one may say that the therapist must let himself or herself be contaminated by the patient.) Benjamin also asserts that the other is given a language, which means that he or she will only verbalize the symptoms through identification with the speaking subject, the therapist. The patient is in danger of losing himself or herself as an "other". Benjamin (1998) says: "If the patient must 'become' the analyst, the analyst must also 'become' the patient" (p. 116). This double identification leads to a breakdown of complementarities such as "knower and known, active and helpless, subject and object" (p. 116). She goes on to say that these thoughts are crucial in the reformulation leading to the intersubjective and relational revision that has taken place within psychoanalysis (Benjamin, 1998; Binder, Holgersen, & Høstmark Nielsen, 1998). Benjamin (1998) says that the objective is to "formulate a space in between suggestion and objective distance, which encompasses the analyst's emotional response to the patient [and which] takes account of her or his involvement in the complementary transference action as well as the means for extricating herself or himself from it" (p. 129). In this process, the patient becomes less objectified and the therapist more subjectified. The main point when dealing like this with complementarities or opposites is to transform them into "dialectic tension, into tolerable paradox instead of into antinomies that compel dangerous choices" (p. 129). This implies that going through dilemmas, living with or in them, is at the core of psychotherapy. I interpret this as being identical with the above-mentioned metaphor for deconstruction.

The movement in the meaning of the concept of transference has, in my story, moved its focus towards a mutuality between the therapist and the patient; this story is trying to illustrate that when something is brought into the centre, it is, at the same time, important to grasp what it marginalizes. This will clarify existential tension, dilemma, or paradox. Mutuality will, for example, always exist in a relation of tension when faced with lack of mutuality. The danger with these new intersubjective and relational formulations is that one may believe that mutuality between the therapist and the patient makes them similar. This will cover up and conceal the obvious differences in power and control that are implicit in the positions of therapist and patient. The relationship is precisely characterized by both mutuality and non-mutuality.

## *Family therapy*

Let us now have a look at family therapy. Can the above-mentioned story have any significance for family therapy? Is there anything in the described movements within the concept of transference that can direct one's attention towards movement within the field of family therapy? Can a clarification of opposites and their interpretation as dilemmas be of any importance for family therapy? If the dichotomy and the establishing of binary opposites are part of the Western discourse, how does this present itself within the field of family therapy as a part of this discourse?

Kirkebøen (1993) reprimands the field of family therapy by pointing out that the field has not incorporated the metaphorical character of its concepts. In one particular field, which had earlier taken the statement "the map is not the terrain" (Bateson, 1972b) as one of its central statements, one discovers that forgetting metaphors has a tendency to come about, especially when new formulations are launched. One of the main ideals in our Western science-orientated culture has been "hard science". In order to avoid being branded as a charlatan or quack, one has to place one's therapeutic activities within this scientific domain. Within this domain, it has become increasingly clear that language is not a neutral tool for communication. "The linguistic turn" (Pålshaugen, 1997) within philosophy and science demonstrates that the topics and concerns of science never come unmediated (Haraway, 1991). The implications of this are, of course, expressed in different perspectives on science. In the field of family therapy, social constructionism (McNamee & Gergen, 1992) has been a central formulation of these circumstances. On the other hand, there are formulations showing that traditional science has included these aspects in its activities and that the perspective and critical comments of social constructionism are irrelevant to science today. These comments are incorporated in modern science (Grenness, 1998). I do not wish to continue this debate here but would like to indicate that the hunt for scientific legitimacy often seems to lead to the search for equality between, on the one hand, modern technology and formulations within the traditional "hard sciences" and, on the other, concepts and explanations one uses in terms of human and interpersonal conditions. It is as if by turning mankind into an example of what the machine is, one legitimizes the concepts one uses precisely for humanity. The paradox, however, is that quantitative ("hard") science makes it clear that something is qualitative ("soft" science), linguistic, and metaphorical. The sciences that have been traditionally associated with "soft science" sometimes seem to forget this more easily than those associated with "hard science". This is most evident when one introduces a time perspective. The further away in time, the easier it is to recognize the metaphorical character of the concept, while the metaphorical character of current concepts can be easily overlooked. Concepts such as text, narrative, and deconstruction used in a family therapy context are as much metaphors as information, feedback, and system.

Our look at psychoanalysis in this chapter has revealed two positions: first, a movement from a focus of understanding or insight into how former relationships and experiences control or decide reactions here and now to the fact that it is actually the fantasies and conflicts in what one might call the emotional here-and-now that are influenced and changed through the interaction here-and-now. In this movement, one can sense a displacement from linguistic insight to new, factual relational experiences. The second position deals with the way in which some concepts become central elements and how others are thrust out or "repressed". Let us now have a closer look at the dichotomies or conceptual opposites that have dominated the field of family therapy.

Hansen, Johnsen, and Sundet (1994) indicate different dichotomies in the history of the field. Based on a debate connected to what was termed first- and second-order cybernetics (Maruyama, 1968), both Speer (1970) and Hoffman (1971) raise the question of whether the models used by family therapy are only useful in terms of describing stability. No satisfactory presentation is given of what generates change. Bateson (1980) formulates the relation between stability and change by using the metaphor of the tightrope walker. A tightrope walker has to make a change in the form of his movement in order to keep himself on his tightrope. Stability is not an either/or, but a both/and.

The metaphorical use of deconstruction which I have chosen here encourages me to look upon dichotomies as existential fields of tension. The relationship between client and therapist places both in dilemmas. The experience of being in these dilemmas is characterized as existential fields of tension. Furthermore, my interpretation of this metaphor suggests that these dilemmas are often not solved—they have to be lived. Sundet (1997) uses psychiatric diagnostics as an externalization of problems (White, 1989) to help persons with psychotic symptoms or those needing help for modes of functioning that are described by diagnoses of personality disorders. In my work, I was continually confronted with the question of whether the symptom should be changed or learnt to be lived with. In the case of a patient where the borderline diagnosis was used as an externalization, our discussions circled around the issue of whether we should work with his tendency to place people in the category of "only good" or "only bad". We shifted constantly between accepting this tendency, and thus finding ways of preventing that it had too many negative consequences, and exploring paths that might dissolve or remove this tendency. For the therapist, it felt like moving around in an existential field of tension that would not go away and in which one had to find ways of living.

Development in the field of family therapy has in many ways kept up with developments and debates in the sciences, and these have been a source of inspiration. Within cybernetics, Heinz von Foerster (1984) presented the expression "the cybernetics of cybernetics". This concept is derived from Margaret Mead (Keeney, 1982). Together with Gregory Bateson she had worked in, among other places, Bali and New Guinea. Also, they were married to each other. For them, and also in a number of other contexts, their professional, personal, and private relationships were strongly interwoven. This makes me see clearly that the purely professional and the purely personal—for example, as expressed by concepts such as objectivity and subjectivity—also has to be regarded as an existential field of tension. This is what the expression "the cybernetics of the cybernetics" calls attention to. One could say that a brain studies a brain. What is true for the studied brain must also be true for the brain that is studying. Aspects in the studied brain say something about what causes the studying brain to bring forth what is brought forth. Qualities in the studying or observing system blend into or contribute to what the studied or observed system represents (von Foerster, 1984). During the 1980s, this was expressed in the distinction between first-order and second-order cybernetics (Hoffman, 1985; von Foerster, 1984). The focus was moved from the study of interaction and communication in families to how therapists and family members regard and have come to regard this interaction.

In many ways, there were in fact two focuses in the point of departure for family therapy: one was on interaction, the other on communication. All behaviour was looked upon as communicative, while at the same time the interactional patterns were also of interest. One could in some ways say that the field existed between these two. Communication was primarily about influence; this influence sometimes resulted in changes in interaction, which again implied a communication about the relationships of the family members. One could change communication and/or interaction therapeutically (Watzlawick, Beavin, & Jackson, 1967).

An important concern in Watzlawick, Beavin, and Jackson's well-known book from 1967 was to show that meaning is not a central concept in their work. They write: "'meaning', a notion that is essential for the subjective experience of communicating with others, but which we have found to be objectively undecidable for the purposes of research in human communication" (p. 44). Their central concern is: "a search for pattern in the here and now rather than for symbolic meaning, past causes, or motivation" (p. 45). In addition to suspecting a clash of interests with the psychoanalytic tradition, with its emphasis on symbolization, past history, and motivation, one sees the field's attention directed at behaviour and interactional patterns.

Campbell and Draper, in their book from 1985 about the applications of systemic family therapy, express the following about the relationship between meaning and action: "In our view, meaning and action are two sides of the same coin" (p. 6). Campbell, Draper, and Huffington (1988), furthermore, write that "Meaning and behaviour have a recursive or circular relationship. We voluntarily behave as we do because we have certain beliefs about the context we are in, and our beliefs are supported or challenged by the feedback from our behaviour" (p. 16).

The concept of meaning, which was refuted in the 1960s and 1970s, had—as we can see—its renaissance in the 1980s. In my reading of history, this is precisely connected to the above-mentioned dichotomy between the objective and the subjective, between the shifting of focus from the observed to the observing system. During this period, Humberto Maturana became a central theoretician for the field of family therapy. He placed "objectivity in parentheses", in the sense of forbidding himself to refer to objectivity as a legitimation of his presentations and explanations (Sundet, 1988). When findings and explanations were presented, he wished to legitimize them through the actions he carried out,. What is brought to the fore is brought to the fore through language (Maturana, 1978; Sundet, 1988). Through Maturana, the focus of family therapy is on language. One aspect of this was that, for Maturana, meaning was not a central concept for specifying language. His focus was on language as the coordination of actions (Maturana, 1978).

Parallel with the field's interest in developments within the systemic sciences, it moved on further in terms of practical innovations in the therapeutic space. One important example of this is the Milan group's subsequent development of the one-way mirror and team positions, as a movement away from focusing on intervening interaction and towards explorative conversation through questioning and generating hypotheses (Selvini-Palazzoli et al., 1980). Here in Norway, the Tromsø group (Andersen, 1987b) expanded this work by making use of the reflecting team. In addition to this clinical work, Tom Andersen has played an important part in presenting the thinking and practice of others, especially the work of Harry Goolishian. The work of Goolishian stands on its own two feet, of course, but Tom Andersen's consistent referring to Goolishian as an inspiration and important conceptual enthusiast as regards the reflecting team has, in my opinion, contributed to Goolishian's renown in the field.

In 1988, Tom Andersen enthusiastically arranged a conference, "A Greek Kitchen in the Arctic", in Sulitjelma. At this conference, Harry Goolishian proclaimed that family therapy should bet on a different horse. With the introduction of language, one had to distance oneself from the field's main preoccupation with systems theory, cybernetics, and the machine metaphors used in these theories. Language, in his opinion, was about creating meaning and about interpretation. The new metaphors should now come from hermeneutics, literary theory, and linguistic philosophy (Goolishian, 1988). From this point, family therapy's interest in language seems to have exploded, and there have been a number of formulations focusing on the importance of language. In connection to these formulations, new practices and techniques are specified and old ones have again come into their own. The fact that Carl Rogers's practice and formulations have gained new relevance (Miller, Duncan, & Hubble, 1997) can serve as an example.

Let us now take one step back and look at this chapter's specification of dichotomies. I have chosen to start my story with the problematization of the relationship between stability and change that took place during the 1960s and 1970s. A different dichotomy emerges in this work within cybernetics. The relationship between subjectivity and objectivity is problematized through concepts such as first- and second-order cybernetics (von Foerster, 1984) and radical constructivism (von Glasersfeld, 1984). In this work the role of language gradually becomes more important. Family therapy of the 1990s can in many ways be regarded as bringing language and meaning into focus. The postmodern approach to therapy is a concept that keeps on turning up in this context. It is represented by Harlene Anderson, Harry Goolishian's collaborator of long standing. For Anderson (1997), the centrals parts of therapy are "language, conversation and relationship . . ." (p. 1). She also says that "a therapy system is one kind of relational language system in which people . . . generate meaning with each other" (p. 72). The production of meaning is, for her, the central element in therapy. Meaning denotes our interpretations and our understandings. These are "linguistically and jointly constructed through spoken and unspoken language" (p. 206).

We have seen that in psychoanalysis, one movement is from linguistic formulations through interpretation of the transferred there-and-then, to interplay within the emotional here-and-now. In family therapy, we can sense an opposite movement, from the behavioural here-and-now to the linguistic here-and-now, but where the focus is on generating meaning. It is not my task to challenge or change any of these perspectives on therapy. They have produced and are still producing a series of exciting formulations around therapy. Within family therapy, I have concentrated on Harlene Anderson's book. A number of other authors could be mentioned (e.g. Freedman & Combs, 1996; Lundby, 1998; Parry & Doan, 1994; Riikonen & Madan Smith, 1997; White, 1995, 1997). The matter I am pursuing here is that we are immersed in a cultural practice and discourse that has a tendency to produce conditions and events such as dichotomies and opposites. Moreover, one aspect or part of such a dichotomy has a tendency to be pushed into the background, or simply to be forgotten. Strong emphasis on language and meaning implies marginalization of non-language and non-meaning. This, to my mind, clarifies the language/non-language, and meaning/non-meaning dichotomies.

### *Non-language and non-meaning*

Let us now look at what non-language and non-meaning can be. By doing this, we are entering into the field of tension of this dichotomy, because it is also through language that we seek to approach it. What we are seeking to grasp is conveyed through language, and it is marked and tinted by this language while at the same time being non-language. Perhaps one should not talk about this. One might perhaps interpret this as something almost divine, where, for example, only "fools rush in, and where angels fear to tread" (Bateson & Bateson, 1987), or in any case, that what one cannot say anything about, one ought to keep one's mouth shut about. I do not intend to turn this into a theological or philosophical issue but, rather, into a practical one. My point as a therapist is to direct attention to dilemmas and dichotomies and to what these can make me forget or overlook. The language/non-language and meaning/non-meaning dichotomies might make one tone down events in situations of being together that cannot be conveyed through the first two concepts in the conceptual pairs. What, then, can non-language and non-meaning actually signify in a therapeutic context?

I have earlier mentioned language as a coordination of action. A more precise way of expressing this is that language arises when one has a coordination of coordinations of action. Coordinated action is not language, but when one has such a coordination and this leads to a coordination of action, then one can speak of language (Maturana, 1978). The important point here is that meaning does not have a central place in this kind of understanding of language. Dance is a good metaphor for coordination. What characterizes dance is that the movement of the one becomes the point of departure for the movement of the other. It is what takes place in contiguity to action which is the point of departure for further action. For me, in therapy, it is this temporal closeness that non-meaning is about. When psychoanalysts speak of the emotional here-and-now, family therapists speak of interaction, and developmental psychologists speak of interplay, proto-dialogue, and preverbal dialogue (Hansen, 1991a; Stern, 1985), then one of the central events here will be occurrences taking place in temporal closeness.

Focusing on contiguity leads one to look at interplay here and now—how actions are chained together and how they can be specifically evolved. The therapist becomes an agent acting together with the clients. One may speak of a joint action developed by client(s) and therapist(s). The description in chapter 7 of therapy with adolescents can exemplify these thoughts. The important point here is that one does not need to speak of meaning, even though these joint actions are almost inevitably given meaning. By focusing on what takes place in temporal closeness to an action, one has taken a step forward into learning psychology and back to the former orientation in family therapy towards interaction. My particular interest in the ongoing development of therapy in our culture leads me to observe the implications of this aspect of therapy. Therapy implies not only generating meaning and reflection but also close participation, where one floats along without necessarily knowing where one is going and, even if one does know, it is not certain that one will arrive there. As meaning-generating human beings, we can always generate meaning from these movements. We can create narratives about them, but perhaps this movement is based just as much on what happens at the moment as on the meaning we ascribe to what is happening. For this reason, the therapist needs to be a participant who is embedded in a togetherness of action with his or her clients, just as much as in a togetherness of meaning. This also implies letting clients be participants of this kind, and not always moving them towards generating meaning. Non-meaning is not meaninglessness but, perhaps, only experiential togetherness. We live our dilemmas together, we feel and experience them, and we can—but do not always need to—create narratives about this togetherness.

CHAPTER TWELVE

# To know or not to know— or how do we know that we know?

## Some remarks on the relevance of theories of knowledge for clinical practice

*Vigdis Wie Torsteinsson*

The paraphrase, in the chapter title, of one of the most famous quotations in world literature is a living example of the fact that this is not only a "modern" problem. Throughout the entire drama, Hamlet is preoccupied, even engrossed, in the question of how one can have true and certain knowledge about others. In one of the scenes we meet the king and the queen, Hamlet's stepfather and mother, who are worried because Hamlet is still grieving over the loss of his father. The queen asks:

> If it be,
> Why seems it so particular with thee?
> Hamlet: Seems, madam! Nay, it is; I know not "seems."
> 'Tis not alone my inky cloak, good mother,
> Nor customary suits of solemn black,
> Nor windy suspiration of forc'd breath,
> No, nor the fruitful river in the eye,
> Nor the dejected 'haviour of the visage,
> Together with all forms, moods, shapes of grief,
> That can denote me truly. These, indeed, seem,
> For they are actions that a man might play . . .
>
> [Act I, ii: 74–84]

This short passage can be read as a comment on one of the constantly recurring questions about the nature of knowledge. Is it sufficient to observe the exterior characteristics of a person's conduct, the observable dimensions that are accessible to all, or must we take into account something that can be called "an interior", something that is only accessible from the "inside" of a person's consciousness or body? Hamlet expresses here *his* understanding of what is needed to have a true and certain knowledge of others—for him, the inner, subjectively experienced world is the only reality. And this is a position easily recognized by therapists.

Under the word "science" in the *Norsk Riksmålsordbok* [The Norwegian Dictionary of Standard Language] the following can be read: the study, examination, exploration (of nature, individuals, society, culture) undertaken to reach a greater understanding of reality, built on objective, systematic, methodical compilation and sifting of single phenomena and the adaptation of these to generally valid laws or principles. The *Riksmålsordbok* has taken a different stand from Hamlet on what knowledge is. Here it is the knowledge *from the outside* that is central—nothing is understood or explained before it can be understood as something applying to us all as common laws representing the ways of human beings.

## The current debate on the nature of knowledge

Two key concepts form the framework for this presentation—namely, *truth* and *knowledge*. We are constantly reminded of the need for more knowledge in today's professional debate. Increased knowledge is called for from different quarters as a means of presenting more competent, productive, or effective treatments to our clients. No one will question this, even though one can heartily disagree about how to solve this issue in order to find the best answers. As an example, I would here like to quote from an editorial in the *Journal of the Norwegian Psychological Association*: the editor, Geir Høstmark Nielsen, says that both nationally and internationally one speaks a great deal about *knowledge-based health services*:

> The disagreement deals more with the issue of what is valid and relevant knowledge for clinical practice (predominant research perspective), and which research methods, procedures, and instruments are most suitable to procure this knowledge. This debate clearly shows, in my opinion, that clinical psychology (as well as psychiatry) is still moving in the special and demanding field of tension between natural science, social science, and humanities—between naturalism and hermeneutics, between positivism and hermeneutics, between classical and constructivistic concepts about truth, between absolutistic and contextual understanding, between quantitative and qualitative forms of documentation. If one does not include this fact in one's considerations, then "knowledge-based practice" can easily be used as an argument for a limited perspective on knowledge and dubious imperialism regards method.
>
> . . . It is, however, neither original nor helpful merely to demonstrate that there are alternative and competing ways of regarding the world, science, and our field. The practical consequences of the diversity of perspectives will first appear with full strength at the moment when *someone* shall decide which epistemological and methodological foundation should be applied to . . . an evaluation scheme. [Høstmark Nielsen, 1997, pp. 857–859; translated for this edition]

Høstmark Nielsen points here to the necessity of maintaining a nuanced perspective on the concept of knowledge. However, in concrete discussions it often seems that we have to take sides: that the alternative paradigms represent mutually precluding ways of thinking. It *is* important to see the differences, to be aware of what different paradigms define as knowledge. But perhaps it is just as important to maintain a diversity of perspectives, precisely to keep an open mind about the consequences of our choices.

The debate in the same journal between John Rønning (1997a, 1997b) and Gert Henrik Vedeler (1997) about standardized diagnostic procedures is an illustration, among others, of a current and concrete variant of this discussion. The topic of the debate is that some Norwegian outpatient clinics have introduced what is called "standard documentation procedures" in order to—as it is expressed—strengthen the identity and professionality of the field of child and adolescent psychiatry.

The intention is definitely good: they wish to make a point of assessing whether the clients' problems have diminished in the course of their contact with the psychiatric services, and whether they are satisfied with what they were offered. The underlying assumption is that these requirements will be guaranteed by standard procedures on admission and termination. The procedures consist of standard questionnaires to be filled in, where the results are quantifiable and thus comparable.

Criticism of these procedures is first and foremost directed at placing instruments like standard questionnaires between oneself and the client in the first session. This fails to

> take into consideration the unique situation which in every single case should be established between a client-system and a therapist-system. The way in which one meets the client, the family and the child, is totally decisive for the subsequent course. Having to place a number of "instruments" between oneself and the person one meets, will hardly ensure quality, rather the opposite. [Vedeler, 1997]

Implicit in these formulations is also a criticism of the specific theory of knowledge which is represented by standardization thinking, where one does not take into account that the way the question is formulated does, in a sense, also constitute the answer. From the opposite point of view, the argument is that clients appreciate being met with a professional seriousness that implies that their problems are thoroughly examined (Rønning, 1997a, 1997b).

For me, this is an example of the importance of the theory of knowledge for our "everyday clinical life". When taking a stand in this kind of debate, one can of course also take one's point of departure in the common sense of ordinary experiences and preferences. But it can also be useful to have knowledge about the options and limitations in the various positions of the epistemology debate. As Jean-Paul Sartre might (possibly) have put it: "If one chooses one thing, then one fails to choose another thing." If one chooses standardized forms as the basis for one's knowledge and understanding of a client family, then one possibly fails to choose the realization that this knowledge is a kind of co-production between what one as a therapist and the clients are contributing (Andersen, 1987a). The dialogue between a different therapist with other ideas and other questions would have "co-produced" a different family. On the other hand, if one is exclusively preoccupied with "co-producing", one may overlook the difference between situation-specific topics and general topics in different contexts, which may be an important factor. I shall return to this later.

To my mind, the theories of knowledge represent, first and foremost, rituals for guiding one's curiosity. I have a question, I am wondering about something. And the theories of knowledge try to give me an answer about what to do in order to find something that can be called an *answer* to what I am wondering about.

The theories of knowledge are therefore important *both* for establishing the knowledge we use in our practice *and* for evaluating the usefulness of our contributions to our clients. However, the theories of knowledge can also be seen as systematizing and refining more general ways of thinking and arguing when we are to give reasons for something we believe to be true or correct (Midgley, 1989). In this respect, it is not essentially different from a logic we all use in different contexts. For this reason, it is also important in the encounter with clients where we are supposed *both* to use already established knowledge *and* become acquainted with a new world, a description of reality unknown until that very moment of dialogue. I hope the examples I have chosen will make these options more explicit.

## *Knowledge and truth*

The fact that we need knowledge is, in a way, a non-controversial assertion. But when one problematizes the relationship between *truth* and *knowledge*, as one does in today's postmodern debate, the concept of knowledge becomes an extremely controversial dimension. In the world of scientific theory, one distinguishes between realism and relativism. The realist believes that there is a world around him of which he can have true and certain knowledge. For the relativist, everything is literally relative: no world exists beyond our constructions of it, or, alternatively, it is possible that there is a world beyond our constructions, but we cannot know anything about this (Potter, 1996). In this type of debate, a social constructionist will, for example, say that "there is no objective truth, there is nothing in the world which in a way forces us to conceive of it in definite ways". And it is certainly not difficult to agree to this—on one level. Because if one asks two persons who have just had a meeting with each other to describe this meeting, it would surprise most of us if we were given two identical descriptions. And which one of them is most "correct", most true? In family therapy, it is precisely concepts like neutrality that are signposts for the therapist in terms of giving equal validity to all the different descriptions of a situation or a problem. The different *perspectives* are thus providing depth and variation as an aid in the work of change and contribute to deconstructing the dominant narrative, opening up to the alternatives, the exceptions. In this context, one may call the differences useful without having to worry whether some of the versions are "more truthful" than others. The concept of usefulness has in this understanding taken the place of the earlier concept of truth (Gergen, 1994).

For me, however, this is in many ways an unsatisfactory solution. To my mind, at least, *usefulness* is not a good replacement for what the concept of truth was meant to take care of. In other professional contexts, truth is still a persistent problem. This applies, for example, to cases where there is a question of whether a child has been exposed to sexual abuse, or where there is a question of a deficit in parental care. In these context, one's conclusions as a professional as to whether it can be called true or not play an enormous role. Here one can *not* argue that one version is as good as the other, or that the concept of usefulness should be an adequate description of the intention to ascertain whether an abuse has actually taken place. My most important argument advocating that we as professionals ought to relate to and take interest in the theories of knowledge lies in this range between the fact that different descriptions of reality are equally good and the fact that there are descriptions that are truer than others. First, we need to answer in which sense and in which way the issue of truth is important or significant. Second, in continuation of this, we need to take a stand on how we can find out something about what are the true or valid answers to the questions we pose.

There are two additional comments to be made on the concept of truth. It is as if the word has become too big for us, that we are reluctant to use it because it involves more unalterable and universal factors than we wish to represent. The favourable aspect of this is that it forcibly generates a humility in us in relation to the limited perspective that each one of us, at any given time, can have. The problematic part, in my opinion, is that we can risk shirking our responsibility to choose and prioritize between different descriptions.

When someone asserts that the extinction of six million Jews during World War II is a falsification of history, it is easy to dismiss this as an assertion made by crazy people—in this area we know what is *true*. We can even say that this is an *objective truth*, even though these are words that we would otherwise never take into our mouths.

The concept of truth is often used synonymously with "objective truth"—something that is true at all times, in all contexts, and from all viewpoints. Thomas Nagel (1986) has called this "the view from nowhere". This usage probably arises from the fact that the scientific debate about truth has been dominated and defined by a quantitative and empirical perspective. Far too much thinking about scientific method has asserted that the only way of producing truth is by way of observations that are not dependent on who asserts them or where they are at any given time. It *is* the earth that turns around the sun—and this is true, irrespective of whether it is you or I asserting it, or whether one of us happens to be in China when the observations are made. But in my opinion it is a misunderstanding to believe that the qualitative researcher is less concerned with *truth*, even if the truth she or he is looking for is local and perhaps even unique. If, for example, one chooses to expose me to a qualitative and partly self-directed interview about my therapeutic practice instead of sending me a quantifiable questionnaire, the reason for this will be that the qualitative interview gives a more correct—or truer—picture of my therapeutic practice. And when we as family therapists do *not* want to operate with general theories about "sick" and "healthy" families, or proclaim ourselves as observers of the families we meet, is not part of the reason always that this gives a more truthful picture of what is actually going on?

What the philosopher of science calls *the pretension of truth*—meaning the wish to attain true and valid knowledge—follows all scientific activity and, thus, also all that we call *knowledge*. The theories of knowledge are precisely this giving of guidelines about how to acquire reliable and valid knowledge. And for us practitioners, this is especially important—for, each time we make a diagnosis, give an evaluation, or draw a conclusion, what else are we doing other than saying that we have a certain type of knowledge about the individual or the people it concerns and the situation in which they find themselves? We can be more or less certain, we can be preoccupied with our own role in presenting this knowledge, we can call it situational—but it is always a kind of knowledge. And perhaps one may also say that in a certain sense it is precisely this that the clients are asking for—an understanding, a knowledge that they feel they need but are themselves unable to produce?

### *Is empiricism useful?*

I personally have given some thought to the fact that traditional empirical research in many contexts is of great significance in both the large and the small context. One example from my own practice as both a child therapist and a family therapist is the change that has taken place during the last ten years in the understanding of the child's earliest development. The developmental psychology that has dominated clinical psychology has traditionally consisted of variations related to Freudian theories. These have largely been based on experiences with the childhood memories of adult clients, and they have then been included in understanding therapeutic processes with children. It is not easy, as we know, to question infants, so the development of theory in this area has come about by, for example, pointing to measurable changes in the attention or recognition patterns that one has decided to *understand* as an answer.

Daniel Stern, one of the central persons in the field of developmental psychology, has used new empirical observations of children's earliest relationships to evolve an alternative theory for the understanding of the child's earliest developmental process in relation to its care persons. This theoretical framework offers new possibilities both for individual therapy with children and for family therapy (Stern, 1985, 1995; see also Hansen, Johnsen, & Sundet, 1994).

Judy Dunn is another researcher studying children's development. Among her many contributions that are relevant in this context, only her empirical studies of children in their normal home environment will be mentioned (Dunn, 1988, 1993). By changing the premises for the study, she demonstrates, for example, that children are *not*—as Piaget claims—egocentric until about the age of 7 years. According to Dunn, small children have a natural keen interest in their close relationships, including in the sense of trying to understand how the world is experienced by others. And for a family therapist who has been taught to think that "the whole is more than the sum of its parts", and that the predominant communication pattern or family premise is the element controlling each member's understanding and experience of reality, it is useful to see Dunn's concrete documentation that, in a certain sense, children in the same family do, in a way, grow up in different families. Her empirical indications make it possible to understand the family premises *both* as something common to all and as something unique, where each family member in a sense maintains his or her own perspective on the predominant whole. This point is also underlined by Jerome Bruner in *Actual Minds, Possible Worlds* (1986). However, the application of this knowledge must also have its roots in the concrete therapeutic dialogue about perspectives. As Bruner demonstrates in his book, it is only the dialogue with clients that decides whether this knowledge will result in suggestions that will develop into important clinical contributions.

In all clinical work, an empirical basic attitude is inevitable. A very great number of our evaluations are small empirical studies. If a mother cries in our first session, I can look upon it as a situational phenomenon; if she is still crying in the ninth session, I will certainly have different thoughts about it. The *quantitative* difference makes a *qualitative* difference for the way in which I understand her crying.

A simple seminar evaluation is also a small empirical study. One or two members of a group may be dissatisfied, but it is regarded as a different phenomenon if *everyone* in the group is dissatisfied.

These are examples of one of the characteristics of all empirical thinking—namely, that "together we are strong" and "the majority is always right". By its very nature, democracy is a purely empirical phenomenon. This means a great deal to us in very many contexts. If, in a team discussion, one hears the argument "but is it not like this in families with anorexia", then for me, at least, it will make a difference if the person saying this has worked with just one or with a hundred of families with an anorectic child.

## *What do we understand by empiricism?*

Empirical knowledge begins with a hypothesis that is operationalized—that is to say, it is transformed into distinct units that can be measured or counted. Concretely, it is often formulated as a question or a statement with fixed response alternatives. This means that my possible responses have to fit into fixed categories that, again, can be compared to the responses of others. Each time I fill in these quantifiable questionnaires, I feel frustrated. Let me illustrate this with an example. Some time ago I took part in an investigation into the "living conditions" of therapists. One of the questions was: "How often have you been ill during the last year?" Ill and ill—in how many ways can a simple word like that actually be understood? If I have gone to work with a cold—is that ill? If I have a headache after having been up all night working with something that I should have done a long time ago—is that ill? The end of it was, of course, that I decided that it meant "to stay home from work", so I answered no. Consequently, my answer did not, on another level, give a true and accurate picture of what my life had been like these last months. I started having problems because I was uncertain whether my categories for "ill" were concurrent with those of the inquirer—I would have needed several specifications in order to give proper answers. At the same time, I also know (I suppose) that, if the inquirer really is interested in the state of health of therapists, it would have been interesting for him or her to know something about my actual health—because the answer he or she gets is more about my bad conscience about staying away from work than about being a sick or healthy person. For *my* need, this definition—just the word "ill"—became too simple. This frustration often occurs when one is asked to categorize answers on the basis of a conceptualization that one is not certain is in agreement with one's own. This can happen because the topics are difficult to operationalize precisely, or because the definition splits up something that for the person replying is a part of a story or context where one needs to understand the whole in order to know how to understand the part. And when this happens, the only thing that helps is to clarify that every single answer only has meaning as part of a story, a context, a way of *using* the word. This meaning will disappear completely when all one can do is to tick off a category or underline a word that one is not quite certain is in accordance with one's own ways of categorizing. The stories become examples of how one uses the word in relation to the phenomenon one is asked to categorize. They are therefore absolutely necessary, though implicit, premises in every operationalization process, no matter how descriptive it may seem at the start. Both the original categorization and my efforts to find "my" category consist of what we call qualitative or hermeneutic interpretative processes.

Operationalizing a hypothesis also means that one operationalizes on the basis of what is important for the *hypothesis* or problem, and not on the basis of what is important for the person who responds. This is not *always* an argument against empiricism, since the inside of one's skin sometimes is not a privileged position in terms of understanding oneself. Sartre makes a big point of a similar argument in his philosophical basic attitude: what other people give me is an outside, which, in a sense, can never become accessible to me. It is the others who are the experts on how I seem to others, or what I look like from the outside, even though I can have more or less well-founded hypotheses about it (Vetlesen, 1993). The other day I spoke to a father who had tiny tics that he himself was not at all aware of. No one else had pointed them out to him either. But his son was referred to the psychiatric clinic for assessment of a possible attention deficit hyperactivity disorder (ADHD) diagnosis. In this connection there are strong empirical indications that the hereditary component is important, and this was also why the physician examining the child drew the father's attention to this. In the microchip on my bank ID card, there is a lot of information about how I use my money. Maybe—or certainly—there are a lot of patterns that I am totally unaware of or consider insignificant, but that might play a role if I were aware of them. My shopping habits could therefore also be compared to others' and, perhaps, give both me and a number of marketers some ideas about how to influence these habits in different ways.

This last part—the possibilities of comparison—is the basis, for example, for all testing, be it intelligence/functional tests or personality tests. Both the Weschler Intelligence Scale for Children (WISC) and Rorschach represent tests that give a standardized stimulus—it is equal for all—and have norms for the evaluation of the responses we give, though on different precision levels. And it is the deviation from a norm that indicates that something is difficult or at least deserves extra attention. It clearly makes an important difference for a child that one has realistic expectations about what it can achieve in different areas. Comparisons are central phenomena in many interpersonal contexts. Among other things, we expose our children to it through many years of school attendance. Comparison is also a crucial part of the evaluations we make in our thinking about justice.

It can sometimes also be therapeutically useful to train clients to be able to clarify their own situation empirically. This is often used, for example, with bulimics, where one simply asks them first to register when and where they eat, and when and where they throw up (Røer, 1996). Gradually the "thin" descriptions—indications of time and place—are filled out with "thicker" descriptions of the contexts in which this takes place (Geertz, 1973; Sørhaug, 1996). This always supplies useful ideas about the contexts—for example, "it definitely always happens when I have been together with her", or "if I start thinking about . . .". The main point, at any rate, is that both the client and I, the therapist, in a certain sense now have *new* information, on the basis of which we can set up very different hypotheses. In therapy, the client's validation of the hypotheses is of importance, in contrast to situations where one only hands over information without having any control of how it is interpreted.

One difficult point for professionals in this connection is that being *too* confident of one's own theories—which one does not necessarily share with the client—can be just as uncomfortable and "alienating" as unsatisfactory empirical categorizations, because it is the theory and not the client who decides how we understand

and interpret what he or she is telling us. And it is easy to interpret the client's protest about our interpretations as, for example, resistance. In the systemic tradition, one seeks to counteract this by insisting that the therapy process or the use of hypotheses should depend on feedback from the family. But it can be a problem that the more enthusiastic one becomes about one's analytic tools, the less attentive one may become to alternative conceptions. On more than one occasion, one has let oneself be frustrated by clients who most of all would have liked to see "an expert".

## *The difficult concept of objectivity*

The concept of objectivity is again connected to the observation of simple dimensions that in one respect are visible to all in the same way. Some will also claim that there is a connection between how concretely one defines what one should observe and how little or how much theory is implicit in the observations. The purpose of diagnostic systems in psychiatry is to be as descriptive and thus as "theory-free" as possible. But this is a dubious idea. Perhaps this can be illustrated by an example from the area of sexual child abuse. In reports about abuse, an important reference for our observations is the empirical studies undertaken in relation to this group. Improving the empirical basis is regarded as a premise for gaining more and better knowledge about the consequences of abuse, so that one may be better able to deduce definite causes from the observed consequences in a child (see e.g. Furniss, 1991). The crucial issue is, of course, whether it is possible to use this type of empirical knowledge to confirm or invalidate hypotheses about sexual abuse in concrete cases. One type of empirical connection often used in abuse investigations is that of forms of sexualized behaviour in the child. On one level, this type of behaviour can readily be identified as definable units suitable for categorization and quantification. In this domain, one also has empirical data confirming that this is a mode of reaction in a great majority of children who have been exposed to abuse. Sexualized behaviour can be described as different activities or words linked to the genitals. But as soon as we use the word "sexualized", we have moved to a new level of abstraction. We presuppose an intention in the child: that it wishes to stimulate others in ways that we define as sexual. Therefore, the theory we have about children's sexuality will be decisive for what we categorize as sexualized conduct.

The advantage of having indicated an empirical link between sexualized behaviour and abuse is, first, that it says something about a *likely* link also in the concrete cases we are dealing with. Second, we can, if we agree on an understanding of sexualized behaviour, observe this in many different contexts. Because, if this phenomenon only makes its appearance in *one* context, one ought to—as a good empiricist—pose the question of whether this response is generated by situational variables more than by the child's earlier experiences.

I believe that empirical reasoning is an important part of every assessment. One part of every clinician's horizon is precisely the experience and knowledge about the various consequences of sexual abuse. And *without* this help to categorize important bits of the total amount of information, these categorizations— categorizations that we *have to* make in order to keep track of a great bulk of information and distinguish between important and not important—are based on our own, partly contingent experiences. Some of the discipline that calls for pointing at concrete and definable phenomena that one has emphasized in one's evaluations is not only useful for oneself in terms of learning a great deal about how one is thinking—it can be of vital importance also to others.

The first step in an empirical examination is therefore to agree what one shall search for. But a descriptive similarity is not sufficient proof for anything. Sexualized conduct in a child does not necessarily imply that it is a consequence of a certain type of experience. The crucial point is the rationality in the way in which one argues and the possibility of intersubjective agreement about the validity of the indicated connections. Jon Elster (1989) formulates it thus: "Explaining an event is to give an account of why it happens. Normally this comes about in such a way that we point to a previous event as the cause of the event we wish to explain" (p. 13).

So, *both* choosing events and actions that let themselves be categorized under the operationalization we have chosen *and* linking them to earlier events or actions are in a certain sense consensus-based, interpretative processes.

Empirical reasoning is therefore something other and more than pointing out that a child displays sexualized behaviour. We need to show, with the aid of both general knowledge and knowledge about the concrete child, that there is a connection between this and earlier events in the child's life—in this context, experiences of abuse. Automatic translation procedures do not exist. The knowledge we have about other children must always be made relevant in relation to the concrete child and the concrete family we work with. And this can, in my opinion, best be described as a hermeneutic process, where the significance of what we observe is a result of a comprehensive process of creating meanings in relation to the concrete context in which we work.

### *The limitations of empiricism— or the hermeneutic assumptions in empiricism*

It often happens that the phenomena we are dealing with are not easy to define or categorize. A quote from the novel *Naiv. Super* (1996) by Erlend Loe can illustrate this point. His hero is making an unsuccessful attempt at making an empirical analysis on the theme of "important and unimportant things in life".

> Yesterday I made a list of what I have and do not have.
>
> This is what I have:
>
> —A nice bicycle
> —A good friend
> —A bad friend
> —A brother (in Africa?)
> —Parents
> —Grandparents
> —A big student loan
> —A Bachelor's degree
> —A camera
> —A handful of (borrowed) money
> —A pair of almost new trainers
>
> This is what I do not have:
>
> —A plan
> —Enthusiasm
> —A lover

—The feeling that things are connected, and that things will finally turn out well
—Charming manners
—A clock

When I looked at the list today, I noticed that I have more than I do not have. I have 11 things. I lack 6 things. This ought to be a source of optimism.

But after having done some close reading of the list, it has become clear to me that it is all together a fairly unbalanced and bad arithmetic problem. It does not work out.

Some of what I have, I could easily have done without, and several of the things I do not have, seem crucial to me for being able to live the way I want to live.

I would, for example, anytime have exchanged my bad friend with a bit of enthusiasm.

Or a lover.

Anytime.

But I know as well as all the others that it does not work that way.

I made a game of adding the numbers in the lists. 11+6.

Is 17. Quite a large number in terms of essential things in a person's life.

For a few seconds I was a little proud. But it does not give any meaning at all. It is idiotic to add things one has, and things one does not have. And besides, some of the things are less essential. The clock for example. I would like to have a clock, but I will not assert that it is essential. I just feel like having one. In order to keep better track of time. As I have said, I have problems coping with time, and I believe it is better to confront one's problems than flinching from them. But is the clock essential? Hardly.

It is the same with the trainers. They are not essential either, but I have them. Maybe I can say that the clock and the trainers cancel each other out. Then it will be 10+5. That is 15. Also a fairly high figure in this context. But unfortunately just as useless and just as devoid of meaning as 17.

I have to try to think of something else.

[translated for this edition]

The author carries out a small empirical study and concludes that even though these "things" can be classified in two categories, it gives no meaning to do it in this way. The meaning of individual phenomena does *not* lie in themselves but in a story, a context, *and* in a person's evaluation of what the different phenomena mean for him or her. As figures and comparisons they become as meaningless to the person as the outer signs of grief are for Hamlet. This again emphasizes the point that theory-less observations are an impossibility—that is to say, descriptions that are not linked to a theory or an understanding binding together the individual phenomena. Here one suggests hermeneutics as an alternative: The understanding of human action always requires an interpretation of meaning and context.

From a hermeneutic point of view, an empirical approach is an ever-present problem since it does not necessarily include my self-understanding, even if I am the object of the study. What I *mean* with what I am saying, and what I am doing, is, in one way, of less interest. And if I choose to relate to another person with a standardized questionnaire, then I can lose the context in which the responses exist—the evaluations, choices, and values that are possibly the underlying reason for concrete actions. Family therapists have actually emphasized this very point: without the *context*, in a certain sense all phenomena become meaningless. The hermeneutic tradition has always relied on this, and its main thesis is that the parts can only be understood in terms of the whole.

A postmodern alternative to this could be that the meaning with my statements is not a private phenomenon; it lies in the dialogue, in the context. It is the language and the words' relationship to other words that is meaningful, not the words' relationship to a nonverbal "reality" or to my thoughts or reactions. This is also the point of departure of social constructionism.

But this generates a difference in relation to hermeneutics which I would like to underline. For the point of departure for hermeneutics is that there is a fundamental *difference* between the one who understands and the one who is to be understood. Originally, hermeneutics was a historical science whose challenge lay in interpreting texts that originated in a totally different period. Gradually it evolved to becoming a way of relating to all meaningful material—in other words, to all human actions and expressions. In terms of a client, this means that I meet her with my understanding, and the client meets me with her understanding. The fact that I understand this client does *not* mean that I shall take over the client's self-understanding with the help of some kind of empathy. Nor is the objective that the client shall take over my understanding, but that a kind of third position will develop—a new, more elaborated perspective containing both my perspective and hers. An understanding of the subject as generating meaning is important in a hermeneutic perspective.

Hermeneutics also makes a point of underscoring that processes of establishing knowledge must not be reduced to pure subjectivity. The problem of hermeneutics, however, is that everything, in a way, must be understood from within and outwards—I always have a meaning or intention with what I am doing. My actions cannot be understood without this from-within-perspective. It is what distinguishes human action from other events in the world (Henriksen, 1997). Action always takes place within the frames of historical and cultural practices, which are then interpreted by a subject. And it is here that social constructionism and hermeneutics part company, up to a certain point. The chief concern of a social constructionist is not the from-within perspective. Others may just as well have an opinion about the way in which I participate in various interactions. My actions and my self-understanding must be interpreted on the basis of what is given in the practice or interaction in which I participate. My intentions only have meaning as a product of an interactional process (Gergen, 1994).

If we choose to comprehend the subject as something more than a discursive product, then Hamlet points to an extremely complicating factor. Will we ever be really able to understand what concerns *another* person? Implicit in these theories there is actually also an understanding of the nature of the relationships. Taking a stand on how to acquire knowledge about others implies, first and foremost, taking a stand on what kind of relationship we have to each other as human beings, and what the similarities and differences between us are. Within an empirical frame, one presumes that we are similar in such a way that we can always be compared to each other, without always having to explain or interpret what we give out as information. A part of what I perceive when I am with clients gives meaning without my needing to ask what it means. A hermeneutic perspective presupposes a difference, but a difference that can be bridged or that can be resolved by creating a mutual understanding, a third perspective. Each one of us has an interior that gives meaning and intention to every action. This interior undergoes changes in communication between my world and that of the other. But the subject has a different status here from that in the social-constructionist conception. Even though hermeneutics also takes its point of departure in the individual as "being-in-the-world", it is mostly an understanding of how one builds a sense of community between subjects who *also* always experience and understand the world differently. The social constructionist Gergen strongly asserts that it is a misunderstanding to give the subject a status as a producer of meaning. The subject is a discursive product, and the meaning belongs to the relationship.

## *Concluding remarks*

In this chapter I have primarily wanted to indicate that theories of knowledge do not imply anything fundamentally different from the strategies we all use when we think we know or understand something in different concrete situations. Gaining knowledge about the implications of these different positions has made me take myself more seriously, in the sense that I have become more precise in explaining—both to myself and to others—how I think and what I base my evaluations on. These problems are simply too important not to be taken seriously, in terms both of their possibilities and of their limitations.

Also, I definitely do *not* wish to reinforce the conflict emphasized by many regarding the distinction between qualitative and quantitative method, or between empiricism and hermeneutics. A good quantitative analysis requires hard hermeneutic work both by the person questioning and by the one who is questioned. Nor does a qualitative analysis have to be immune against quantitative elements in what it tries to understand the meaning of. In his book *Actual Minds, Possible Worlds* (1986), Jerome Bruner asserts that we as a species operate with two different systems in order to generate meaning. One way of thinking he calls propositional, which corresponds to what characterizes logical/empirical analysis. The other way is the narrative, which deals with wholeness and contexts. Renouncing the one would then mean renouncing half of one's cognitive resources! And surely none of us is so smart that we can afford that.

The concept of truth may finally turn out to be an ethical concept. The despised concept of objectivity is meant to be, when one comes across it in its "natural" home environment, a kind of "antidote" against subjectivity, randomness, unjustifiable statements.

Tranøy (1986) calls the commitment to truth a constitutive norm that, in itself, cannot be true but is based on values. Another philosopher of science, Mary Midgley (1989), puts it this way: "Officially, this move to neutrality is itself just a formal one, undertaken purely in the interests of clear thinking. But the reasons . . . for making it were moral reasons, reasons concerned with the danger of taking sides" (p. 160). When one presents something as truth or a piece of knowledge, the demand for objectivity here means neutrality as an ethical demand to represent something more than one's own, private standpoint. As such this is an expression of what is important between people, more than a relation between an observation and an outer reality. The commitment to truth must lie in the relation *between* the one inquiring and the one responding—not only in the inquirer.

When one thinks of knowledge-based practice in our line of business, it is always linked to a relationship. Either it is a matter of *using* general knowledge with real other people, or it concerns having a relationship as the point of departure for *establishing* general or local knowledge. In both contexts the *quality* of the relationship is important for the kind of knowledge we can produce. And it is not possible to illustrate the good relationship, either by epistemological aids or by ontological aids. This is the domain of ethics.

A philosopher of high standing in today's ethical debate is Emmanuel Levinas (1991). He remains the leading exponent for the view that relationships are basically ethical. In his understanding, the other is always a total otherness. The relationship to the other must consequently be fundamentally ethical, and *not* based on knowledge. Turning the relationship to the other into a question of knowledge is to make him or her equal to me, thus denying the other's radical difference. Zygmunt Bauman (1993), who has nominated Levinas as "the ethicist of postmodernism", says that knowledge can be a detour around the obstacle of strangeness. "The stranger carries a threat of wrong classification, but—more horrifying yet—she is a threat to classification as such, to the order of the universe, to the orientation value of social space—to my life-world as such . . ." (p. 150). More explicitly, one can say that using or generating knowledge without regard to the quality of the relationship in which it operates will invalidate the knowledge. Knowledge does not generate good relationships, but good relationships lead to the possibility of producing and using knowledge.

Levinas can also stand forth as a radical example of something that is a fundamental topic in all ethical theory. The subject is constituted—as accountability—in this encounter with something totally alien, something that actually cannot be understood. "The premise of imagining the individual as an ethically reflecting and moral being, capable of being responsible for its own actions, and at the same time being held responsible by others for what it does, is the reason why one regards it as a subject" (Henriksen, 1997, p. 22). Consequently it becomes problematic to "decentre" the subject in such a way that one no longer sees it as the source of meaning-based and meaning-generating action. Based on ethics, we need an understanding of the subject that enables it to relate to its initial conditions. There is thinking to be done here in terms of our social-constructionist inclinations. Gergen (1994) concludes in the following way: "The individual is removed as the central concern of moral deliberation: More explicitly, if the narratives in which we are embedded are products of ongoing interaction, then problems of moral action may be separated from issues of mental state" (p. 103). Here too we find an either/or set of problems, the limits of which we should attempt to transcend.

A focal point for further thinking around this topic will have to be how to distinguish—with a point of departure in the relational totalities we all are a part of—among data that are observed, interpreted, and constituted in dialogue.

This is a challenging but important problem in relation to concrete interactional situations with children and families, since the lack of distinction creates problems for the way in which we *make use of* knowledge.

It may seem as though there is an important aspect of control in all acquisition of knowledge about other people. This is not primarily about having control over other people, but about attempts to control one's own subjectivity, perspective, and standpoint. All the methods outlined here, irrespective of which type of data they believe interactional situations can supply, have a level of intersubjectivity, universality, distance, or a priori ethical obligation as "the good" in their approach. In the same way, the instructions about articulated rationality ensure a possibility of control over the way in which one makes use of knowledge, so that it can actually function in terms of achieving benefits in practice.

Being able to give an account of both the knowledge one makes use of and the knowledge one secures in encounters with other people will imply greater frankness about how we think and what kind of ideas our actions are based on. But just as important as it is to see the epistemological reasoning for this is to focus on the *ethical* point that is emphasized here. Postmodern, family-therapeutic notions such as "not-knowing positions" (Anderson & Goolishian, 1988) and "the reflecting team" (Andersen, 1987a) express in my opinion first and foremost the same *ethical* perspective: as a therapist, I take knowledge and experience with me into the therapy-room, but I know little about the client's understanding of himself or herself and his or her reality. And regardless of how much I learn and understand, the client's perspective can never be reduced to what I comprehend.

CHAPTER THIRTEEN

# On understanding relation and ethics: an ethical perspective on the narrative self

*Vigdis Wie Torsteinsson*

'Tis writ, "In the beginning was the Word!"
I pause, perplex'd! Who now will help afford?
I cannot the mere Word so highly prize;
I must translate it otherwise,
If by the spirit guided as I read.
"In the beginning was the Sense!" Take heed,
The import of this primal sentence weigh,
Lest thy too hasty pen be led astray!
Is force creative then of Sense the dower?
"In the beginning was the Power!"
Thus should it stand: yet, while the line I trace.
A something warns me, once more to efface.
The spirit aids! from anxious scruples freed,
I write, "In the beginning was the Deed!"

Johann Wolfgang Goethe, *Faust*

We are daily confronted with situations that challenge us in different ways. What does one say to Anna, who is 16 years old, worn out, unhappy, and pregnant and who cannot even think of the possibility of being able to share her misery with the child's father or her own mother? Or what does one say to Siri, mother of a girl with severe anorexia, who secretly has read her daughter's diary? She is worried about her daughter's utterances about death, but she does not want to talk to her daughter about her concern. What is it that guides our choice of actions when we stand face to face with another person—whether client or not? Some of our pre-understanding we call knowledge in a traditional sense--about the problems we are presented with, about adequate and not-so adequate relationships, about processes of change, and about premises. However, knowledge can be so many things. It need not always seem either relevant or beneficial to the person we relate to, however adequate the empirical documentation. How can we take care of this, so that what we are offering can really be beneficial to the person who is asking for our help?

Some of this is dealt with by reflecting on the epistemological situation in which we find ourselves. Irrespective of the methods we are using, we must always consider whether it is the person we are relating to as "the object of the investigation" who eventually will have to validate what we call knowledge about the other and say whether what we call knowledge is valid in the context in which we try to use it. However, ethical problems are also constantly held forth as something important to relate to, something that takes care of human relationships *in a different way* from our knowledge-based thinking. The family therapist Harlene Anderson says that her "ideas come from an ethical position" (quoted in Holmes, 1994, p. 156). So what does this imply? Well, according to her, it means "genuinely respecting people, allowing people to experience dignity in their relationship with you and in their lives, to have responsibility for their own lives—that is an ethical base" (quoted in Holmes, 1994, p. 156). But how, then, do we distinguish between a knowledge-based and an ethical perspective on the relationship between therapist and client?

The word "ethics" is originally a Greek concept. The word "ethos" means custom or habit; the equivalent in Latin is "morals". Today, a number of authors make a distinction between these concepts in the sense that morals are ideas of what is right or wrong, connected to one's own actions or those of others, while ethics is systematic reflection on moral conduct, hence a theory of morals (Aadland, 1998). In this chapter, I have chosen to alternate between these concepts. The problematic part about maintaining this type of distinction is reflected in the way in which different ethical theories consider the relation between an individual and a relational focus. Traditional ethical theory has largely an individual focus, in which the understanding of how one can attend to the interests of another person is linked to individual qualities or skills. The ethics of the profession bears ample testimony to this. This is in stark contrast to family therapy, with its focus on the relationships as the constitutive element in the understanding of what characterizes us as human beings.

Thus the catchword for today's trend-setting family therapists is "relational responsibility". The responsibility lies in the relationship, not in the individual. However, the focusing on narratives in the current understanding of therapy opens up new possibilities of an ethical perspective that, in a certain sense, transcends the discord created by the sharp distinction between an individual and a relational approach.

## *Professional ethics*

Professional ethics is usually an outline of some important principles that one believes should be taken care of in the professional encounter. In "Ethical Principles for Nordic Psychologists" this is formulated in the following way: "the area of work is often a field of tension between dependence and autonomy, between coming in touch with the individual's integrity and boundaries, and taking care of the individual's autonomy." The first of the four basic principles is "respect for the person's rights and dignity", which is defined as follows: "The psychologist shows respect and promotes the development of each person's rights, dignity and integrity. He or she respects *the individual's right to a private life, self-determination and autonomy* in conformity with the psychologist's other commitments and the law" (emphasis added). According to the Norwegian Union of Social Educators and Social Workers' "Ethical Principles in Social Work", the first principle is independence, which is defined in the following way: "Social work is based on the value of independence. The aim of social work is therefore to enable individuals and groups to work with their own lives and living conditions, to take care of themselves and to develop independently and together with others" (Norsk Sosionomforbund, 1989/1992).

Professional thinking is therefore built on a clear understanding that the individual is the basic entity that the principles are meant to take care of. Concepts such as independence, integrity, and dignity clearly point to a historical tradition in which the individual is the focal point, at the centre of all our endeavours to take care also of what happens *between* us.

In a philosophical context, ethics represents precisely the understanding of how we take care of each other, what enables us to have consideration for each other in our interactions. An ethical perspective turns others into persons who affect us in a fundamental way (Beauchamp, 1982; Williams, 1985). Seen from a historical perspective, we may say that the more our theories about human behaviour have focused on the individual, the greater the mystery that we are able to relate to the needs and wishes of others and be attentive in relation to another person's perspective and interests.

How, then, are we to combine this with a relational understanding in which the individual is part of a common reality? We use words like "autonomy" and "integrity" in the context of ethics without so much as batting an eyelid. But in a relational context, where the sense of community is a common dimension, the client is part of a greater whole that also constitutes him or her as a person. In a certain sense, the therapeutic relationship is thus also individuality-constituting, in the sense that two different therapy contexts can create widely different images of the client or the clients we are dealing with. Implicit in the ethical principles lies a theory about the relation between the individual and his or her relationships which, in many ways, is extremely different from the relational understanding we as therapists operate with.

Therapeutic understanding, on its part, must contain a level where speaking about respect for the client's integrity will not be an unproblematic formulation.

How has this been resolved? Two classical formulations in the literature of family therapy can, for the time being, serve as examples of how the relational perspective in family therapy had an impact on our ethical thinking. First of all, I would like to mention von Foerster's introduction to "Ethics and Second-Order Cybernetics" at the family therapy conference in Paris in 1990 (von Foerster, 1991). Here he underlined that, in his view, ethics is not about pointing to the one correct alternative action, but about *increasing* the client's alternatives to act. This means that the therapeutic relationship constitutes an arena for experiencing and understanding new, alternative ways of acting. This is an ethical project in itself. But there is also another aspect in von Foerster's presentation which is interesting in this context. His justification lies in the metaphysical principle of choices connected to what he calls "undecidable questions"—questions to which there are no answers. As examples of "undecidable questions", he uses concepts such as freedom of choice and accountability, and he claims that they apply to each one of us. In these situations, it is up to "each one of us to make this decision and take responsibility for it". Individual accountability for the context in which one is a part is here a precondition for creating a greater number of action possibilities.

In line with this, Harold Goolishian and Harlene Anderson (1991) also point to the fact that a changed theoretical position implies new ways of thinking ethics. We are only ethical when we are able to cope with what is threatening our efforts to maintain openness in the dialogues. In addition, it is of decisive importance that we are able to maintain several contradictory dialogues simultaneously, without concluding any of them (Goolishian & Anderson, 1991, p. 10). Here the relationship is the focal point. The open, always unconcluded dialogue is the essence and character of ethics. But can one say that the individual makes a contribution to this? The choice is between thinking that it is the relationship itself that generates this openness as a response from the participants, or thinking that it is the individual person who contributes to this in ways that makes this openness possible. The fact that the individual can have an influence on this just by being able to make a closure, to terminate the dialogue, makes it important to focus on different ways of conceptualizing the relationship between individual and relational ways of thinking about these questions. Consequently, the individual's contribution to the keeping up of the dialogue still becomes a topic.

So the question we have to take along with us is as follows: to what extent is it the way we speak about these topics, the theoretical frames within which we find ourselves, that limits us in terms of being able to maintain a double perspective on ethics?

## *A story about ethics*

The ethical theories have their developmental history. In ancient Greece, the society was comparatively simple, and being part of the social community was not problematized in the way we have now become used to. Man, for Aristotle, was a social being who could only realize his or her potentials within a social community. "The smallest parts of society are not individuals, but two people", says Trond Berg Eriksen (1999) in his introduction to Aristotle's *The Nicomachean Ethics*. Yet he emphasizes the individual's accountability to the community. The citizens must do their very best to make the community function optimally. Consequently, one does not —as is our tendency today—make a contrast between thinking individual responsibility and good relationships.

The great change in this viewpoint occurred when, in a large number of areas, the culture had to re-assess its understandings. "The Copernican turning point", as this shift in epistemology is often termed, implied the insight that even though it *looks as though* the sun is revolving around the earth, the opposite is actually the case. The senses deceive us—we cannot rely on their telling us how things really are in our environment. All we have to go by is our own notions about what is taking place. Consequently, one is obliged to give reasons for both knowledge and morals with the help of qualities in or characteristics of the individual human being. There were too many elements of uncertainty in the relationship between man and his environment to justify any final conclusions about the external world.

What are the qualities, then, that have been extracted throughout the ages to justify our having consideration for others, our understanding of the other's well-being? The two great alternatives have been reason or feelings. For a rational thinker—for example, Immanuel Kant—reason is humanity's common property, and only reason can prevent random moods and irrational feelings from becoming the basis for our actions. Reason operates within certain categories that we simply cannot do without in our perceptions and thoughts about the world that surrounds us. We cannot relate to the "real" reality, *"das Ding an sich"*. Our categorizations are implicit in all our observation. Ethical theory becomes a combination of the categories of reason and our freedom to choose between alternative actions. Our freedom results in self-imposed rules—we agree to whatever reason shows us to be the best universal principle.

Another approach is to take one's point of departure in our inborn capacity for feelings for other people.

With reference to David Hume, this viewpoint suggests that feelings are the motivation for action. It is mostly feelings that make us act. Hume assumes that we have a kind of altruistic or universally human feeling of sympathy in us which constitutes the moral sense. One example of how this thinking is expressed today can be found in what is called the ethics of closeness, where the emphasis on *empathy* as a condition for showing consideration for others (Vetlesen & Nordtvedt, 1994) is an important element. Is it our kindness towards others, our empathic sensitivity, that enables us through our actions to focus on the well-being of others? Or does it concern the understanding of what, of necessity, is the right action, and then the choice among several possible alternatives?

The result of the breach in the natural unity between individual and community is that both knowledge and ethics have to find their justification inside the individual. Both the traditions that have been mentioned have this in common. Yet they refer to immensely different qualities of the individual—or, rather, they bring out different sides of us as aspects of something universally human. This becomes important because these qualities offer us the best opportunity for transcending our limitations, which will enable us to look beyond our little parish-pump and take care of the interests of others to the same degree as our own. Kant and Hume see our limitations in different areas. Kant sees limitations in our ability to have sympathy with anyone not close to us, so that moral evaluations based on feelings would be casual and different according to how closely connected we are to the people our actions are directed at. Hume sees our limited rationality as a greater hazard. But common to them both is the wish to find a position where every one of us can make moral choices without these choices being marked by partiality and coincidences. In brief, they wish to describe a position where the individual can transcend his or her limitations and represent a universally human perspective on the world.

We are still living with this problem. How do we react to the fact that all of us have only a partial perspective on the world and our fellow human beings and that, in order to act ethically, we must transcend it in one way or another? As specialists today, we also to a greater degree take it for granted that all we have is perspectives on the world and accept that every perspective also includes an evaluating attitude (Tranøy, 1986).

## *The postmodern criticism— and an alternative formulation*

This dilemma has a clear connection to postmodern criticism of all traditional ethical theory. The point of departure in these theories is that the focus is on the individual, and that the individual consciousness or psyche is the centre for ethical evaluations. On the subject of ethical issues, Western people are psychologists, says Kenneth Gergen (1994, p. 94). The arguments against the ethical traditions deal naturally with the fact that as long as ethics is about the relationship between people and not about the individual consciousness, we need a relational language that can be a reflection of this. From the standpoint of social constructionism, Gergen wants to reconstruct the moral language "in terms of linguistic forms for a common life", as he rather sweepingly expresses it. In other words: take our point of departure in a language describing relationships and, on the basis of this, reformulate the ethical issues.

But Gergen's social-constructionist interpretation of traditional moral language leads him to question whether we actually need a language for moral deliberations. In *Realities and Relationships* (1994, p. 106), he refers to a study by Felson, published a decade previously, of convicted assailants and the factors that had triggered the episodes of violence they had been involved in. In his commentary on this study, Gergen concludes that when ethical principles were introduced into social situations, it made the interpersonal situation *worse*, not better. He understands this as a consequence of the ethical language functioning as "a language for moral superiority". It is as though he were saying that every ethical reflection contains an "I know best, and all you do is wrong". This perspective is even more pronounced in the book *Relational Responsibility* (McNamee & Gergen, 1999). Here, the ethical language is quite simply defined as a language for accusing others. Again, the point is a profound criticism of the individual focus in all ethical theories. The ethical language is thus described as a language that puts an end to dialogue instead of holding it open. Nor does it ensure that dialogues can continue. Speaking about ethics in an individual language terminates the possibilities of further dialogues.

These reflections on this topic are, in turn, based on severe criticism of subject philosophy, especially the concept of individual responsibility. According to these authors, this focus promotes both egoism and isolation and a feeling that others can neither understand nor feel with us (McNamee & Gergen, 1999, p. 8). They state in the same spirit that this focusing has caused our culture to think of relationships as being "artificial and repressive" (p. 29).

This might have had the result that an alternative thinking would totally exclude the individual or the subject as a necessary element in an ethical theory. And yet it does not seem like it. Instead, one wishes to come to *a different understanding of* subjectivity and individuality—an understanding of the subject where relationships and belonging have an important place. They join Henry Miller, who says that "We must die as egos and be born again in the swarm, not separate and self-hypnotized, but individual and related" (quoted in McNamee & Gergen, 1999, p. 5)—a manifesto to which most of us will give unconditional support.

Therefore, on closer examination, a number of apparent opposites will disappear. But there are still important differences, since a key point in this version of a postmodern ethics is to remove the belief in individual power to act, an initiative for which each person is responsible or assumes responsibility. Or, expressed metaphorically: do we float down the river of history or of contexts without any possibility of manoeuvring on our own initiative, or are we equipped with paddles which, to a certain degree, enable us to position ourselves in relation to the medium in which we find ourselves?

There is also another problem. It is not only I as an individual who disappears independent of the relational context—so does the other as otherness. In a way, the other disappears as a concrete, living other who cannot be understood as a product of my interaction or the interactions of others with her.

Zygmunt Bauman (1993) says that the postmodern perspective is widely conceived of as embracing a total relativism. One almost celebrates the downfall of ethics and replaces ethics with aesthetics. Ethics is looked upon as a modern straitjacket that one has now thrown into the "rubbish bin of history", as an illusion that postmodern people can very well do without (p. 2). His alternative answer is that postmodern thinking does not reject the problems that were also the concern of modernity, but that it can offer new answers. For not even a postmodernist can get away with what he defines as the fundamental moral dilemma—namely, the evaluation that precedes every choice of action. Evaluation is inextricably connected to choice of action and to decisions. Bauman continues to say that what characterized the modern approach to moral issues was that one believed in the possibility of a non-ambivalent moral code, a code that gave clear and unambiguous answers. The recognition that this kind of clarity is impossible is the point of departure for postmodern ethics.

Bauman thus introduces *choice* as a central element in the dialogues and interactions of which each of us is a part. When the therapist and the client speak to each other, the course of the dialogue also turns them into subjects, as individuals. But this also offers them possibilities or commitments that are not only determined by their positions in these dialogues. Or, said differently, the positions through which they are created are ambiguous in such a way that choices and decisions, reflections on the part of the individual participant, are necessary preconditions for understanding the content of the dialogue.

One of the issues we are left with is whether this matter of choice gives scope to what we may call personal responsibility in these contexts. Is there in these interactional situations an unclarification, an indetermination, that causes us to say that reflection and responsibility in terms of our own actions are meaningful elements in our efforts to understand what happens when we interact with other people?

The point that can easily be lost in a social-constructionist context is, therefore, that the ethical language is not only a language for condemning others, but a language for reflection on one's own actions and on one's own mode of conduct in the world.

## *An understanding of a narrative self—Paul Ricoeur*

Today's therapy theory is characterized by different narrative understandings. The narrative metaphor has had a great impact in different theoretical contexts, from psychoanalysis (e.g. Schafer, 1992; Spence, 1982) to family therapy (e.g. White, Epston) (see chapter 5). It has become especially important in terms of the concept of the self, perhaps because it renders it possible to refer to individuality through a cultural and linguistic focus. In a certain sense, this has solved a difficult point in a postmodern understanding of the self: the notion of a socially and linguistically constructed self, which also includes temporal permanence, intentionality, and vigour. These qualities are linked to the narrative, *not* to the self.

A philosopher who has written extensively on this topic is the French philosopher Paul Ricoeur. Through his book *Time and Narrative* from 1981, he turns the focus onto topics dealing with the distinction between fictive and historical narratives. What is the difference between telling something that has actually happened and an entirely fabricated story? The same question arises in therapy contexts when we ask ourselves whether any kind of alternative story is good enough as a substitute for the problem-story that people bring to therapy. In which way must an alternative story have its roots in factual events, and how do we decide what are factual events when all we have are different stories about what has been?

In Ricoeur's book *Oneself as Another* from 1992, this topic is further developed in terms of understanding the connection between self-experience/self-understanding, ethics, and narrative. This connection is complicated and not always easy to understand.

However, important issues are clarified, and it is worth the attempt even if it puts one's patience to the test.

An important premise lies in how this philosopher is often characterized. Ricoeur is called the "philosopher of detour" (Nicolaysen, 1997). This is perhaps most explicit in his efforts to grasp the human self-experience through his analyses. For the emphasis lies all the way on "self" being a reflexive concept, in the sense of the reflexive element in all the personal pronouns: one says both "myself" and "himself". In this context, it means that we have to make a detour around the different cultural manifestations in order to comprehend the phenomenon of being someone, which we here want to concretize.

## *"When I say this, then I stick to it"*

But let me attempt to illustrate the problems with an example. In this case, they date back to a dialogue with a 14-year-old girl, Heidi, and her mother. The family is being assessed by Child Welfare after Heidi's stepfather was arrested on suspicion of liquor smuggling and violent behaviour.

Heidi's mother was also interrogated in this connection, but the police found no grounds for suspecting her of participation. Heidi has a younger sister for whom she has taken much responsibility because the mother is receiving partial-disability benefit on account of arthritis. For a short period of time, mother had been married to Heidi's biological father, who originally came from South America. He moved back again later on, so that Heidi has little contact with him and his family. Even though Heidi takes on a lot of responsibility, it does not mean that she just sits at home and does her "job". She has gradually made friends who are a good deal older than she, and she has had several sexual affairs. Mother is afraid of Heidi being involved in drug abuse and criminal activities through these connections.

Child Welfare's main concern is to reduce Heidi's responsibility towards her family. They maintain that it is too much for a 14-year-old to be responsible for a mother who is dependent on getting a great deal of help and a sister who is still so young that she is dependent on a well-functioning adult to take care of her. Mother realizes this too and tries to tell Heidi that she wants Heidi to get more care for herself and take less responsibility. On this basis she tries, to the best of her ability, to establish a dialogue with Heidi.

One might think that for many reasons it would be a relief for Heidi to have a mother who will, far more than previously, consider Heidi from an adult perspective and thus let her daughter be a child. But Heidi reacted with enormous rage to this invitation to a new type of dialogue. She accused her mother of a number of unpleasant things, but mostly of being a liar. "But you know me—you *know* you are telling lies." "If you think you are being kind now, you are all wrong!" "I know how everything is, and how it should be, you can't make me change my mind!" "I know what is right—you mustn't try to change that!" All these statements were presented by Heidi in answer to her mother's attempts and those of Child Welfare and the outpatient clinic to provide Heidi with more age-adequate care. And yet one can understand Heidi's protests in view of the fact that her history is a history of problems, loyalty, and mastery, in which she has seen herself as an essential contribution to the family's common life. However, one might have thought that the repeated offers to take part in new dialogues, even with her mother and her little sister, would have gradually diminished her need to hold on to this *single* description of the world. But in spite of all this, none of the involved therapists succeeded in creating conditions for dialogues on these terms.

One way of understanding Heidi was to realize that it was important for her that the dialogue between herself and her mother should be rooted in something beyond the words themselves. By using concepts such as truth and lies about her mother's descriptions, she gives us indications of being someone who holds on to a referential understanding of language, as if what really matters is the fact that there is only one true description of reality, which is hers. She does not, in any case, wish to renounce her ideas about how things are connected, even though everyone around her does. On the other hand, Heidi's protests are closely connected to her self-experience. It would therefore not be right to take from her the right to formulate her perspectives in her own way. The contact with Heidi and her family was a reminder that understanding a narrative merely as a summing up of something that has been is in no way adequate for what the narrative represents to her. Which is to say, that on Heidi's part the narrative was not only a description of something that had been, including a demand for representing the "true story", but just as much an ethical project, an articulation about the future, about who she is and will continue to be. Convincing Heidi that it is not "like this" any more would be of limited significance as long as focusing on the future—and with it also the ethical perspective implied in a narrative—is not also a part of our understanding.

## *The action—a beginning in the world*

Relating to Heidi's self-experience therefore also means relating to ethics. This is linked to the connection between narratives and ethics. The reason for this viewpoint is based on a discussion about different approaches to an understanding of the self. "The concept of self is an answer to four different questions," says Ricoeur. In order to understand self-experience we must include all these modes of analysis or reflection. Language, action, narrativity, and ethics are therefore all necessary elements for grasping the self.

As regards the answer to the question of "Who speaks?" Ricoeur says that an understanding of this is only possible through the grammatical and semantic limitations imposed by our attempts to analyse the self. This is where the focus of a social-constructionist perspective has been placed. The I does not exist outside the language, outside the dialogue—it is created and maintained in the dialogue, says Harlene Anderson (1997, p. 219). Language both creates and maintains the experience of a self. But "the privileged point of perspective on the world which each speaking subject is, is the limit of the world and not one of its contents", is Ricoeur's reply to this (1992, p. 51). There are limitations in the picture we can have of Heidi through the way in which she speaks of herself, through the way in which she uses the words "I" and "me" in our talks. At the same time, she *is* what she is talking *about*—and what she is cannot be reduced to the content of her statements.

There are also limitations to an understanding of Heidi through the possibilities offered by theories of action—because the limitation of the theories of action is, says Ricoeur, that they end up by giving equal status to both action and event. When Heidi does something with regard to her family, one can with the help of the theories of action point out which actions Heidi carries out (ascription). However, these theories are incapable of ascribing the responsibility of these actions to Heidi, as though there were an accidental connection between the action and Heidi, as though in a way it did not matter that it is precisely Heidi who is doing what she is doing. At this point, Ricoeur's understanding is essentially different from the social-constructionist ethics outlined earlier. For MacNamee and Gergen, the dissolution of the connection between subject and accountability is a condition for the "new" ethics that they wish to inspire. For Ricoeur, an action theory must be able to explain the way in which the ability to act involves an initiative that, in a way, interrupts ongoing processes while at the same time being dependent on them. Heidi does not act in a vacuum, but in a context. Yet it is important that it is Heidi who is doing what she is doing. The social-constructionist criticism takes its point of departure in the thought that ascribing the ability to act to Heidi is the same as saying that Heidi acts in a vacuum, as though she could choose freely, independent of the context in which she finds herself. In Ricoeur's conceptual world, this means "a beginning *of* the world". He himself speaks of "a beginning *in* the world" (1992, p. 105). Heidi's actions are, of course, an *answer* to what she conceives as essential in the context in which she finds herself. But there is also an initiative on the part of Heidi, an initiative that she expresses as, for example, "I *know* that you have said that I should be more adolescent. And you think that I am doing this only in order to. . . . But it *is* not like this! I *want* it!" Relating to the world is both an answer and an initiative, reaching a decision.

In Ricoeur's vocabulary, one refers to two different ways of understanding the fact that in a sense we remain the same, despite the vicissitudes of life. In order to describe these different ways of being the same, he introduces the concepts of *idem* and *ipse* (1992, p. 2). Both concepts are linked to how we reflect on personal identity extending over time. *Idem* can perhaps be translated with "sameness" or "likeness". It is this form of self-constancy that has been the dominating factor in our attempts to understand the phenomenon of identity. It deals with the relationship between past and present—that is to say, whether I can say that I am the same as I have been. In one sense, Heidi is the same Heidi as she was last year or the year before that. A popular variant of this issue is the question of whether I return to port with the same boat if I have systematically changed all its parts underway. If we do call it the same boat, then we must say that it is the design, the connections, or the relationship between the parts that is the same. The same constancy can therefore also be found in us (Madsen, 1991).

However, Ricoeur emphasizes that this understanding lacks something essential. He shows that we use two ways of referring to ourselves that point to two different forms of temporal permanence. The other form of permanence is about keeping one's word, about promises—about continuing in a sense to be the person one has said one should be. Here, too, Nietzsche has been a source of inspiration: "To raise an animal with the right to make promises—is this not the paradoxical task that nature has set itself in the case of man?" (Nietzsche, 1967, p. 57). Being able to promise is about articulating oneself as the future, not because we are not *able* to do something different, but because we decide to want what we once wanted, to be the one we once were. This form of self-constancy is termed *ipse* by Ricoeur, or "selfness". While *idem* is the answer to the question of *what* I am, *ipse* is the answer to the question of *who* I am. But *ipse* does not contain any assertion about a permanent core in the personality (Ricoeur, 1992, p. 2).

All this has to be seen in terms of Ricoeur's intention to take his point of departure in our actions, not only in what we are *saying* about what we are doing: "The implicit axiom that 'everything is language' has often led to a closed semanticism, incapable of accounting for human actions as actually *happening* in the world, as though linguistic analysis condemned us to jumping from one language game to another, without the thought ever being able to meet up with actual action" (p. 301).

We therefore speak of two forms of temporal permanence that are implicit in these two ways of understanding the self. We need unifying concepts so that this difference in meaning will not constitute a division, a difference. This can only be taken care of by a narrative understanding of identity. The narrative identity becomes an intermediary between these two forms of permanence. Heidi has her habits too, her ways of doing things, her fixed patterns. In this way, she is different from her sister and her girlfriends. "This is typically Heidi," says her little sister. But the wishes that Heidi formulated for herself and her family are not a product of this characterization. The connection between the person she has been and the person she promises to be is a *narrative* connection, woven together in the stories she tells, as a cord between the past and the future.

The reason for thinking identity as a narrative phenomenon is connected to the relationship between what is and remains the same and what changes all the time. This is a complicated point in terms of a postmodern understanding of the subject. On the one hand, one speaks of the multiple self that is constituted in relation to the context and the relationships in which it finds itself. But when a social constructionist like Harlene Anderson comments on what may look like a fragmentation of the self-experience, she agrees with the social anthropologist Hermans that "multiplicity of the self does not mean that the self is fragmented, since it is the same I moving between different positions (Anderson, 1997, p. 221).

Ricoeur's perspective is that it is only by understanding the self as a narrative phenomenon that one can understand the self as a kind of synthesis of similarity and difference. It is the plot of the story which makes it possible to integrate the temporal permanence of the self with what looks like the opposite of permanence—namely, differences, discontinuity, and instability. The process of configuration taking place when one tells about events that are a part of a narrative generates connections between order and coherence and splitting and breakdown. The narrative process consequently creates a synthesis of the heterogeneous. What may take place as a coincidence is recreated by the narrative as a necessity. But the necessity—and therefore also the meaning—is understood backwards. The unexpected is transformed into necessity by means of narrative time. The narrative operation has thus created a concept of identity that includes both identity and difference. Or, in the words of Bengt Uggla (1994): "Narrative activity and its intrinsic dynamics can function as a model for thinking of identity as something beyond change as well as absolute identity. . . . Through the narrative fantasy's ability to explore possible combinations of permanence and change in personal identity, the play between the 'is' of similarity and the 'is not' of difference, will become rooted in the very heart of personal identity" (p. 445). In this way, Uggla resolves what for Harlene Anderson looks like an insoluble dilemma.

However, the most important point in this context is that ethical considerations are also included in the very act of narrating (Ricoeur, 1992). Between the experience connected to the past and the expectation connected to the future, the narrator action expresses what is called the responsible engagement (Kemp, 1999). This engagement is exemplified by another of Ricoeur's concepts: *attestation* (1992, pp. 21–23). In terms of Heidi, the attestation is the confirmation that it is Heidi and no one else who expresses herself—what she says, she stands for. The attestation underlines the simple fact that what one says is not "only words".

Another way of shedding light on this phenomenon is to think that, in a way, both culture and language represent the context within which we express ourselves, which is a condition for what we are saying and doing being meaningful. Knowing who I am is somehow the same as knowing where I stand in terms of these cultural norms. These norms must—using a term from the world of therapy—be internalized. Through language and action, we formulate our attitude and, in a certain sense, create ourselves as subjects (Taylor, 1989, p. 510). Even if the overriding cultural context existing prior to and independent of the subject carries the meaning-generating sources, these will only be accessible through a subjective resonance.

Other important concepts in connection with attestation are suspicion, trust, and confidence. These concepts point directly to the relational context in which the statements are formulated. Heidi herself gives an example of how important this is. What happens with her when she is not heard or taken seriously is that she no longer knows what to do. She somehow loses her strength. "If another were not counting on me, would I be capable of keeping my word, of maintaining myself?" (Ricoeur, 1992, p. 341). Heidi's experience makes this into more than a rhetorical question. It also shows clearly how Heidi's reflections about her own situation contain an element of subjectivity, as a "beginning *in* the world", an activity of her own that cannot be reduced to a product of the analysis that has preceded it.

As already mentioned, an important point for Ricoeur is to hold on to the connection between language and the practical world, the world of action. To express this connection, he introduces the concept of mimesis, which he gives three different meanings. Mimesis means miming and is used in contexts where one attempts to say something about the relationship between the word and the experience. As a point of departure, Ricoeur points to connections that he calls "narrative inductors". In the world of action, understood as practice, there already exist structures that resemble the structures in a narrative. One of these structures is the fact that we always conceive human action as purposeful, that one has a purpose with what one is doing. He shares this conviction with Jerome Bruner (1990a). Another form of structure is temporal. In many ways, infant psychology corroborates Ricoeur in his conviction that these are fundamental structures in our dealings with the world (Stern, 1995).

This is connected to the fact that language always points beyond itself, though not in an uncomplicated and one-to-one-mode. "The language cannot be about anything but reality" (Uggla, p. 396). The reference has only been given a more indirect character. Or, rather, instead of using the word "reference", Ricoeur wishes to replace it with the word *re-figuration*. Re-figuration is interpreted as "the revealing and transforming force of narrative configurations when they are 'used' on the actual action and suffering" (1987, p. 44). Language gives comments on reality, not by describing it, but by re-describing it. All these complicated formulations are necessary for emphasizing that every presentation of a course of events by using words is precisely not only a repetition, but also a transformation of the same course of events. But reference to a lived story is still important. It is expressed by *traces*—"as 'no longer' and as 'still'". What we are telling about no longer exists, yet it is present in the presence as traces (Ricoeur, 1987, p. 53). Heidi also has historical references supporting her interpretation of herself and her relational belonging. A short autobiographical history aims both at being a reconstruction of the past and a re-description directed at the context in which we find ourselves at any time. It is not possible to re-establish the past and the events Heidi speaks of, nor are they gone in the sense that they are unrecognizable or impossible to say anything about. The narratives make it somehow impossible to distinguish between what is revealed and what is made up. Heidi's version of the common narrative is, in this context, neither true nor false—it offers a gateway to the real through the possible. Heidi's narrative describes something that has happened, but not in such a way that the narrative creates a copy in words. The narrative changes and transforms what it represents. Consequently, it naturally also contains elements of fiction. And at the same time it confronts a factual, jointly lived world of action. It binds us to these joint experiences, while also separating us and our own perspective on the same experiences. The statement has a kind of generating reference to reality. What is conceived of as real is changed by the statement, but without our losing sight of the traces of the historical events.

But the narrative's relationship to action is also twofold in another way. On the one hand, the narrative transforms the actions that have already taken place; on the other, it has a progressive function as part of the actions that are now taking place. Expressing oneself through a narrative also means presenting oneself as an ethical subject, with a perspective on both what has been and what will come. It represents the responsible engagement in relation to the common world.

Heidi's formulations of her own narrative remain meaningful in many different ways. She tells her story, and with it she says something about how she has understood the past as a basis for her understanding of the present and what is important in our dialogues. But the narrative does not only represent aspects of knowledge that can be confirmed or invalidated. There is also this responsible engagement, a message to us all that she is present as herself and actively interested in the progress of the dialogue. In addition, the narrative also points to the future, who—as it were—she commits herself to be, even if conditions should change. And identity develops with the help of an ethical structure (Uggla, 1994).

Other researchers have formulated similar connections. Morson (1994) believes that all thinking around the self contains implicit assumptions about time. He criticizes the current conception of narratives that makes too much of use of the time axis for describing a necessary, closed process. To some extent, this too is an understanding that characterizes use of narratives by therapists. Clients come with a "problem narrative", and the task of therapy is to transform it into a narrative about mastery and success. Focusing on narratives prepares the ground for this type of understanding in many ways. Events are linked together with the aid of the plot in the story. The logic of the narration is a glance of retrospective necessity—the narrative has to be closed in a way in order to be coherent. With his concept of "sideshadowing", Morson points to features in narratives one does not focus on: they also contain a "mid-realm" of real possibilities—things that could have happened even though they did not happen. He refers to Dostoyevski who indicated that this understanding of narratives provides an image of human freedom and therefore also of accountability. If we emphasize the openness of time, every "now" becomes a number of possibilities that we choose or do not choose.

So then we are left with a theory telling us that our ability to symbolize and our use of language does not remove us from the actual world of events by having a casual relationship to it—but makes us to an even greater extent responsible for our actions. The fact that there are actually different ways of describing the same experiences connects what we can call acts of representation to accountability (Newton, 1995, p. 19). In order to understand the narrative process, we must include the ethical aspect, which implies being able to take an initiative, being a beginning *in* the world. Moreover, each narrative—however autobiographical—contains narratives about important persons in our lives. Therefore, the ethical perspective also points to the commitments linking every narrator to the person or persons one tells about. Heidi, at least, stuck to her narrative and fought for it until we who were her helpers finally understood the implications of her story.

# REFERENCES


Aadland, E. (1998). *Etikk for helse- og sosialarbeidarar.* Oslo: Det Norske Samlaget.

Alexander, F., & French, T. M. (1946). *Psychoanalytic Psychotherapy.* Lincoln, NB: University of Nebraska Press.

Andersen, T. (1987a). *Family Process, 26*: 415–428.

Andersen, T. (1987b). The reflecting team: Dialogue and meta-dialogue in clinical work. *Family Process, 26.*

Anderson, H. (1997). *Conversation, Language, and Possibilities: A Postmodern Approach to Therapy.* New York: Basic Books.

Anderson, H., & Goolishian, H. (1988). *Family Process, 27*: 371–393.

Andersson, M. (1995). Mother–daughter connection: The healing force in the treatment of eating disorders. *Journal of Feminist Family Therapy, 6* (4): 3–19.

Andersson, M. (1997). *Mor–datter relasjonen som helbredende kraft i behandling av spiseforstyrrelser.* Seminar ved Nic Waals Institutt i Oslo, 28 February.

Bakhurst, D., & Sypnowich, C. (1995). *The Social Self.* London: Sage.

Bateman, A., & Holmes, J. (1995). *Introduction to Psychoanalysis: Contemporary Theory and Practice.* London: Routledge.

Bateson, G. (1972a). Cybernetics of self. In: *Steps to an Ecology of Mind.* New York: Ballantine.

Bateson, G. (1972b). *Steps to an Ecology of Mind.* New York: Ballantine.

Bateson, G. (1980). *Mind and Nature: A Necessary Unity.* New York: Bantam Books.

Bateson, G., & Bateson, M. C. (1987). *Angels Fear: Towards an Epistemology of the Sacred.* New York: Macmillan.

Bauman, Z. (1993). *Postmodern Ethics.* Oxford: Blackwell.

Beauchamp, T. (1982). *Philosophical Ethics.* New York: McGraw-Hill.

Benjamin, J. (1988). *Bonds of Love: Psychoanalysis, Feminism, and the Problem of Domination.* New York: Pantheon Books.

Benjamin, J. (1998). The primal leap of psychoanalysis, from body to speech: Freud, feminism and the vicissitudes of the transference. In: A. Elliot (Ed.), *Freud 2000.* Cambridge: Polity Press.

Berg Eriksen, T. (1999). Innledende essay. In: Aristoteles, *Den nikomakiske etikk.* Oslo: Bokklubben Dagens Bøker.

Binder, P.-E., Holgersen, H., & Høstmark Nielsen, G. (1998). Psykoanalytisk psykologi ved Århundreskiftet. Fremveksten av de relasjonelle perspektivene. *Tidsskrift for Norsk Psykologforening, 35.*

Boalt Böethius, S., & Berggren, G. (1998). *Forskning om barn- och ungdoms- psykoterapi. En oversikt.* Stockholm: Ericastiftelsen.

Boscolo, L., & Bertrando, P. (1992). The reflexive loop of past, present and future in systemic therapy and consultation. *Family Process, 31:* 119–130.

Boscolo, L., & Bertrando, P. (1993). *The Times of Time: A New Perspective in Systemic Therapy and Consultation.* New York: W. W. Norton.

Boscolo, L., & Bertrando, P. (1996). *Systemic Therapy with Individuals.* London: Karnac.

Boscolo, L., Cecchin, G., Hoffman, L., & Penn, P. (1987). *Milan Systemic Family Therapy.* NewYork: Basic Books.

Boston Change Process Study Group (2002). Explicating the implicit: The interactive microprocess in the analytic situation. Report Number 3. *International Journal of Psycho-Analysis.*

Boston Change Process Study Group (2003). The "something more than interpretation": Sloppiness and co-construction in the psychoanalytic encounter. Report Number 4 (in preparation.).

Bowen, M. (1978). *Family Theory in Clinical Practice.* New York: Jason Aronson.

Bradley, B. S. (1989). *Visions of Infancy: A Critical Introduction to Child Psychology.* Cambridge: Polity Press.

Bråten, S. (Ed.) (1999). *Intersubjective Communication and Emotion in Early Ontogeny.* Cambridge: Cambridge University Press.

Bruch, H. (1985). Four decades of eating disorders. In: D. Garner & P.

Garfunkel (Eds.), *Handbook of Psychotherapy for Anorexia Nervosa and Bulimia*. New York: Guilford Press.

Bruch, H. (1988). *Conversations with Anorexics*. New York: Basic Books.

Bruner, J. (1986). *Actual Minds, Possible Worlds*. Cambridge, MA: Harvard University Press.

Bruner, J. (1990a). *Acts of Meaning*. Cambridge, MA: Harvard University Press.

Bruner, J. (1990b). Autobiographies of self. In: *Acts of Meaning*. Cambridge, MA: Harvard University Press.

Buber, M. (1958). *I and Thou*. New York: Charles Scribner's Sons.

Buber, M. (1974). *Between Man and Man*. London: Collins.

Burbatti, G., & Castoldi, I. (1994). *A Case of Severe Anorexia*. Unpublished manuscript, Milan.

Burman, E. (1994). *Deconstructing Developmental Psychology*. London/New York: Routledge.

Burr, V. (1995). *An Introduction to Social Constructionism*. London: Routledge.

Byng-Hall, J. (1990). Attachment theory and family therapy: A clinical view. *Infant Mental Health Journal, 11* (3): 228–236.

Byng-Hall, J. (1991). An appreciation of John Bowlby: His significance for family therapy. *Journal of Family Therapy, 34*: 5–16.

Byng-Hall, J. (1995a). Creating a family science base: Some implications of attachment theory for family therapy. *Family Process, 34*: 45–58.

Byng-Hall, J. (1995b). *Rewriting Family Scripts*. New York: Guilford Press.

Campbell, D., & Draper, R. (1985). *Applications of Systemic Family Therapy: The Milan Approach*. New York: Grune & Stratton.

Campbell, D., Draper, R., & Huffington, C. (1988). *Teaching Systemic Thinking*. London: DC Associates.

Cecchin, G. (1987). Hypothesizing, circularity and neutrality revisited: An invitation to curiosity. *Family Process, 26*: 405–413.

Chaiklin, S. (1992). From theory to practice and back again: What does postmodern philosophy contribute to psychological science? In: S. Kvale (Ed.), *Psychology and Postmodernism*. New York: Sage.

Claude-Pierre, P. (1997). *The Secret Language of Eating Disorders*. New York: Times Books, Random House.

Crossley, N. (1998). *Intersubjectivity*. London: Sage.

Culler, J. (1989). *On Deconstruction: Theory and Criticism after Structuralism*. London: Routledge.

Cushman, P. (1991). Ideology obscured: Political uses of the self in Daniel Stern's infant. *American Psychologist, 46* (3): 206–219.

Danziger, K. (1990). *Constructing the Subject*. Cambridge: Cambridge University Press.

Darwin, C. (1872). *The Expression of the Emotions in Man and Animals*. Chicago, IL: University of Chicago Press, 1965.

Dawes, R. M. (1994). *House of Cards: Psychology and Psychotherapy Built on Myth*. New York: Free Press.

Deleuze, G., & Guattari, F. (1996). *Hvad er filosofi?* Oslo: Gyldendal.

Derrida, J. (1976). *Of Grammatology*. Baltimore, MD: John Hopkins University Press.

Derrida, J. (1981). *Dissemination*. London: Athlone Press.

de Shazer, S. (1988). *Clues: Investigating Solutions in Brief Therapy*. New York/London: W. W. Norton.

de Shazer, S. (1994). *Words Were Originally Magic*. New York: W. W. Norton.

Dreyfus, H., & Wakefield, J. (1987). Alternative philosophical conceptualization of psychopathology. In: S. B., Messer, L. A., Sass, & R. L. Woolfolk (Eds.), *Hermeneutics and Psychological Theory: Perspectives on Personality, Psychotherapy and Psychopathology*. New Brunswick, NJ: Rutgers University Press.

Duncan, B. L., Solovey, A. D., & Rusk, G. S. (1992). *Changing the Rules: A Client-Directed Approach to Therapy*. New York: Guilford Press.

Dunn, J. (1988). *The Beginnings of Social Understanding*. Cambridge, MA: Harvard University Press.

Dunn, J. (1993). *Young Children's Close Relationship. Beyond Attachment*. London: Sage.

Dunn, J., & Plomin, R. (1990). *Separate Lives: Why Siblings Are So Different*. New York: Basic Books.

Dunn, J., & Plomin, R. (1991). Why are siblings so different? The significance of differences in siblings' experiences within the family. *Family Process, 30*: 271–283.

Eakin, P. J. (1992). *Touching the World*. Princeton, NJ: Princeton University Press.

Eliot, T. S. (1963). *Collected Poems (1909–1962)*. London/Boston: Faber & Faber.

Elster, J. (1989). *Nuts and Bolts for the Social Sciences*. Cambridge: Cambridge University Press.

Engelstad, I. (1976). *Fortellingens mønstre: En strukturell analyse av norske folkeeventyr*. Oslo: Univeritetsforlaget.

Erikson, E. H. (1994). *Identity and the Life Cycle*. New York: W. W. Norton.

Ferreira, A. (1963). Family myth and homeostasis. *Archives of General Psychiatry, 9*: 457–463.

Fivush, R. (1993). Emotional content of parent–child conversations about the past. In: C. Nelson et al. (Eds.), *Memory and Affect in Development*. Hillsdale, NJ: Lawrence Erlbaum.

Fivush, R. (1994). Constructing narrative, emotion and gender in parent–child conversations about the past. In: U. Neisser & R. Fivush (Ed.), *The Remembering Self*. New York: Cambridge University Press.

Flaskas, C. (1997). Engagement and the therapeutic relationship in systemic therapy. *Journal of Family Therapy, 19*: 263–282.

Foucault, M. (1972). *The Archaelogy of Knowledge*. London: Routledge.

Foucault, M. (1977). *Language, Countermemory, Practice*. Ithaca, NY: Cornell University Press.

Freedman, J., & Combs, G. (1996). *Narrative Therapy: The Social Construction of Preferred Realities*. New York: W. W. Norton.

Freeman, M. (1993). *Rewriting the Self: History, Memory Narrative*. London/York: Routledge.

Freud, S. (1973). *New Introductory Lectures on Psychoanalysis*. Harmondsworth: Penguin.

Friedman, S. (Ed.) (1993): *The New Language of Change: Constructive Collaboration in Psychotherapy*. New York: Guilford Press.

Frosh, S. (1995). Time, space and otherness. In: S. Pile & N. Thrift (Eds.), *Mapping the Subject: Geographies of Cultural Transformation*. London: Routledge.

Frosh, S. (1997). *For and Against Psychoanalysis*. London: Routledge.

Furniss, T. (1991). *The Multi-Professional Handbook of Child Sexual Abuse*. London: Routledge.

Geertz, C. (1973). *The Interpretation of Cultures*. New York: Basic Books.

Geertz, C. (1995). *After the Fact: Two Countries, Four Decades, One Anthropologist*. Cambridge, MA: Harvard University Press.

Gergen, K. J. (1992). Toward a postmodern psychology. In: S. Kvale (Ed.), *Psychology and Postmodernism*. Thousand Oaks, CA: Sage.

Gergen, K. J. (1994). *Realities and Relationships*. Cambridge, MA: Harvard University Press.

Gilligan, S., & Price, R. (Eds.) (1993). *Therapeutic Conversations*. W. W. Norton.

Goethe, J. W. (1956). *Faust*. London: Penguin Books.

Goolishian, H. (1988). Paper presented at the Greek Kitchen in the Arctic Conference, Sulitjelma, Norway.

Goolishian, H., & Anderson, H. (1991). *AFTA Newsletter* (Winter).

Grenness, C. E. (1998). Vitenskaplig ansvarlighet. Kvalitetssikring, vitenskapelighet og etikk. *Tidskrift for Norsk Psykologforening, 35*.

Griffiths, M., & Whitford, M. (1988). *Feminist Perspectives in Philosophy.* New York: Macmillan.

Gullestad, S. E., & Theophilakis, M. (Eds.) (1997). *En umulig profesjon? Om opplæring i intensiv dynamisk psykoterapi.* Oslo: Universitetsforlaget.

Haley, J. (1977). *Problem-Solving Therapy.* San Francisco, CA: Jossey-Bass.

Hansen, B. R. (1991a). *Den første dialogen: En studie av spedbarnets oppmerksomhet i samspill.* Oslo: Solum Forlag A/S.

Hansen, B. R. (1991b). Intersubjektivitet—et nytt utviklingspsykologisk begrep? *Tidsskrift for Norsk Psykologforening, 28*: 568–578.

Hansen, B. R. (1996a). Den affektive dialogen i psykoterapi med barn: Implikasjoner fra nyere spebarnsforskning. In: M. Kjær (Ed.), *Skjønner du? Kommunikasjon med barn.* Oslo: Kommuneforlaget.

Hansen, B. R. (1996b). "Implications of Daniel Stern's Model on Child Therapy: Some Suggestions Concerning the Therapeutic Relationship and Communication." Soria Moria conference, Oslo.

Hansen, B. R., Johnsen A., & Sundet, R. (1994). Daniel Stern og familieterapi. *Fokus på Familien,* 22 (2): 94–108.

Haraway, D. J. (1991). *Simians, Cyborgs, and Women: The Reinvention of Nature.* London: Free Association Books.

Harré, R. (1998). *The Singular Self.* London: Sage.

Harré, R., & Parrott, W. G. (1996). *Emotions: Social, Cultural and Biological Dimension.* London: Sage.

Hartmann, E. (1997). Joseph Lichtenberg: Selvpsykolog eller motivasjonsteoretiker? In: S. Karterud & J. Monsen (Eds.), *Selvpsykologi: Utviklingen etter Kohut.* Oslo: ad Notam Gyldendal.

Havnesköld, L., & Mothander, P. R. (1995). *Utvecklingspsykologi. Psykodynamisk teori i nya perspektiv.* Stockholm: Liber Utbildning.

Henriksen, J.-O. (1997). *Grobunn for moral.* Oslo: Høyskoleforlaget.

Hoffman, L. (1971). Deviation-amplifying processes in natural groups. In: J. Haley (Ed.), *Changing Families.* New York: Grune & Stratton.

Hoffman, L. (1981). *Foundations of Family Therapy: A Conceptual Framework for Systems Change.* New York: Basic Books.

Hoffman, L. (1985). Beyond power and control: Toward a "second-order" family systems therapy. *Family Systems Medicine, 3.*

Hoffman, L. (1992). A reflexive stance in family therapy. In: S. McNamee & K. Gergen (Eds.), *Therapy as Social Construction.* London: Sage.

Hoffman, L. (1993). A reflexive stance. *Exchanging Voices.* London: Karnac.

Holmes, S. (1994). A philosophical stance, ethics and therapy. *Australia & New Zealand Journal of Family Therapy, 15* (3): 155–161.

Høstmark Nielsen, G. (1997). Kunnskapsbasert praksis. *Tidsskrift for Norsk Psykologforening, 34* (10): 857–859.

Hougaard, E. (1995). *Psykoterapi. Teori og Forskning*. København: Dansk psykologisk forlag.

Hoyt, M. (1997). Postmodernism, the relational self, constructive therapies, and beyond, a conversation with Kenneth Gergen. In: M. Hoyt (Ed.), *Constructive Therapies, Vol. 2* (pp. 347–368). New York: Guilford Press.

Irigaray, L. (1985a). *Speculum of the Other Woman*. Ithaca, NY: Cornell University Press.

Irigaray, L. (1985b). *This Sex Which Is Not One*. Ithaca, NY: Cornell University Press.

Johnsen, A. (1995). *Vendepunkter: Om familieterapi ved spiseforstyrrelser*. Oslo: Tano As.

Johnsen, A. (1996). Selv og de andre. En presentasjon av Helm Stierlins systemiske selvmodell of relevansen av denne for klinisk praksis. *Fokus på familien, 24*: 127–139.

Johnsen, A. (1997). Familieterapi og psykologi. *Fokus på familien, 25*: 166–172.

Johnsen, A., Tømmerås, S., Hundevadt, L., & Haavardsholm, B. (1987). *Harde knuter og brutte bånd: Om binding og utstøting i familier*. Oslo: Tano As.

Johnsen, A., & Torsteinsson, V. W. (1997). Å forstå hverandre—hva er det? Om affektinntoning, selvopplevelse og samspill. In: *Familieterapi i Nordisk lys*. Kongressbok. Stockholm: Mareld Bøcker.

Johnsen, Anne (1998). Semistrukturert følelsesbevissthetsintervju tilrettelagt for parterapi. *Fokus på familien, 26*: 21–32.

Johnson, B. (1981). Translator's Introduction. In: J. Derrida, *Dissemination*. London: Athlone Press.

Karterud, S., & Monsen, J. (Eds.) (1997). *Selvpsykologi. Utviklingen etter Kohut*. Oslo: ad Notam Gyldendal.

Keeney, B. P. (1982). What is an epistemology of family therapy. *Family Process, 21*.

Keeney, B. P. (1983). *Aesthetics of Change*. New York: Guilford Press.

Kemp, P. (1999). *Tid og fortælling: En introduktion til Paul Ricoeur*. Aarhus: Aarhus Universitetsforlag.

Killingmo, B. (1971). *Den psykoanalytiske behandlingsmetode*. Oslo: Universitetsforlaget.

Kirkebøen, G. (1993). Fra naken keiser til bare klær: Konstruksjon og "dekonstruksjon" av Kybernetisk familieterapi. *Fokus på Familien, 21*: 75–99.

Kugiumetziakis, G. (1999). Neonatal imitation in the intersubjective companion space. In: S. Bråten (Ed.), *Intersubjective Communication and Emotion in Early Ontogeny*. Cambridge: Cambridge University Press.

Kundera, M. (1998). *Identitet*. Oslo: J. W. Cappelens Forlag.

Kvale, S. (Ed.) (1992). *Psychology and Postmodernism*. London: Sage.

Kvale. S. (1994). Profesjonspraksis som erkjennelse: Om dilemmaer i terapeutisk forskning. In: S. Reichelt (Ed.), *Psykologi i forandring*. Oslo: Norsk Psykologforening.

Laplanche, J., & Pontalis, J.-B. (1980). *The Language of Psycho-Analysis*. London: Hogarth Press.

Lennon, K., & Whitford, M. (Eds.) (1994). *Knowing the Difference: Feminist Perspectives in Epistemology*. London: Routledge.

Levinas, E. (1991): *Ethics and Infinity*. Pittsburgh, PA: Duquesne University Press.

Loe, E. (1996). *Naiv. Super*. Oslo: Cappelen.

Lundby, G. (1998). *Historier og terapi. Om narrativer, konstruksjonisme og nyskriving av Historier*. Oslo: Tano As.

Madsen, C., & Tygstrup, F. (1996). Om Gilles Deleuze og Hvad er filosofi? In: G. Deleuze & F. Guattari (Eds.), *Hvad er filosofi?* Oslo: Gyldendal.

Madsen, K. (1991). *Daimon*. Oslo: Aschehoug.

Madison, G. B. (1982). *The Phenomenology of Merleau-Ponty: Search for the Limits of Consciousness*. Athens, OH: Ohio University Press.

Marshall, B. K. (1992). *Teaching the Postmodern: Fiction and Theory*. London: Routledge.

Maruyama, M. (1968). The second cybernetics: Deviation-amplifying mutual causal processes. In: B. Buckley (Ed.), *Modern Systems Research for the Behavioral Scientist*. Chicago, IL: Aldine.

Maturana, H. (1978). Biology of language: The epistemology of reality. In: G. A. Miller & E. Lenneberg (Eds.), *Psychology and Biology of Language and Thought. Essays in Honor of E. Lenneberg*. New York: Academic Press.

Mauss, M. (1990). *The Gift*. London: Routledge.

McCall, C. (1990). *Concepts of Person*. Aldershot: Avebury/Gower Publishing Group.

McEwan, I. (1995). *The Daydreamer*. London: Vintage Books.

McLeod, J. (1997). *Narrative and Psychotherapy*. London: Sage.

McNamee, S., & Gergen, K. J. (1992) (Eds.). *Therapy as Social Construction*. Thousand Oaks, CA: Sage.

McNamee, S., & Gergen, K. J. (1999). *Relational Responsibility*. Thousand Oaks, CA: Sage.

Meltzoff, A., & Moore, K. (1995). Infant's understanding of people and things: From body imitation to folk psychology. In: J. L. Bermudez, N. Eilan, & A. Marcel (Eds.), *The Body and the Self*. Cambridge, MA: MIT Press.

Midgley, M. (1989). *Wisdom, Information and Wonder*. London: Routledge.

Miller, G. A., & Lenneberg, E. (Eds.) (1978). *Psychology and Biology of Language and Thought. Essays in Honor of E. Lenneberg*. New York Academic Press.

Miller, S. D., Duncan, B. L., & Hubble, M. A. (1997). *Escape from Babel: Towards a Unifying Language for Psychotherapy Practice*. New York: W. W. Norton.

Mills, S. (1997). *Discourse*. London: Routledge.

Minuchin, S. (1977). *Families and Family Therapy*. London: Routledge.

Minuchin, S., Rosman, B., & Baker, L. (1978). *Psychosomatic Families: Anorexia Nervosa in Context*. Cambridge, MA: Harvard University Press.

Moi, T. (1985). *Sexual/Textual Politics: Feminist Literary Theory*. London: Routledge.

Monsen, J. (1997). Selvpsykologi og nyere affektteori. In: S. Karterud & J. Monsen (Eds.), *Selv-psykologi: Utviklingen etter Kohut*. Oslo: Ad Notam Gyldendal.

Moore, H. (1994). *A Passion for Difference*. Cambridge: Blackwell.

Morson, G. (1994). *Narrative and Freedom: The Shadows of Time*. New Haven, CT: Yale University Press.

Nagel, T. (1986). *The View from Nowhere*. Oxford: Oxford University Press.

Nelson, K. (1996). *Language in Cognitive Development*. Cambridge: Cambridge University Press.

Newton, A. Z. (1995). *Narrative Ethics*. Cambridge, MA: Harvard University Press.

Nicolaysen, B. K. (1997). *Omvegar fører lengst*. Oslo: Samlaget.

Nietzsche, F. (1967). *On the Genealogy of Morals*. New York: Vintage Books.

Nordby, T. T. (1998). Følelse og tanke, individ og system. *Fokus på familien, 26*: 213–223.

Norris, C. (1987). *Derrida*. London: Fontana Press.

Norsk Sosionomforbund (1989/1992). *Erklæring om etiske prinsipper i sosialt arbeid—med kommentarer* [Declaration of ethical principles in social work—with commentary]. Norwegian Union of Social Educators and Social Workers. <www.ifsw.org/Publications/4.4.1.nor.pub.html>

Øvreeide, H., & Hafstad, R. (1996). Marte meo-metoden: Styrking av foreldres kompetanse. In: S. Reichelt & H. Haavind (Eds.), *Aktiv Psykoterapi*. Oslo: Ad Notam Gyldendal.

Pålshaugen, Ø. (1997). *Kritikk av den ene fornuft: Adorno, Derrida og Wittgenstein contra Habermas*. Oslo: Spartacus.

Papp, P., & Imber-Black, E. (1996). Family themes: Transmission and transformation. *Family Process, 35*: 5–20.

Parry, A., & Doan, R. E. (1994). *Story Re-visions: Narrative Therapy in the Postmodern World*. New York: Guilford Press.

Partridge, E. (1979). *Origins: A Short Etymological Dictionary of Modern English*. London: Routledge & Kegan Paul.

Peterfreund, E. (1978). Some critical comments on psychoanalytic conceptualizations of infancy. *International Journal of Psychoanalysis, 59*: 427–441.

Pocock, D. (1997). Feeling understood in family therapy. *Journal of Family Therapy, 19*: 283–302.

Potter, J. (1996). *Representing Reality*. London: Sage.

Priest, S. (1998). *Merleau-Ponty*. London: Routledge.

Reichelt, S. (1995). Hvilken nytte praktikere har av epistemologi. *Fokus på familien, 3*.

Reichelt, S., & Haavind, H. (Eds.) (1996). *Aktiv psykoterapi: Perspektiver på psykologisk forståelse og behandling*. Oslo: Ad Notam Gyldendal.

Reiss, D. (1981). *The Family's Construction of Reality*. Cambridge, MA: Harvard University Press.

Ricoeur, P. (1981). *Time and Narrative*. Chicago, IL: University of Chicago Press.

Ricoeur, P. (1987). Den fortalte tid. *Slagmark, 10*.

Ricoeur, P. (1992). *Oneself as Another*. Chicago, IL: University of Chicago Press.

Riikonen, E., & Madan Smith, G. (1997). *Re-Imagining Therapy: Living Conversation and Relational Knowing*. Thousand Oaks, CA: Sage.

Røer, A. (1996). *Nattemennesker: Systemisk, narrativ og lingvistisk tilnærming til bulimi*. Oslo: Kommuneforlaget.

Rønning, J. A. (1997a). Regionsenteret I barne- og ungdomspsykiatri: Akkulturasjon mellom forskning og klinisk virksomhet. *Tidsskrift for Norsk Psykologforening, 34* (3): 204–213.

Rønning, J. A. (1997b). Dette skjer I Nord-Norge. *Tidsskrift for Norsk Psykologforening, 34* (6): 513–519.

Schafer, R. (1992). *Retelling a Life: Narration and Dialogue in Psychoanalysis*. New York: Basic Books.

Schjødt, B., & Egeland, T. A. A. (1991). *Fra systemteori til familieterapi*. Oslo: Tano As.

Schrag, C. O. (1997). *The Self after Postmodernity*. New Haven, CT: Yale University Press.

Seller, A. (1994). Should the feminist philosopher stay at home. In: K. Lennon & M. Whitford (Eds.), *Knowing the Difference: Feminist Perspectives in Epistemology*. London: Routledge.

Selvini-Palazzoli, M. (1974). *Self-Starvation*. London: Human Context Books.

Selvini-Palazzoli, M., Boscolo, L., Cecchin, G., & Prata, G. (1980). Hypothesizing—circularity—neutrality: Three guidelines for the conductor of the session. *Family Process, 19*: 73–85.

Sheehan, J. (1998). Die Befreiung von Erzählstilen in der systemischen Therapie. *Zeitschrift für systemische Therapie, 16*: 84–98.

Sommer, D. (1997). *Barndomspsykologi*. Oslo: Pedagogisk Forums Forlag.

Sørhaug, T. (1996). *Fornuftens fantasier*. Oslo: Universitetsforlaget.

Speed, B. (1997). Editorial: Might psychoanalysis be of use to systemic therapies? *Journal of Family Therapy, 19* (3): 233–239.

Speer, A. (1970). Family systems: Morphostasis and morphogenesis. *Family Process, 9*.

Spence, D. (1982). *Narrative Truth and Historical Truth: Meaning and Interpretation in Psychoanalysis*. New York: W. W. Norton.

Spence, D. (1987). *The Freudian Metaphor: Toward Paradigm Change in Psychoanalysis*. New York: W. W. Norton.

Stern, D. N. (1985). *The Interpersonal World of the Infant: A View from Psychoanalysis and Developmental Psychology*. New York: Basic Books.

Stern, D. N. (1990). *Diary of a Baby: What Your Child Sees, Feels, and Experiences*. New York: Basic Books.

Stern, D. N. (1992). The "pre-narrative envelope": An alternative view of "unconcious phantasy" in infancy. *Bulletin of the Anna Freud Centre, 15*: 291–318.

Stern, D. N. (1995). *The Motherhood Constellation: A Unified View of Parent–Infant Psychotherapy*. New York: Basic Books.

Stern, D. N. (1996). *Who Is the Mother, Who Is the Child*. Seminar, Nic Walls Institutt, Oslo.

Stern, D. N. (2000). New Introduction. In: *The Interpersonal World of the Infant: A View from Psychoanalysis and Developmental Psychology*. New York: Basic Books.

Stern, D. N. (in press). *The Present Moment in Psychotherapy and Everyday Life*. New York: W. W. Norton.

Stern, D. N., Sander, L. W., Nahum, J. P., Harrison, A. M., Lyons-Ruth, K., Morgan, A. C., Bruschweiler-Stern, N., & Tronick, E. Z. (1998). Non-interpretive mechanisms in psychoanalytic therapy. The "something more" than interpretation. (Boston Change Process Study Group, Report No. 1). *International Journal of Psycho-Analysis, 79*: 903–921.

Stierlin, H. (1974). *Separating Parents and Adolescents*. New York: Quadrangle.

Stierlin, H. (1981). *Separating Parents and Adolescents* (2nd edition). New York: Jason Aronson. .

Stierlin, H. (1994). *Ich und die Anderen*. Stuttgart: Klett Cotta.

Stierlin, H., Rucker-Embden, I., Wetzel, N., & Wirsching, M. (1980). *The First Interview with the Family*. New York: Brunner/Mazel.

Stierlin, H., & Weber, G. (1989). *Unlocking the Family Door: A Systemic Approach to the Understanding and Treatment of Anorexia Nervosa*. New York: Brunner/Mazel.

Stierlin, H., Wynne, L. C., & Wirsching, M. (Eds.) (1983). *Psychosocial Intervention in Schizophrenia*. Berlin: Springer-Verlag.

Sundet, R. (1988). Objektivitet i parentes. Presentasjon av og betraktninger rundt Humberto Maturanas arbeider. *Fokus på familien, 16* (1).

Sundet, R. (1993). Familieterapi—fra endring av mønster og struktur til samskaping av nye beretninger. In: B. S. Haugland & P. Rosenquist (Eds.), *Familie-behandling innen rusomsorgen i Norden*. Helsingfors: NAD, publikasjon no. 25.

Sundet, R. (1997). Bruk av psykiatrisk diagnostikk som eksternalisering. *Fokus på familien, 25* (3–4).

Taylor, C. (1989). *Sources of the Self*. Cambridge: Cambridge University Press.

Taylor, C. (1992). *The Ethics of Authenticity*. Cambridge, MA: Harvard University Press.

Torsteinsson, V. W. (1995). Relasjon og selvopplevelse: Sentrale begrep i arbeidet med spiseforstyrrelser. In: A. Johnsen (Ed.), *Vendepunkter: Om familietrapi ved spiseforstyrrelser*. Oslo: Tano As.

Tranøy, K. E. (1986). *Vitenskapen—samfunnsmakt og livsform*. Oslo: Universitetsforlaget.

Trevarthen, C. (1999). The concept and foundation of infant intersubjectivity. In: S. Bråten (Ed.), *Intersubjective Communication and Emotion in Early Ontogeny*. Cambridge: Cambridge University Press.

Tronick, E. Z., Bruschweiler-Stern, N., Harrison, A. M., Lyons-Ruth, K., Morgan, A. C., Nahum, J. P., Sander, L. W., & Stern, D. N. (1998). Dyadically expanded states of consciousness and the process of therapeutic change. *Infant Mental Health Journal, 19*: 290–299.

Uggla, B. K. (1994). *Kommunikation på bristningsgränsen*. Stockholm: Brutus Østling.

Vedeler, G. H. (1997). Hva skjer i Nord-Norge. *Tidsskrift for Norsk Psykologforening, 34* (5).

Vetlesen, A. J. (1993). *Relations with Others in Sartre and Levinas*. Unpublished manuscript, Oslo.

Vetlesen, A. J., & Nordtvedt, D. (1994). *Følelser og moral*. Oslo: Ad Notam Gyldendal.

von Foerster, H. (1984). *Observing Systems* (2nd edition). Seaside, CA: Intersystems Publications.

von Foerster, H. (1991). "Ethics and Second-Order Cybernetics." Opening address for the International Conference on Systems and Family Therapy: Ethics, Epistemology, New Methods, Paris, 1990. <www.stanford.edu/group/SHR/4-2/text/foerster.html>

von Glasersfeld, E. (1984). An introduction to radical constructivism. In: P. Watzlawick (Ed.), *The Invented Reality*. New York: W. W. Norton.

Watzlawick, P., Beavin, J. H., & Jackson, D. D. (1967). *Pragmatics of Human Communication*. New York: W. W. Norton.

Wetherell, M., & Maybin, J. (1996). The distributed self: A social constructionist perspective. In: R. Stevens (Eds.), *Understanding the Self*. London: Sage.

White, M. (1989). *Selected Papers*. Adelaide: Dulwich Centre Publications.

White, M. (1993). Deconstruction and therapy. In: S. Gilligan & R. Price (Eds.), *Therapeutic Conversations*. New York: W. W. Norton.

White, M. (1995). *Re-Authering Lives: Interviews, & Essays*. Adelaide: Dulwich Centre Publications.

White, M. (1997). *Narratives of Therapists' Lives*. Adelaide: Dulwich Centre Publications.

White, M., & Epston, D. (1990). *Narrative Means to Therapeutic Ends*. New York: W. W. Norton.

Whitford, M. (1988). Luce Irigaray's critique of rationality. In: M. Griffiths & M. Whitford, *Feminist Perspectives in Philosophy*. New York: Macmillan.

Wilden, A. (1972). *System and Structure: Essays in Communication and Exchange*. London: Tavistock Publications.

Wilden, A. (1977). *System and Structure: Essays in Communication and Exchange* (2nd edition). London: Tavistock Publications.

Wilkinson, M. (1992). How do we understand empathy systemically?. *Journal of Family Therapy, 14*: 195–205.

Williams, B. (1985). *Ethics and the Limits of Philosophy*. New York: Fontana.

Wirsching, M., & Stierlin, H. (1982). *Krankheit und Familie*. Stuttgart: Klett.

Wittgenstein, L. (1958). *Philosophical Investigations*. Oxford: Blackwell.

Wrangsjø, B. (1993). *Ungdomsutveckling och ungdomsterapi i ljuset av Daniel Sterns sjalvteori*. Stockholm: SFPH, monografiserie no. 36.

Yeatman, A. (1994). Postmodern epistemological politics and social sciences. In: K. Lennon & M. Whitford (Eds.), *Knowing the Difference: Feminist Perspectives in Epistemology*. London: Routledge.

Zachrisson, A. (1997). Terapeutisk holdning. In: S. E. Gullestad & M. Theophilakis (Eds.), *En umulig profesjon? Om opplæring i intensiv dynamisk psykoterapi*. Oslo: Universitetsforlaget.

# INDEX


Aadland, E., 279
abuse:
  child, parental, 231
    sexual, 268
  sexual, 123, 192, 261, 268–269
accessibility, therapist's, 216
accountability, 276, 283, 292, 298
  concept of, 282
acknowledgement, concept of, 171
activation contours, 93
"acts of meaning", 28
adaptation, issues of, in adolescent therapy, 160
adolescent(s), therapy with [clinical examples], 155–179
adultomorphization, 32
affect(s):
  attunement of, 5, 16, 22, 30, 50, 60, 100–101, 104–106, 112–113, 167, 169, 194, 206, 233, 234
    concept of, 32, 91, 94–98, 105, 160, 207
    criteria of, 170–171
  concept of, 90, 92
  fundamental patterns of, 238
  -laden experience, 127, 140, 146
  matching, concept of, 91
  regulation, 5, 16, 19–20, 101, 151, 169, 216, 229
  theory(ies), 90–91
  vitality, 17–18, 24, 28, 30, 52, 91–100, 113, 159, 205–206
    and categorical affects, 14, 27, 93–94
    concept of, 100
affective attunement, 106
affective being-together, 172
affective component of key experience, 140
affective dialogue, 91, 205–208
affective states, sharing of, 21
affectivity, 19–20, 52, 165–166
Age of Enlightenment, 43, 243
Alexander, F., 230, 231
amodal perception, 17, 24, 159, 233
analogous apperception, 68–69
Andersen, T., 162, 252, 259
Anderson, H., 40, 45, 48, 65, 226, 228, 233, 253, 277, 279, 282, 291, 294, 295

Andersson, M., 211
Anna O. (O. Pappenheim) [Freud's case], 246
anorexia/anorexic(s), 38, 62, 186, 199, 202, 205, 208, 210, 211, 265, 279
*see also* bulimia/bulimic(s); eating disorder(s)
anthropological attitude, concept of, 96
anxiety:
issues of, in adolescent therapy, 160
neurosis, 115–116
apperception, analogous, 68–69
Aristotle, 283
assumed actual point of origin, 139
atomistic individualism, 45
attachment, 5, 166
and autonomy, 203
and detachment, 203
research, 5
role in development, 5
and separation, 141, 199–201, 204
social, 26
theory, 4, 137
attention, 166
deficit hyperactivity disorder (ADHD), 266
attestation, concept of, 295
attunement, 95, 206
affect, *see* affect attunement
concept of, 246
Augustine, St, 132
autonomy, 14–15, 42–43, 138–141, 159, 201, 203–204, 211, 226, 245, 280–281
concept of, 63
issues of:
in adolescent therapy, 160
with eating disorders, 197
patients', 226
awareness, invariant patterns of, 51

backshadowing, concept of, 131
Baker, L., 102, 185, 194, 198
Bakhurst, D., 43, 45
Barthes, R., 56
Bateman, A., 238–241
Bateson, G., 38, 40, 45, 65, 129, 136, 185, 228, 248–250, 254
Bateson, M. C., 79, 254
Bauman, Z., 276, 287
Beauchamp, T., 281
Beavin, J. H., 65, 251
behavioural genetics, xx, 6, 182–184
Benjamin, J., 242, 245–247
Berg Eriksen, T., 283
Berggren, G., 12, 50
Bertrando, P., 4, 132
Betrando, P., 115
Binder, P.-E., 238, 239, 247
binding families, 185, 194
Boalt Böethius, S., 12, 50
borderline diagnosis, 250
Boscolo, L., xxiv, 4, 102, 115, 132, 136, 137, 199
MIlan group, 65
Boston Change Process Study Group, xvii
Boszormenyi-Nagy, I., 89
boundary(ies), 53
family, 103
and eating disorders, 198
in therapy, 280
clinical example, 223–228
Bowen, M., 102
Bowlby, J., 4
Bradley, B. S., 31
Bråten, S., 76, 78, 79
breadth:
vs depth, 222, 239
-psychology, 222–223
Bremond, H., 131, 132
Brontë sisters, 195
Bruch, H., 199, 207
Bruner, J., 5, 24, 28, 52, 57–58, 76, 77, 113–115, 130, 134, 137, 181, 209, 264, 274, 296
Buber, M., 67, 69–72, 78, 82
bulimia/bulimic(s), 97, 99, 100, 199, 202, 208, 210, 211, 267
*see also* anorexia/anorexic(s); eating disorder(s)
Burbatti, G., 207
Burman, E., 158
Burr, V., 46, 48
Byng-Hall, J., 4, 137, 141

calendar time, 129
Campbell, D., xxiv, 251

"Caroline" [clinical example: loneliness], 141–144
Castoldi, I., 207
categorical affect(s), 52, 91, 97, 205
  and vitality affects, 14, 27, 93–94
causal thinking, linear, 114, 199
Cecchin, G., 65, 137, 199
centrifugal family, 102
Chaiklin, S., 157
checking behaviour, adolescents', 169
child, egocentric, 5
Child and Adolescent Psychiatric Outpatient Clinic, Drammen, 179
choice, freedom of, 282
circular questioning, 137, 142, 145, 154, 185, 188
Claude-Pierre, P., 207
Cleese, J., 168
clinical psychology, xxii, 258, 263
close social world, 18–20
closeness, issues of, in adolescent therapy, 160
closure, 228–229, 282
  concept of, 225, 226
  and narratives, 114, 125, 129
cognitive development:
  of siblings, similarities in, 196
  theories of, 27
cognitive involvement, 166
cognitive psychology, 24
cognitive theory, 64, 90
coherence:
  and meaning, 28–29, 106
  and organization, nonverbal experience of, 233
Colorado Adoption Study, 186
Combs, G., 253
communication(s), 236
  and dialogue, concepts of, 66
  of feelings, nonverbal, 97
  focus on in family therapy, 251
  nonverbal/affective, 29
  theories of, 65
  therapeutic, 7
  verbal/narrative, 29
companion, evoked, 20, 30, 162, 166–167, 177
concept(s):
  formation, 232–234
    in therapy, 215–234
  self, 1, 34–60, 288
    autonomous, independent, 20
    Cartesian, 43–45
    context-based, chameleon, 49
    essentialistic, 39
    and identity, 37, 40
    language-based, 56
    Ricoeur, 291
    self-sufficient, 39
    social-constructionist, 47
    Stern, 13, 37, 81
    vs subjectivity, 48
    traditional, as cultural prejudice, 38
conceptual development, 2, 235
conceptual opposites, 241, 249
conceptual pairs, 245, 254
conceptual schemas, 27
conceptualization:
  and thinking, 216–234
  variations in understanding of, 266
concretization, 59
confidence, concept of, 295
consciousness, 20, 43–44, 67–69, 95, 130, 134, 241–242, 257
  feeling-, 91–92
  individual, 78, 83, 285
  landscape of, 130
  self as introspective phenomenon of, 44
constructionism, xx, 47
  social, *see* social constructionism
constructivism, xx, 233, 253, 258
  Maturana's, 44
containment, 246
contamination, 228–229, 246
  concept of, 225–226
continuity in time, 19, 164
continuous-construction model of development, 15, 29, 51, 94
control, 5, 14–15, 39, 138–139, 141, 201–205, 208, 211, 238, 247
  issues of, with eating disorders, 197
  and knowledge, 277
conversation, 75–76, 83, 234, 252–253
  concept of, 71
  proto-, 79
  therapeutic, 7

coordination of action, 51–52, 55, 57, 60, 71
concept of, 52, 59
coordination of, language as, 254
Copernican turning point, 283
core self, 16, 23–24, 31, 51, 80–82, 126, 152
as metaphor for therapeutic work with adolescents, 162–167
sense of, 18–20, 25, 105, 138, 151
corrective emotional experience, 230–231
cosmological time, 129
countertransference, 220, 237
criminal behaviour in siblings, similarities in, 196
Crossley, N., 68, 70
Culler, J., 244
culture, role of, in development of feelings, 90
curiosity, 3, 7, 100, 133, 166
concept of, 96
Cushman, P., 31–34, 158
cybernetics, 156, 180, 252
of cybernetics, concept of, 250
first-order, 249, 250, 253
second-order, 6, 249, 250, 253

Danziger, K., 77
Darwin, C., 93
Dawes, R. M., 156
deconstruction, 249
concept of, 244–247
Deleuze, G., 217, 239
delimitation, 37
in therapy [clinical example], 223–228
dependence, 14–15, 75, 138–139, 201, 211, 225–226, 280
and independence, 203–204
issues of, in adolescent therapy, 160
depressed mother, 128
depth, 241, 261
vs breadth, 222, 239
-psychology, 222, 223
Derrida, J., 219, 242, 244
Descartes, R., 40, 43–45, 47
de Shazer, S., 48, 132, 178, 227
determinism, 114, 129
development, continuous-construction model of, 15, 29, 51, 94
developmental process(es), 13, 84, 263
interpersonal, 90
intrapsychic, 90
developmental psychology, xix–xxi, 5, 11, 13, 16, 27, 31–32, 37, 49–50, 58, 76, 80–81, 84, 158, 182, 184, 187, 263
modern, 3, 198, 201, 203–210
developmental theory, xxiii, 2–3, 7, 11, 17, 29, 137, 148, 158, 202–204, 212
Stern's, 12
dialogue(s), 49, 71–72, 272, 276, 290–291, 297
affective, 92, 205–208
and choice, 287
and communication, concepts of, 66
and ethics, 282, 286
with infant, 94
and linguistic development, 22
narrative, 92, 205–212
preverbal, 255
proto-, 255
social, 45–46, 48
therapeutic, 6–7, 37, 84, 100, 115, 158, 264
with adolescents, 157, 159, 161–162, 164, 168, 174, 179
as dance, 60
dichotomy(ies), 34, 241–245, 248, 253–254
as existential fields of tension, 249
between objective and subjective, 251
dignity, concept of, 281
"Dina" [clinical example: sleep problems], 101–107, 113
discourse, 59, 91, 234, 245, 248, 253
concept of, 236–237
displacement, 237, 238
distance, issues of, in adolescent therapy, 160
Doan, R. E., 253
Dostoyevski, F., 298
Draper, R., 251
Dreyfus, H., 222
Duncan, B. L., 226, 253

Dunn, J., 5, 6, 137, 180–196, 209, 264
dynamic shifts, 93
dynamic systems theory, 17

Eakin, P. J., 56
eating disorder(s), xvi, 6, 97, 194
  work with, 197–212
  *see also* anorexia/anorexic(s); bulimia/bulimic(s)
Egeland, T. A. A., 236
ego-mass family, 102
Eliot, T. S., 133–134
Elster, J., 269
emergent self, xv, xvi, 23–25, 82, 151
  as metaphor for work with adolescents, 158–162
  sense of, 16–18, 24
emotion(s), concept of, 90, 92
emotional exchange, 54
emotional experience(s), 22, 89–113, 107, 113, 169
  corrective, 229–232
  shared (inter-affectivity), 14
  supplementary, 229–232
empathic intentionality, 68
empathy, 69, 102, 105, 206, 273, 284
  concept of, 3, 95–97
empiricism, 263–274
  and objectivity, 6
Engelstad, I., 132
enmeshed family, 102
environment:
  concept of, 184
  non-shared, 182
episodic memory, 18, 20, 92
Epston, D., 107, 127, 145, 208, 288
Erikson, E. H., 4, 42
"essential" self, 46
essentialism, 40, 47, 64
ethical aspects of narrative, 133
ethical concept, truth as, 275–277
ethical dilemmas, 135
ethical perspectives, 7
  on narrative self, 127, 278–298
ethical responsibility, 129
ethics, 276
  concept of, Greek, 279
  issues of, 115, 126
    and narrative self, 278–298
  professional, 280–283
  role of, 1, 135, 275
    and recollection, 127
event representation(s), 27, 52
evoked companion, 20, 30, 162, 166–167, 177
existential field(s) of tension, 226, 245, 249–250
expelling families, 185
experience(s):
  affect-laden, 127, 140, 146
  traces of, 114–135
expressiveness, 93

Fairlane, F., 168
families, psychosomatic, 185
family(ies):
  anorectic, 198, 199
  binding, 185, 194
  expelling, 185
  ideology, 141
  legends, 29
  motif, 141
  myth(s), 29, 141, 181
    concept of, 136
  paradigm(s), 29
    concept of, 136
  premise(s), 29, 103, 107, 136–154, 181, 185, 193, 199–200, 209–210, 212, 264
    concept of, 138, 140–141
    Milan group, 136
    rigid or deadlocked, 102
  psychosomatic, 185
  rules, 136, 141, 181
  script, 29
    concept of, 137, 141
  theme, concept of, 136
  therapy (*passim*):
    concept of community in, 64–67
    and concept of transference, 247–254
    historically oriented, 89
    and psychoanalysis, xvii, 235
    social-constructionist, 72
    systemic, xx, xxiii, 3, 90, 136–138, 140, 154, 190, 201
    theory, 66
feeling(s), concept of, 90, 92
feminist philosophy, 245
Ferreira, A., 136

Fivush, R., 53
fixation-regression model of development, 15
Flaskas, C., 3, 97
foreshadowing, concept of, 131
Foucault, M., 217, 236
free association, concept of, 237
free-floating attention, 129
"free-floating feeling", 28
Freedman, J., 253
Freeman, M., 178
French, T. M., 230, 231
Freud, S., 4, 64, 242, 246
Freudian theories, 263
Friedman, S., 178
Frosh, S., 242, 246
Furniss, T., 268

Geertz, C., 157, 171, 267
gender, importance of, 141, 200
Gergen, K. J., 5, 45, 47, 49, 59, 64–65, 90–91, 154, 178, 233, 248, 261, 273–276, 285, 286, 292
  individual consciousness and relational context, 83
  "intersubjective transparency", 83
  meaning and individual significance, 83
  on narratives, 153
Gilligan, S., 178
Goethe, J. W., *Faust*, 278
Goolishian, H., 65, 252–253, 277, 282
gratification, concept of, 171
Grenness, C. E., 248
Griffiths, M., 241, 245
Guattari, F., 217, 239
Gullestad, S. E., 229

Haavardsholm, B., 90
Haavind, H., 229
Hafstad, R., 78
Haley, J., 65
"Hanne" [clinical example: bulimia, sibling relations, vitality affects], 97–101, 113, 189
Hansen, B. R., xxiii, 29, 67, 76–78, 82, 91–92, 204–205, 249, 255, 264
"Harald" and "Sissel" [clinical example], 107–113
Haraway, D. J., 248
Harré, R., 56–57, 90–91
Hartmann, E., 4
Havnesköld, L., 25, 76, 90, 92, 113
healing:
  through encounter, 90
  through systemic change, 90
health services, knowledge-based, 257
"Heidi" [clinical example: personal identity, narratives and meaning], 289–298
Henriksen, J.-O., 273, 276
here-and-now-relationship, 229
Hermans, H., 294
hermeneutics, 48, 252, 258, 272–274
historical point of origin, 127, 135, 139
historical truth, and narrative truth, 3, 125, 135, 139, 153
Hoffman, L., 4, 38, 65, 89, 90, 236, 249, 250
Holgersen, H., 238, 239, 247
Holmes, J., 238–241
Holmes, S., 279
Høstmark Nielsen, G., 239, 247, 257, 258
Hougaard, E., 162
Hoyt, M., 47
Hubble, M. A., 226, 253
Huffington, C., 251
humanities, 258
Hume, D., 284
humiliation, issues of, in adolescent therapy, 160
Hundevadt, L., 90
Husserl, E., x, xv, 67–70, 72, 78
hypnosis, 17
hypothesis, operationalized, 265–268
hypothetical questions, 148

"Ida" [clinical example: similarity and lack of individuation], 186
*idem*, concept of, 292–293
identity, 133
  concept of, 36
  confusion phase, 42
  and subjectivity, 47–49
Imber-Black, E., 136
imitation, 16, 20–22, 50–51, 60, 79, 81, 96, 100–102, 106, 113, 169–170
  concept of, 80, 94–95, 105
independence, concept of, 281

individual self, xvii, 39, 45
individualism, atomistic, 45
individuality, cultural conception of, 39
individualization, 63, 138
individuation, 13, 103, 137, 185–186, 192–194, 204
  related, 13
"Ingun" [clinical example: in search of identity], 121–124, 128, 133–134
instinct(s), concept of, 90
Institute of Family Therapy, Oslo, 198
integrity, 63, 280
  concept of, 281
intentionality, 58, 78, 288
  empathic, 68
intentions, sharing of, 21
interaction, focus on in family therapy, 251
interactive experiences (RIGs), 20, 26, 29, 51
inter-affectivity, 14, 77, 96, 169
inter-attentionality, 21, 77
inter-intentionality, 77
interpersonal interdependence, 22
interplay, 19–20, 23, 31, 89–113, 207, 255
  and senses of self, 155–179
intersubjective self, 96
intersubjective system, 71
intersubjective transparency, 83
intersubjectivity, xv, 18, 51, 94, 229, 233, 277
  Buber, 69–72
  concept of, 7–8
    developmental psychological, 76–79
    limited, 67–69
    philosophical and psychological, 61–85
    Stern, 13
  conveyed to immediate, 82
  Husserl, 67–69, 78
  immediate to conveyed, 82
  Merleau-Ponty, 69–72
  phenomenological foundation, 68
  philosophical context, 67
  primary, 82
    Trevarthen, 78–79
  radical, 69–72
  reflexive form of, 78
  secondary, 80, 82
  and self, xiv
  Stern, 21, 77–82, 94, 96
  and subjectivity, 69, 79–82
  Trevarthen, 78
interview, qualitative, 262
introspection, 44, 96, 112
intuition, 130
intuitive sympathy, 79
*ipse*, concept of, 292–293
Irigaray, L., 242

Jackson, D. D., 3, 65, 251
James, W., 12
Johnsen, A., xi, xiii, xvi, xix–xxiv, 1–8, 11–34, 89–154, 180–212, 249, 264
Johnsen, Anne, 91
Johnson, B., 242
joining, concept of, 96
joint construction of histories, 30

Kant, I., 283, 284
"Kari" [clinical example: feeling of worthlessness], 201–204
"Karl" [clinical example: guilt, parents, and childhood], 115–121, 126–127, 131, 133
Karterud, S., 3, 37, 50, 91, 95
Keeney, B. P., 228, 250
Kemp, P., 75, 295
key experience, affective component of, 140
key therapeutic metaphor, 29, 136–154
  concept of, 115, 126, 138–140
Killingmo, B., 221, 237–238
Kirkebøen, G., 156, 248
Klein, M., 26
knowledge, 44, 51, 279, 297
  -based health services, 257
  Cartesian view of, 43
  concept of, 256–277
  Husserl, 68
  nature of, 257–274
  theories of, relevance to clinical practice, 256–277
  traditional forms of, 6
  and truth, 6, 260–263

"Knut", "Inger", "Tom", "Else", "Ragnhild" [clinical example: togetherness and separation], 144–152
Kohut, H., 3, 4, 37, 50
Kugiumetziakis, G., 80
Kundera, M., 40
Kvale, S., 155, 157, 243

landscape:
of action, 130
of consciousness, 130
language, 22–23
analog, 99
central position of, xx
digital, 99
French philosophy of, 56, 59
as generative, 174
limitations of, 7
and meaning, 65–85
possibilities and limitations of in therapeutic work with adolescents, 172–178
role of, 53–55
Stern, 33
as world or in world, 55–59
Laplanche, J., 238
Laurén, K., 199
Lennon, K., 245
Levinas, E., 275, 276
Lichtenberg, J., 4, 90
"Line" [clinical example: eating disorder], 97, 205–210
linear causal thinking, 114, 199
linguistic construction, self as, 48, 56–58, 60
linguistic meaning, 22–23
"linguistic turn", 248
linguistics, 180
literary theory, 252
Loe, E., 270
logical types, 65
Lundby, G., 253

Madan Smith, G., 253
Madison, G. B., 71, 72
Madsen, C., 217
Madsen, K., 293
manic-depressive illness, 199
map metaphor, 129, 136, 248
Marshall, B. K., 243
Maruyama, M., 249
mastery, 32, 103, 121, 216, 229, 290, 298
issues of, in therapeutic work with adolescents, 162–163, 165
Maturana, H., 44, 251, 252, 254
Mauss, M., 56
Maybin, J., 47, 56
McCall, C., 36
McEwan, I., 62
McLeod, J., 129
McNamee, S., 178, 233, 248, 286
Mead, M., 250
meaning(s) (*passim*):
vs action, 251
and coherence, 18, 23–24, 113, 146, 150
concept of, 251
emergence of latent, 240
and language, 65–85
negotiations about, 30, 172–175
Meltzoff, A., 80
memorabilia, 228, 234
memory(ies), 18–20, 114–135
structure(s), 20, 25
formation of, 19–20
mental landscape, 20
Mental Research Institute (MRI), 132
merger, experience of, 18
Merleau-Ponty, M., 67, 69–72, 82
metaphor(s), xv, xxi, 2, 17, 22, 29, 83, 99–100, 109, 111, 113
key therapeutic, concept of, 115, 126, 136–154
map, 129, 136, 248
narrative, xxi, 114–115, 125, 127, 129, 288
use of, 99
"Mette", "Mari", "Kristina" [clinical example: twin and sibling experiences], 191–193
Midgley, M., 260, 275
Milan group, 3, 65, 103, 145, 199
circular questioning, 137, 185
concept of family premises, 136
one-way mirror and team positions, 252
Miller, H., 286
Miller, S. D., 226, 253
Mills, S., 236

mimesis, concept of, 296
Minuchin, S., 3, 65, 102, 185, 194, 198, 199, 209
mirroring, 100
  concept of, 95
Moi, T., 246
Monsen, J., 3, 37, 50, 90, 91, 95
Moore, H., 51
Moore, K., 80
morals, 283
  vs. ethics, 279–280
Morson, G., 115, 131, 297, 298
Mothander, P. R., 25, 76, 90, 92, 113
mother, depressed, 128
motivation, therapist's, 216
multipartiality, concept of, 96
multiple personalities, 47
mutual attention, sharing of, 21

Nagel, T., 262
narrative(s) (*passim*):
  of abuse, 128
  biographical, 92
  concept of, 249
    as watchword in family therapy, 227
  and construction of social identity, 126
  content of, 153
  and coordination of action, 51
  creating, 175–178
    in family therapy, 200
  ethical perspective, 280–298
  family, 53
    clinical example, 105–107
  fictive, 115
    and truth, 125–129; *see also* narrative truth and historical truth
  and forms of time, 114–135
  individual and shared, 136–154, 192
  interactional, sharing, 175–178
  and intersubjective experiences, 82
  key, 140
  and key therapeutic metaphor, 139
  literary, 127
  ownership of, 115
  personal, 126
  and pre-narrative envelopes, 26
  and proto-narrative envelopes, 28, 30, 52
  real and fictive, 114–115
  and relatedness, 91
  representations of events, 52
  revision of, 123–124, 133–134
  and sense of self, 58, 126
  sharing of, 138
  and significance, 83
  therapeutic, 115
  true, 125
  validity of, 125, 127
narrative dialogue, 91, 205, 208–209
narrative history, 24, 58
narrative inductors, 296
narrative metaphor, xxi, 114–115, 125, 127, 129, 288
narrative mode of thought, 130
narrative point of origin, 127, 139–140
narrative self, 16, 106, 159, 174–178, 278–298
  sense of, 23–34, 149
narrative therapy, significance of time in, 114–135
narrative time, 129, 131, 294
narrative truth, 139
  and historical truth, 3, 125, 135, 153
narrativity, xviii, 60, 291
narrativization, xv
naturalism, 258
nature vs. culture, 33
negotiations about meaning, 172
Nelson, K., 52
neutrality, 145, 275
  concept of, 96, 261
    Milan group, 137–138
Newton, A. Z., 298
Nic Waal Institute, Oslo, xxiii, xxiv, 191, 198
Nicolaysen, B. K., 289
Nietzsche, F., 55, 293
non-shared environment, 182–183, 190–191, 193
nonverbal self-domain, 21
nonverbality, 171
Nordby, T. T., 91
Nordtvedt, D., 284
Norris, C., 242, 244
Norsk Sosionomforbund, 281

"not-knowing position", 6, 96, 277

object-relations theory, 15
objective time, 129
objectivity:
 concept of, 268–270, 275
 and empiricism, 6
 and subjectivity, 253
  concepts of, 250
Oedipus myth, 187
operant analysis, 218
Øvreeide, H., 78
Øyan, J., 36

Pålshaugen, Ø., 248
Papp, P., 136
Pappenheim, O. (Anna O) [Freud's case], 246
paradigmatic mode of thought, 130
parent–child relationship, xxi, 5, 184, 191
 differences in, 186–188
Parrot, W. G., 90, 91
Parry, A., 253
Partridge, E., 244
pathology, parents stigmatized as generating, 231
patient [clinical example: presentation vs transference, closure and delimitation], 219–223
patterned changes, 93
Penn, P., 65
perception, 70–72
perceptual schemas, 27
permanence, temporal, in personal identity, 288, 293–295
person, concept of, 36
personality disorders, 250
Peterfreund, E., 32
phenomenological approach:
 to intersubjectivity, 68
 to therapeutic process, xvi, xvii
phenomenological time, 129
phenomenology, xvi, 37, 50, 67–69
philosophy, xvii, xx, 3, 5, 67, 135, 180, 217, 248, 286
 feminist, 245
 of language, 56
 linguistic, 252
 of subject, 55
 of therapy, 47
physical aggressiveness of siblings, similarities in, 196
Piaget, J., 4, 27, 264
Plomin, R., 6, 180–182, 184–189, 193, 195–196, 209
Pocock, D., 3, 97
point of origin:
 assumed actual, 139
 historical, 127, 135
  narrated, 139
 narrative, 127, 139, 140
Pontalis, J.-B., 238
positivism, 258
postmodern approach to therapy, 253, 277
postmodern criticism of traditional ethical theory, 285–288
postmodern ethics, 286–287
postmodern thinking, xx, xxii, 6, 44, 260, 272, 287–288, 294
 concept of, 243
postmodernism, 276
 concept of, 243
postmodernity, concept of, 243
post-structuralism, xx
Potter, J., 260
practice, concept of, 59–60
Prata, G., 137
predictability, 163
pre-narrative envelope, 26–28, 106
presentation, 229–231, 233, 239, 242, 249, 252, 257, 282, 296
 concept of, 221–222, 235, 241
 linguistic, 178
 vs transference, closure and delimitation [clinical example], 219–223
preverbal dialogue, 255
preverbal self, 50–55
 -domain, 172
Price, R., 178
Priest, S., 72
projection of inner representations, 238
proprioceptive feedback, 163
proto-conversation, 79
proto-dialogue, 255
proto-narrative envelope, 24, 27–28, 30, 52

Proust, M., *A la recherche du temps perdu*, 125
Psychiatric Adolescent Team, Drammen, 179
psychoanalysis, xviii, xx, 3–5, 64, 89–90, 128, 135, 156, 218, 288
  and family therapy, xvii, 235–255
  and systemic family therapy, 3
psychology:
  clinical, xxii
  developmental, xix–xxi, 5, 11, 13, 16, 27, 31–32, 37, 49–50, 58, 76, 80–81, 84, 158, 182, 184, 187, 263
    modern, 3, 198, 201, 203–210
psychopathology, 182–183, 195
psychosomatic families, 185

questions, hypothetical, 148

rationality, concept of, Western, 242
realism vs relativism, 260
recognition, concept of, 171
reflecting team, 252
reflexivity, 59, 71, 82
regression, 238
  fixation-, model, 15
regulation, 18, 30, 50, 60, 81, 100, 104, 166, 175, 207–208
  in adolescence, 159
  affect, 5, 16, 19–20, 101, 151, 169, 216, 229
  of affective states, 94–96
  concept of, 105
  of feelings, mutual, 96
  issues of, in adolescent therapy, 160–162
Reichelt, S., 157, 229
reification, 57
Reiss, D., 136
rejection, issues of, in adolescent therapy, 160
related individuation, 13
relatedness, issues of, with eating disorders, 197
relation-oriented therapy, xiii, xiv, xv, 2
relational perspective, 33, 229, 239, 281
relational responsibility, 280
relational structure, 52, 65
relationship, key concern of therapy, 229
relativism, 40, 43, 49, 287
  vs. realism, 260
repetition, 18–19, 127, 162, 238, 240, 296
  unconscious, 238
representation(s), 13, 15, 18–20, 44–45, 135–136, 172, 238
  concept of, 27
    Stern, 25–30
  event, 27, 52
  formation of, 29
  of generalized interactions (RIGs), 20, 26, 29, 51
  infant's, 30, 51
  internal, 240
  vs. schema, 27
representational entities, 29
repressed:
  parts, 243
  return of, 156, 243
resistance(s), 268
  concept of, 237
respect, concept of, 96, 162
responsibility:
  individual, concept of, 286
  relational, 280
revolt, issues of, in adolescent therapy, 160
Ricoeur, P., x, 5, 53, 57, 115, 126–127, 129, 288, 291–296
  philosopher of detour, 289
RIGs (representations of generalized interactions), 20, 26, 29, 51
Riikonen, E., 253
Røer, A., 99, 208, 267
Rogers, C., 253
Rønning, J. A., 258, 259
Rorschach test, 267
Rosman, B., 102, 185, 194, 198
Rucker-Embden, I., 13
Rusk, G. S., 226
Russell, B., 65

Sartre, J.-P., 259, 266
Schafer, R., 107, 178, 288
schizoaffective psychoses, 199
Schjødt, B., 236
scholastic achievements of siblings, similarities in, 196
Schrag, C. O., 53

science(s), xxii, 236, 250
behavioural, 182
definition, 257
hard, 248
natural, 258
philosophy of, 262, 275
social, 64, 258
soft, 248
systemic, 252
security, 166, 176
concept of, 162
selective attunement, 105–106
self:
-affectivity, 18–19, 32
issues of, in therapeutic work with adolescents, 164
-agency, 18–19
and volition and mastery, 162
-coherence, 18–19, 32
issues of, in therapeutic work with adolescents, 163
concept of, *see* concept of self
core, *see* core self
as cybernetic concept, 38
-delimitation, 185, 194
developmental psychological understanding of, 49–50
-differentiation, 185, 194
emergent, *see* emergent self
essential, 46
-experience(s), xv, 5, 89–113, 136–154, 288–291, 294
in dyads, 85
-history, 18–19, 32, 164
individual, xvii, 39, 45
intersubjective, 96
-invariants, 18–19, 31–32, 162, 165
as linguistic construction, 48, 56–58, 60
narrative, 16, 106, 159, 174–178, 278–298
sense of, 23–34, 149
–other dualism, 80
-with-others experience, 19, 30
preverbal, 50–55
-domain, 172
-psychology, 4, 15, 37, 90
-reflection, 7, 23, 25, 92, 208
sense of, *see* sense(s) of self
social, approaches to, 45–47
subjective, *see* subjective self
symbolic, 23
universal aspects of, 31
verbal self, 16, 24, 145, 159, 171–172
sense of, 22–23, 25, 149–150
Seller, A., 245
Selvini-Palazzoli, M., 38, 137, 185, 252
sensation(s), 232–234
sense(s) of self, xiii, xv, 4, 12–25, 29–30, 37, 40, 43, 45–46, 48–51, 56, 58, 101, 126, 138–140, 146, 149–151, 154, 203–205, 208, 210, 215, 232–233
and interaction, 203
and interplay, 155–179
as "invariant patterns of awareness", 51
issues of, in work with adolescents, 165
language as sole source of, 48–49
sensorimotor schemas, 27
sexes, relationship between, dominance perspective on, 242
sexual abuse, 123, 192, 261, 269
child, 268
Shakespeare, W., *Hamlet*, 256–257, 272
sharing:
of affect, 21, 94, 168
of attention, 21, 167
of experiences, 216
of intentions, 21, 168
of subjective states, 94
Sheehan, J., 115, 125, 127, 129–131
sibling(s), xvi, 1
differences between, 146, 180–196, 209
relationship between, 5, 6, 137, 150, 180–196
differences in, 188–189
Sibling Inventory of Differential Experience (SIDE), 186
sideshadow(ing), concept of, 131, 298
"Signe" [clinical example: concept of self], xv, 41–49, 54–60, 203, 205
social constructionism, xx, 1, 4–5, 15, 31–32, 42–49, 53, 59–60, 72, 82, 90, 134, 248, 260, 272–276, 288, 291–292
American, 63

Anderson, 294
Gergen, 285
social referring, 30
social self, xvii, 43
approaches to, 45–47
socialization, role of, in development of feelings, 90
Solovey, A. D., 226
solution, concept of, as watchword in family therapy, 227
Sommer, D., 47, 49
Sørhaug, T., 267
Speed, B., 3
Speer, A., 249
Spence, D., 3, 5, 107, 115, 125, 129, 139, 156, 222, 288
splitting, through language, 150
"standard documentation procedures", 258
Stern, D. N. (*passim*):
affect attunement, 94
categorical affects and vitality affects, 27
concept of self, 13
developmental model of, xxiii, 12, 15, 153
developmental psychology, 49–50
Foreword, xiii–xviii
interaffectivity, 96
intersubjectivity, 13, 18, 21, 77–82
key therapeutic metaphor, 138–154
model of self-development, 4, 11–34
senses of self, 4, 12–25, 50, 204, 215, 233
and eating disorders, 203–212
five domains of, 138–154, 158–179
temporal feeling shape, 17
theory of self, 4
Stierlin, H., x, 3, 13, 89, 102–103, 185, 194, 196, 198–199
stories, world of, 23–34
subject, concept of, 36
subjective self, 16, 23, 31, 94, 160, 174
-domain, 23, 77
in work with adolescents, 167–172
sense of, 20–22, 25, 105, 139, 150
subjective time, 129
subjectivity, 60, 68, 70, 72, 78–79, 273, 275, 277, 286, 295
concept of, 36, 51
and identity, 47–49
and intersubjectivity, 69
and objectivity, 253
concepts of, 250
and subject, 57
Sundet, R., xi, xiii, xv–xvii, xix–xxiv, 1–8, 11–34, 155–179, 215–255, 264
supplement(s), 218–224
support, concept of, 171
suspicion, concept of, 295
symbiosis, 12, 50, 80–81, 204
and separateness, 12
symbolic play, 22, 159
symbolic self, 23
symbolization, 23, 82, 85, 106, 242, 251
sympathy, intuitive, 79
Sypnowich, C., 43, 45
systemic theory, 1, 3, 29, 90, 156, 196, 218, 236, 252
dynamic, 17

talk, in therapy, 7
Taylor, C., 59, 63, 295
temporal feeling shape, 17, 27–28, 30, 52, 93, 106
Tenfjord, J., 36
terminology, technical:
context-sensitive, 227
problem of, 226–234
text, concept of, 249
theme with variations, 30
Theophilakis, M., 229
therapeutic metaphor, 126, 139–140, 144, 146, 148
key, 29
concept of, 115, 126, 138–140
therapist [clinical example: boundaries and delimitation, contamination, pollution, and contagion], 223–224
therapy, body-oriented, Reichian, 215
thinking, 217–218
identity, as narrative phenomenon, 294
involved, in therapy, 215–234
standardization, 259

time:
  continuity in, 19, 164
  forms of, 129–134
  reflexive and non-linear character of, 132–134
  significance of, in narrative therapy, 114–135
Tomkins, S. S., 90
Tømmerås, S., 90
Torsteinsson, V. W., xi, xiii, xvi, xvii, xix–xxiv, 1–8, 11–85, 89–113, 202, 206–207, 256–298
Tranøy, K. E., 275, 285
transference, 69, 140, 219–221, 227, 229–230, 233
  concept of, 221–222, 235, 237–241, 247
    classical, 239–242
    modern, 239–242
  relationship, 151, 230
Trevarthen, C., 76, 78–80, 82
triadic questioning, 185
triangulation, 198
Tromsø group, 252
Tronick, E. Z., xvii
trust, 14–15, 138–139, 204, 211
  concept of, 295
truth, 261
  concept of, 125, 257, 262, 275
    classical, 258
    constructivistic, 258
  historical, *see* historical truth
  issue of, in narratives, 125
  and knowledge, 6, 260–263
  narrative, *see* narrative truth
  objective, 262
  pretension of, 262
twin(s), 180
  study of, 183, 184
Tygstrup, F., 217

Uggla, B. K., 294, 184, 297
unconscious, making conscious, 241
understanding, 233
usefulness, concept of, 261

Vedeler, G. H., 258, 259
verbal self, 16, 24, 145, 159, 171–172
  sense of, 22–23, 25, 149–150
verbality, 60
verbalization, 7, 51, 164, 178, 234
Vetlesen, A. J., 266, 284
"virtual other", 79
"visual cliff", 168
vitality affects, 17–18, 24, 28, 30, 52, 91–100, 113, 159, 205–206
  and categorical affects, 14, 27, 93–94
  concept of, 100
volition, 19, 49, 216, 229
  issues of, in therapeutic work with adolescents, 162, 165, 176
von Foerster, H., 250, 253, 282
Von Glasersfeld, E., 253

Wakefield, J., 222
Watzlawick, P., 3, 65, 251
Weber, G., 199
Wechsler Intelligence Scale for Children (WISC), 267
Wetherell, M., 47, 56
Wetzel, N., 13
White, M., 107, 127, 145, 178, 227, 234, 249, 253, 288
Whitehead, A. N., 65
Whitford, M., 242, 245
Wilden, A., 156, 243
Wilkinson, M., 97
Williams, B., 281
Wirsching, M., 13, 194, 196
Wittgenstein, L., 65, 66
working alliance, 172
Wrangsjø, B., 159
Wynne, L. C., 196

Yeatman, A., 243
"Yngvild" [clinical example: compulsion problems, shared experience], xv, 62–63, 68–69, 72–76, 81–83

Zachrisson, A., 229, 237

For Product Safety Concerns and Information please contact our EU
representative GPSR@taylorandfrancis.com
Taylor & Francis Verlag GmbH, Kaufingerstraße 24, 80331 München, Germany

www.ingramcontent.com/pod-product-compliance
Lightning Source LLC
Chambersburg PA
CBHW060741150926
51501CB00003B/64
*9780367326784*